Tumor Progression and Metastasis

Edited by Ahmed Lasfar and Karine Cohen-Solal

Published in London, United Kingdom

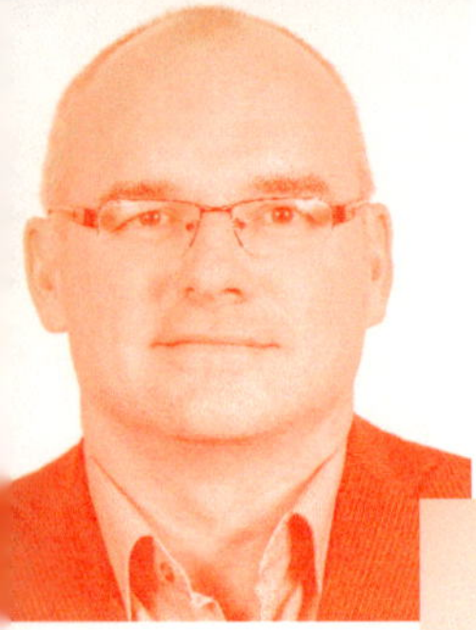
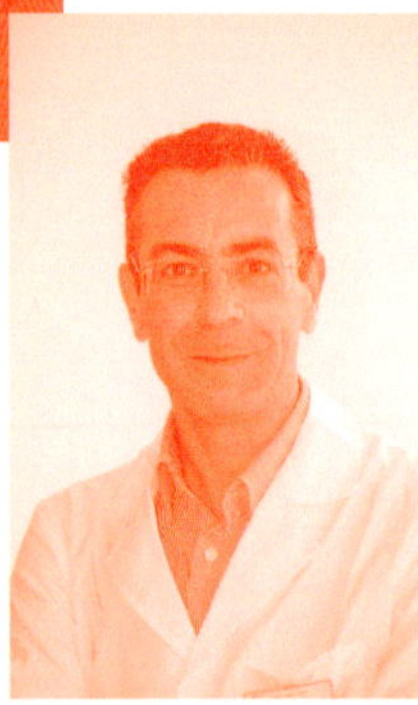
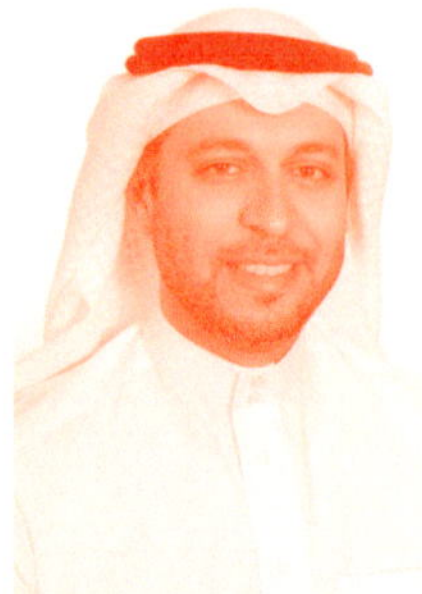
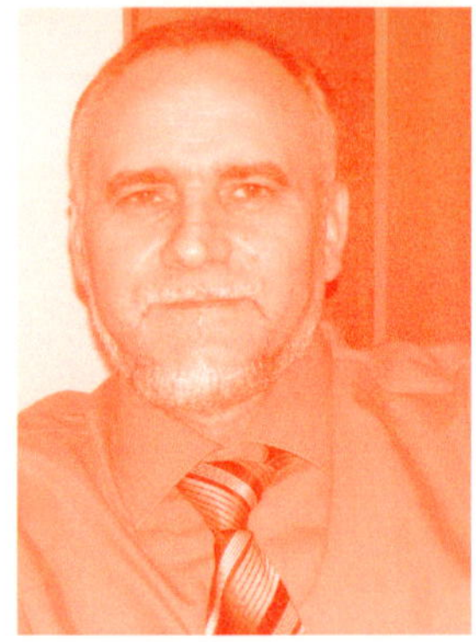
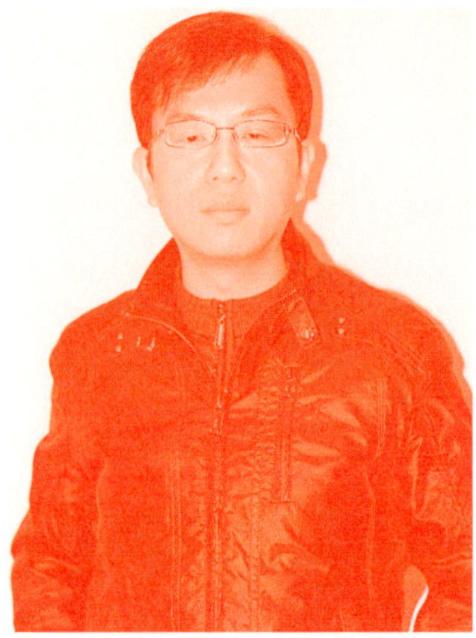
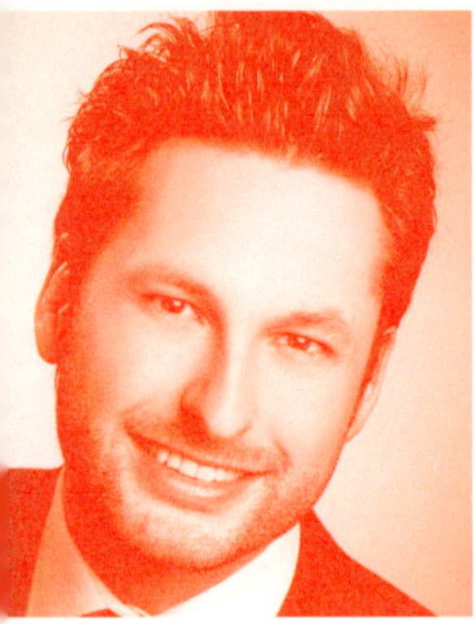
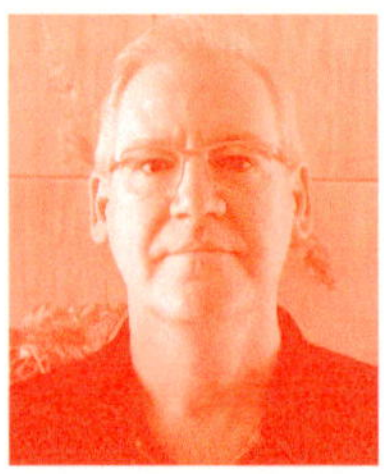

IntechOpen

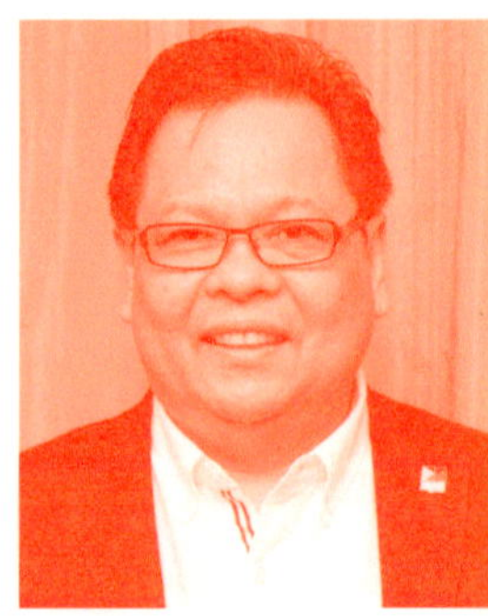
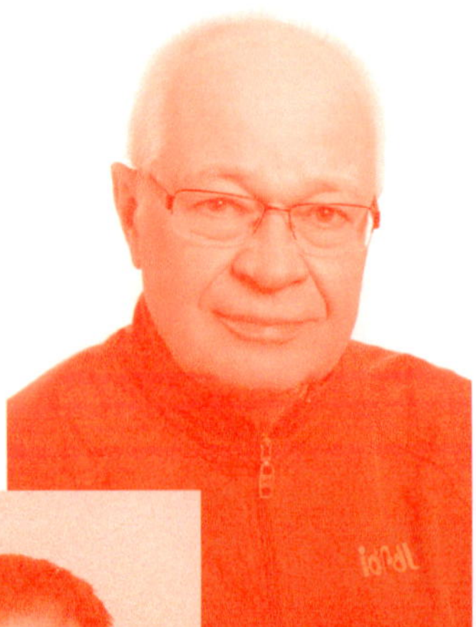
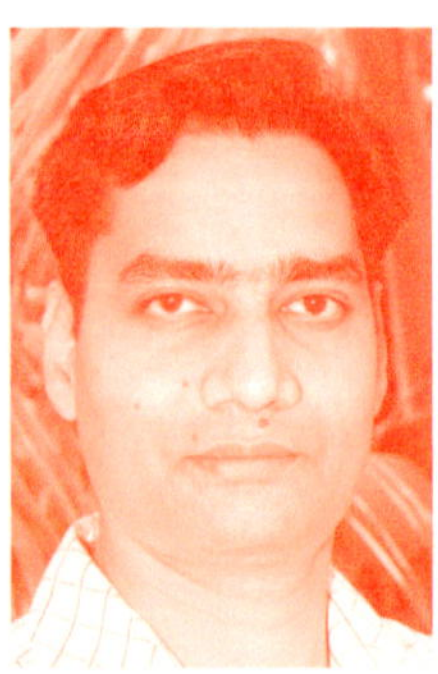
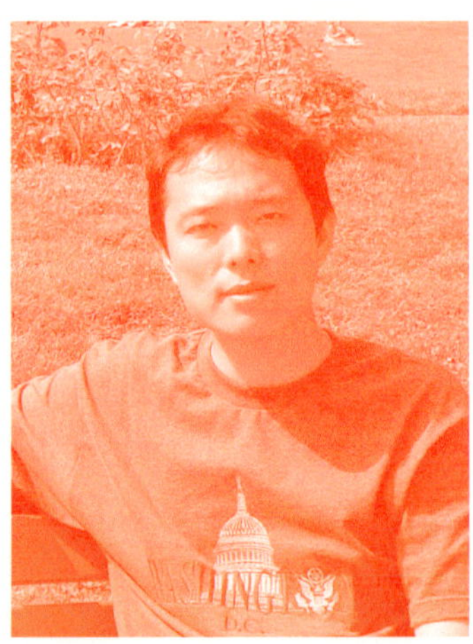
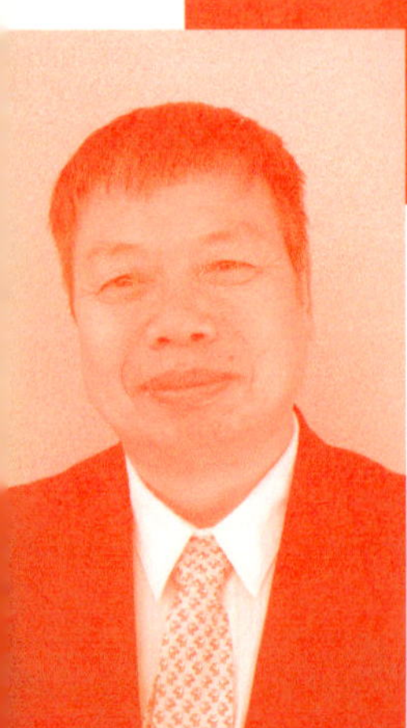
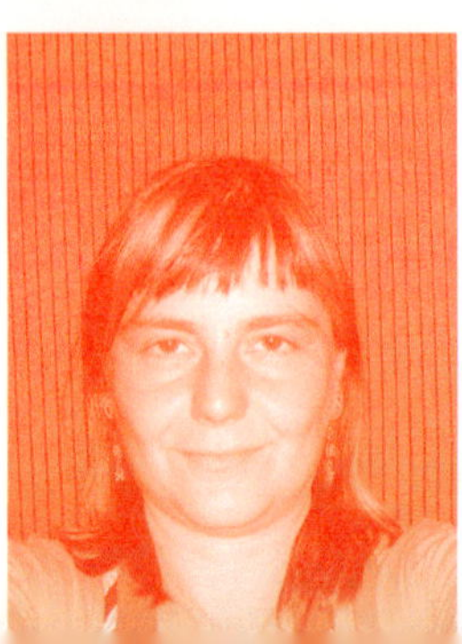

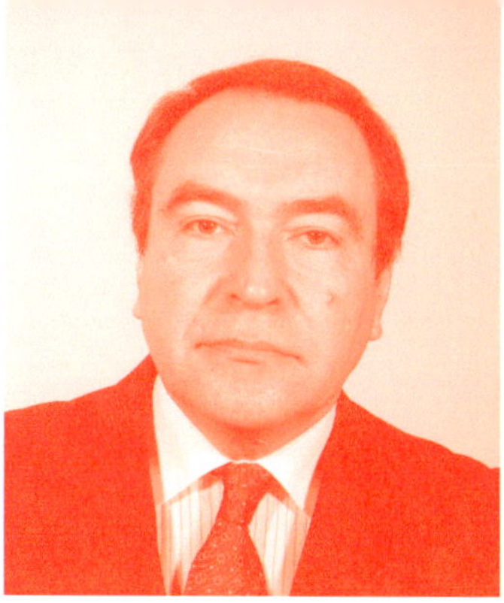
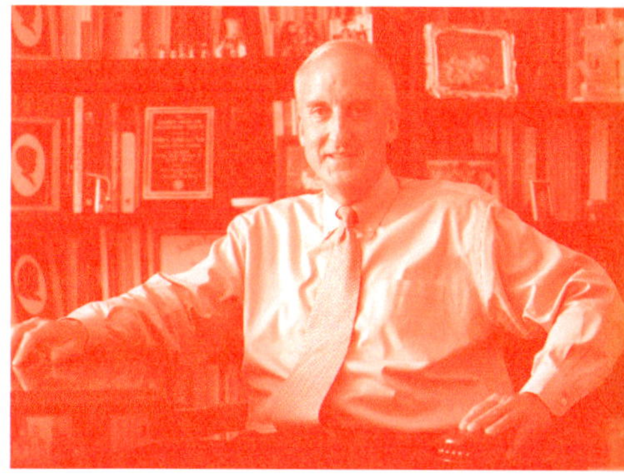
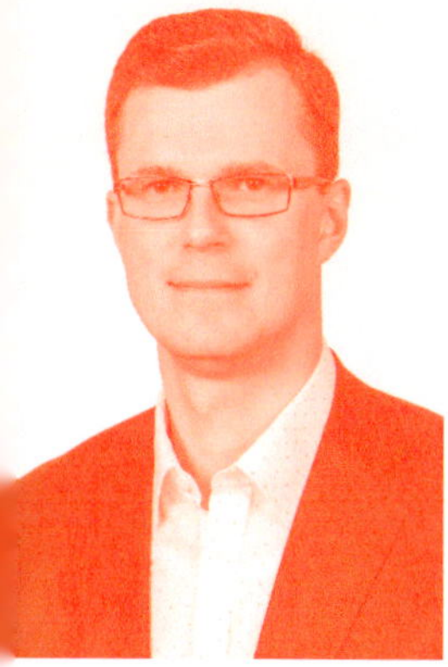
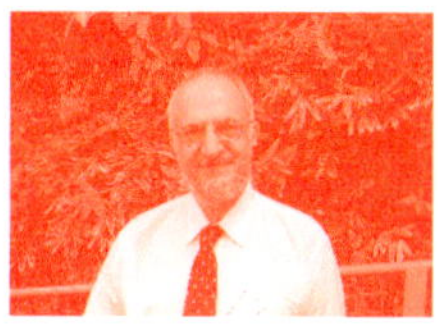
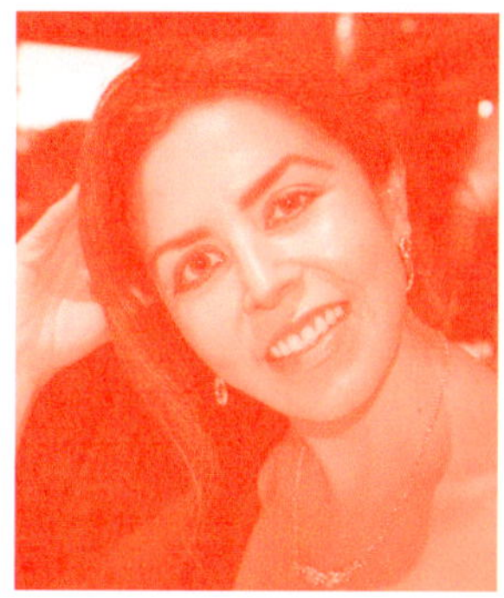

Supporting open minds since 2005

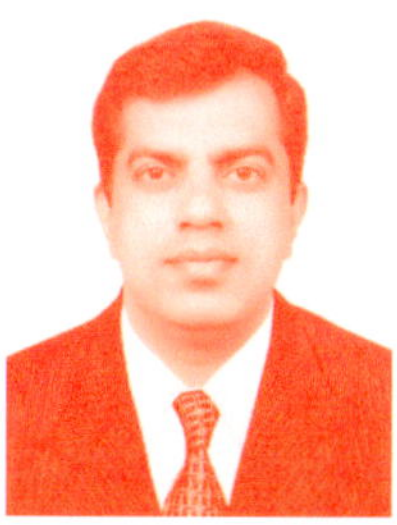
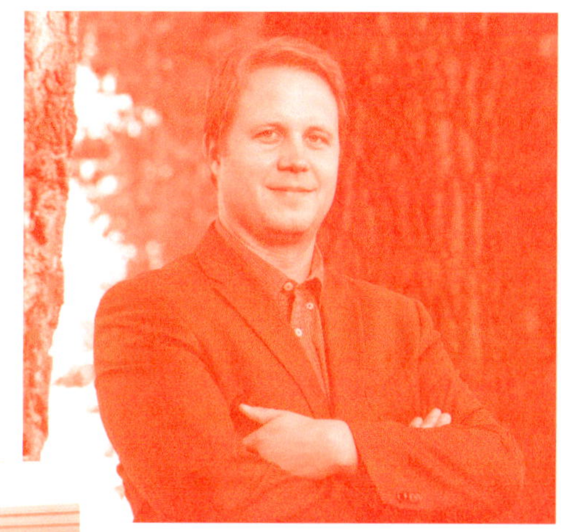
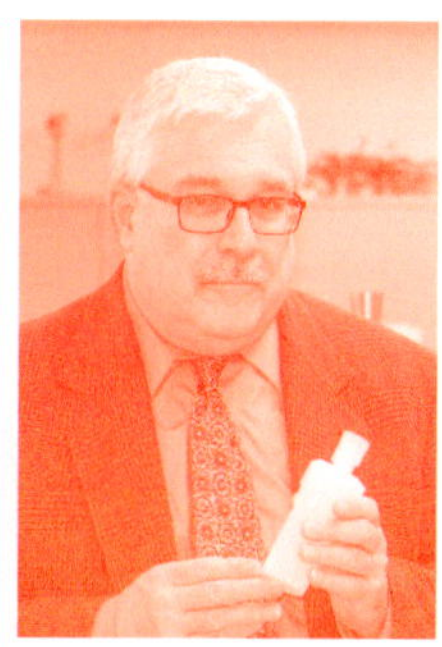
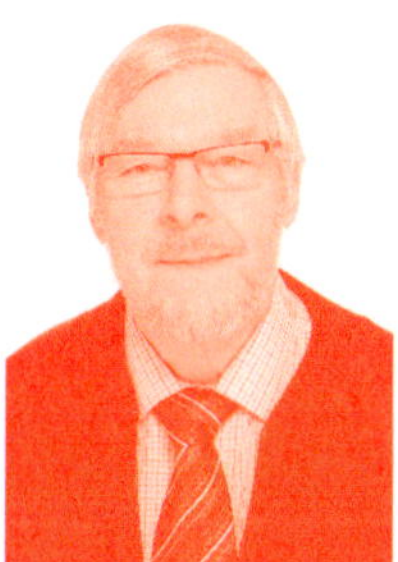
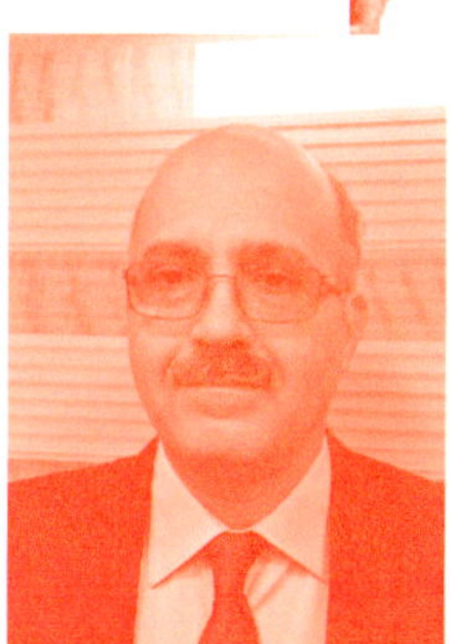
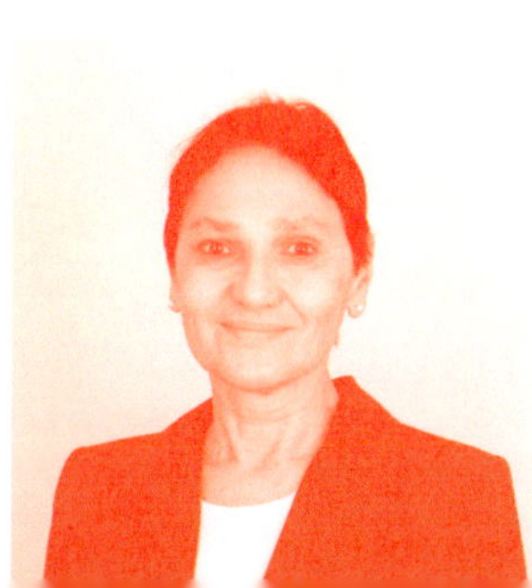
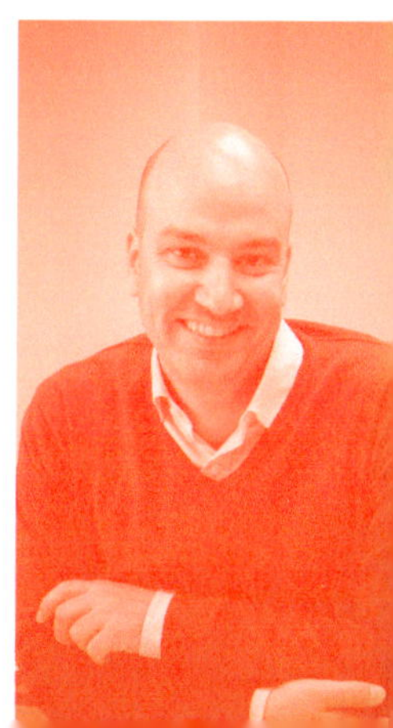

Tumor Progression and Metastasis
http://dx.doi.org/10.5772/intechopen.77832
Edited by Ahmed Lasfar and Karine Cohen-Solal

Part of IntechOpen Book Series: Physiology, Volume 8
Book Series Editor: Angel Catala

Contributors
Marliyya Zayyan, Fernando Yepes-Calderon, Flor Medina, Jose Abella, Pavel Kaspler, Arkady Mandel, Roger Dumoulin-White, Mark Roufaiel, Maitham Khajah, Wabel Albusairi, Beyza Akın, Hülya Yazici, Jorge Morales-Montor, Carmen Ferreira, Alessandra V. S. Faria, Stefano Piatto Clerici, Patrícia Oliveira, Helon Cordeiro, Erica Akagi, Audronė Valerija Kalvelytė, Aurimas Stulpinas, Natalija Krestnikova, Aušra Imbrasaitė, Renato Pietroletti, Marco Clementi, Andrea Ciarrocchi, Guido Rindi, Francesco Carlei, Federica D'Ascanio, Guang-Jer Wu, Cheng-Ta Hsieh, Da-Tong Ju, Nanda Gopal Sahoo, Neha Karki, Himani Tiwari, Anita Rana, Pushpa Negi

First published in London, United Kingdom, 2020 by IntechOpen
IntechOpen is the global imprint of INTECHOPEN LIMITED, registered in England and Wales, registration number: 11086078, 7th floor, 10 Lower Thames Street, London, EC3R 6AF, United Kingdom
Printed in Croatia

British Library Cataloguing-in-Publication Data
A catalogue record for this book is available from the British Library

Additional hard and PDF copies can be obtained from orders@intechopen.com

Tumor Progression and Metastasis
Edited by Ahmed Lasfar and Karine Cohen-Solal
p. cm.
Print ISBN 978-1-78985-349-0
Online ISBN 978-1-78985-350-6
eBook (PDF) ISBN 978-1-78985-146-5
ISSN 2631-8261

For EU product safety concerns:
IN TECH d.o.o., Prolaz Marije Krucifikse Kozulić 3, 51000 Rijeka, Croatia, info@intechopen.com or visit our website at intechopen.com.

IntechOpen Book Series

Physiology

Volume 8

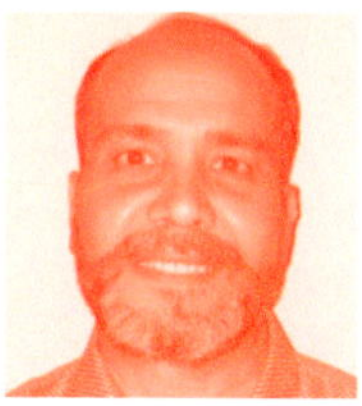

Dr Lasfar is a full member of the Cancer Institute of New Jersey and a Professor at Rutgers University, New Jersey. He is also editor and board member of several international journals and books. Dr Lasfar is a scientific adviser to the pharmaceutical industry and a member of several medical and scientific societies. He is also Head of the Cancer Immunotherapy Laboratory at Rutgers University, funded by the National Cancer Institute. Dr Lasfar graduated in Medical and Applied Science from Paris Rene Descartes University in France. He completed his doctoral studies in Immunology at Paris Diderot University and his postdoctoral training in Cancer Immunology at Robert Wood Johnson Medical, New Jersey

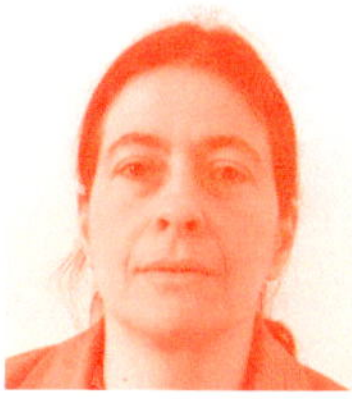

Dr Karine Cohen-Solal graduated from Paris University, France, and has extensive basic and translational research experience in melanoma and cancer metastasis. Dr Cohen-Solal is an expert in receptor-based dysregulated cellular pathways and drug resistance in oncology. Dr Cohen-Solal has received several awards including a Research Scholar Grant from the American Cancer Society, and awards from the New Jersey Commission on Cancer Research and the Melanoma Research Foundation. Currently Dr Cohen-Solal is the Chief Scientific Officer of Lambda Pharmaceutical, an adjunct faculty member at Ernest Mario School of Pharmacy, Rutgers University.

Editor of Volume 8:
Ahmed Lasfar
Ernest Mario School of Pharmacy, Piscataway, New Jersey

Karine A Cohen-Solal
Ernest Mario School of Pharmacy, Rutgers University, Piscataway, New Jersey

Book Series Editor: Angel Catala
National University of La Plata, Argentina

Scope of the Series

Modern physiology requires a comprehensive understanding of the integration of tissues and organs throughout the mammalian body, including the expression, structure, and function of molecular and cellular components. While a daunting task, learning is facilitated by our identification of common, effective signaling pathways employed by nature to sustain life. As a main example, the cellular interplay between intracellular Ca2 increases and changes in plasma membrane potential is integral to coordinating blood flow, governing the exocytosis of neurotransmitters and modulating genetic expression. Further, in this manner, understanding the systemic interplay between the cardiovascular and nervous systems has now become more important than ever as human populations age and mechanisms of cellular oxidative signaling are utilized for sustaining life. Altogether, physiological research enables our identification of clear and precise points of transition from health to development of multi-morbidity during the inevitable aging process (e.g., diabetes, hypertension, chronic kidney disease, heart failure, age-related macular degeneration; cancer). With consideration of all organ systems (e.g., brain, heart, lung, liver; gut, kidney, eye) and the interactions thereof, this Physiology Series will address aims of resolve (1) Aging physiology and progress of chronic diseases (2) Examination of key cellular pathways as they relate to calcium, oxidative stress, and electrical signaling & (3) how changes in plasma membrane produced by lipid peroxidation products affects aging physiology.

Contents

Preface XI

Section 1
Mechanisms of Tumor Progression and Metastasis 1

Chapter 1 3
METCAM/MUC18 Promotes Tumor Progression and Metastasis in Most Human Cancers
by Guang-Jer Wu

Chapter 2 33
Molecular Genetics of Metastatic Breast Cancer
by Hülya Yazici and Beyza Akin

Chapter 3 51
Protein Tyrosine Phosphatases in Tumor Progression and Metastasis: Promoter or Protection?
by Carmen V. Ferreira-Halder, Stefano Piatto Clerici, Alessandra V. Sousa Faria, Patrícia Fernandes de Souza Oliveira, Helon Guimarães Cordeiro and Erica Akagi

Section 2
Tumorigenesis Risk Factors and Role of Neuroimmune Regulations 73

Chapter 4 75
Risk Factors for Ovarian Cancer
by Marliyya S. Zayyan

Chapter 5 103
Appendiceal Neuroendocrine Tumors and Anorectal Melanoma
by Marco Clementi, Renato Pietroletti, Andrea Ciarrocchi, Federica d'Ascanio, Guido Rindi and Francesco Carlei

Chapter 6 113
Neuroimmunoendocrine Interactions in Tumorigenesis and Breast Cancer
by Rocío Alejandra Ruiz-Manzano, Tania de Lourdes Ochoa-Mercado, Mariana Segovia-Mendoza, Karen Elizabeth Nava-Castro, Margarita Isabel Palacios-Arreola and Jorge Morales-Montor

Section 3
Prediction of Response to Therapy and Drug Resistance **145**

Chapter 7 **147**
Recent Approaches Encompassing the Phenotypic
Cell Heterogeneity for Anticancer Drug Efficacy Evaluation
by Aurimas Stulpinas, Aušra Imbrasaitė, Natalija Krestnikova and
Audronė Valerija Kalvelytė

Chapter 8 **195**
The Principles behind Targeted Therapy for Cancer Treatment
by Wabel AL-Busairi and Maitham Khajah

Section 4
New Perspectives for Cancer Diagnosis and Therapy **217**

Chapter 9 **219**
Stereotactic Radiosurgery for Recurrent Glioblastoma Multiforme
by Cheng-Ta Hsieh and Da-Tong Ju

Chapter 10 **237**
Anticancer Photodynamic Therapy Using Ruthenium(II) and
Os(II)-Based Complexes as Photosensitizers
by Pavel Kaspler, Arkady Mandel, Roger Dumoulin-White
and Mark Roufaiel

Chapter 11 **267**
Theranostics Application of Graphene-Based Materials
in Cancer Imaging, Targeting and Treatment
by Neha Karki, Anita Rana, Himani Tiwari, Pushpa Negi and
Nanda Gopal Sahoo

Chapter 12 **293**
Tumor Malignancy Characterization in Clinical Environments:
An Approach Using the FYC-Index of Spiculation and
Artificial Intelligence
by Fernando Yepes-Calderón, Flor M. Medina, Nolan D. Rea
and José Abella

Preface

Tumor metastasis results from the spreading of a primary tumor and establishment of secondary tumors, mostly in vital organs such as the lung, liver, and brain. Tumor metastasis is responsible for the majority of cancer deaths, yet it remains the least understood stage of cancer.

Metastatic tumor cells acquire new biological features allowing them to migrate, invade normal tissues, escape the immune system control, and develop drug resistance. Many mechanisms have been shown to play an important role in the metastatic process, particularly through the tumor microenvironment. Many factors present in the tumor microenvironment have been identified and demonstrated to play either a pro- or anti-metastatic role, allowing the development of new targeted therapies.

However, despite an armamentarium of treatments, patients remain at a high risk for metastasis. Better understanding of the mechanisms leading to cancer metastasis is crucial for the development of novel and more efficacious therapies.

Currently many research areas are involved in the identification of novel biological markers and therapeutic targets. Modern approaches including genomics, molecular biology, immunology, imaging and computational biology, are carried out in cancer research, leading to the development of novel therapeutic options. Many therapeutic options based on the manipulation or modulation of the immune system have shown unprecedented results and have provided new hope to cancer patients. The introduction of targeted and immune-based therapies have significantly improved the cancer survival rate. In addition to discussing relevant options of cancer treatment and ongoing clinical trials, recent breakthroughs in cancer development and metastasis are provided in this book.

Important efforts and collaborations with leading experts in cancer research and clinics were crucial for achieving this high quality book. We thank all the contributors for sharing their expertise, discoveries, and their views and bringing new hopes for cancer patients and their families. The readers will appreciate the excellent and reliable knowledge in this book.

Although the cancer survival rate has significantly improved over the years, the improvement is primarily due to early diagnosis and cancer growth inhibition. Limited progress has been made in the treatment of cancer metastasis due to various factors. Current treatments for cancer metastasis are mainly chemotherapy and radiotherapy, though the new generation anti-cancer drugs (predominantly neutralizing antibodies for growth factors and small molecule kinase inhibitors) also have effects on cancer metastasis in addition to their effects on cancer growth. Cancer metastasis begins with detachment of metastatic cells from the primary tumor, travel of the cells to different sites through blood/lymphatic vessels, and settlement and growth of the cells at a distal site. During the process, metastatic cells go through detachment, migration, invasion, and adhesion. These four essential metastatic steps are inter-related and affected by multi-biochemical events and parameters. Additionally, it is known that the tumor microenvironment (such as extracellular matrix structure, growth factors, chemokines, matrix metalloproteinases) plays a significant role in cancer metastasis. The biochemical events and parameters involved in the metastatic process and tumor microenvironment have been targeted or can be potential targets for metastasis prevention and inhibition. This review provides an overview of these metastasis essential steps, related biochemical factors, and targets for intervention.

This book offers significant coverage of cancer from risk factors to the mechanisms leading to tumor progression and metastasis. It provides new perspectives for diagnosis and cancer therapy. It also includes new technologies and a new basis for current cancer therapies. Although tremendous progress has been made in cancer treatment, cancer metastasis remains a major unmet clinical need. The life and death of many cancer patients hangs on the degree of metastasis. To guarantee the high quality of this book, important topics are included and rigorously discussed in a simple and authentic way. The book includes new mechanisms leading to tumor progression and metastasis and also new answers for promoting both diagnosis and therapy. This book is an important source of knowledge and will be useful for researchers, medical doctors, graduate and medical students, health care and continued medical providers, and all individuals interested in understanding this devastating disease.

Ahmed Lasfar
Full Member of New Jersey Cancer Institute,
Faculty member and laboratory head at Rutgers University,
Department of Pharmacology and Toxicology,
Ernest Mario School of Pharmacy,
Piscataway, New Jersey

Karine A Cohen-Solal
Chief Scientific Officer,
Lambda Pharmaceutical Bridgewater,
New Jersey

Adjunct Faculty at Department of Pharmacology and Toxicology,
Ernest Mario School of Pharmacy,
Rutgers University,
Piscataway, New Jersey

Section 1

Mechanisms of Tumor Progression and Metastasis

Chapter 1

METCAM/MUC18 Promotes Tumor Progression and Metastasis in Most Human Cancers

Guang-Jer Wu

Abstract

In addition to oncogenes and tumor suppressor genes, cell adhesion molecules (CAMs) also significantly contribute to tumor progression and metastasis. For the past two decades, we have demonstrated that METCAM/MUC18, a cell adhesion molecule in the immunoglobulin-like gene superfamily, orchestrates complex interactions of tumor cells with various stromal cells in the tumor microenvironment, resulting in augmentation or reduction of the metastatic potential of carcinoma cells. Here we show that METCAM/MUC18 plays a positive role in the tumor progression and metastasis in most human cancers, such as breast cancer, human melanoma and most mouse melanoma, nasopharyngeal carcinoma type III, prostate cancer LNCaP and DU145 cell lines, and perhaps angiosarcoma, gastric cancer, glioma, hepatocellular carcinoma, non-small cell lung adenocarcinoma, small cell lung cancer (SCLC), osteosarcoma, and human and mouse pancreatic cancer. Possible mechanisms in the METCAM/MUC18-mediated tumor progression and metastasis are proposed. Anti-METCAM/MUC18 antibodies and siRNAs may be used as therapeutic agents to treat these cancers.

Keywords: METCAM/MUC18, Ig-like CAM, tumor promotion, metastasis, breast cancer, melanoma, nasopharyngeal carcinoma, prostate cancer, many solid tumors, mouse models

1. Introduction: cancer and CAM-mediated tumor progression and metastasis

Tumor/cancer is a chronic disease resulting from gradually accumulation of mutations or epigenetic alterations in our genetic material, DNA [1]. Ten to twenty percent cancer risk comes from hereditary factors and 80–90% of cancer risk from environmental factors [2]. The environmental factors in the physical containment include (a) chemically polluted drinking water, air and soil, and diet; (b) irradiation from solar UV, artificial sources, and environmental radioactive elements; (c) pathological agents (tumor viruses, bacteria, and parasites); and (d) the lifestyle (stress, chronic inflammation from obesity, and free radicals from metabolism) [3–5]. These agents aim to attack our DNA in the somatic cells resulting in slow accumulation of mutations and epigenetic alterations in our genes throughout the life span [6]. The question of "Is cancer a metabolic disease or a genetic disease?" cannot be easily answered. Prior to 1970, most cancer researchers thought cancer is a metabolic disease because of the Warburg effect. After 1970 when Warburg died and after 1971 when oncogenes were discovered, most researchers shifted their thinking to view cancer as a genetic disease. After 2010–2015 when cancer was rediscovered as a metabolic disorder, the view was shifted back to "cancer is a metabolic disease." While cancer as a genetic disease looks to be impossibly complex, tumor cells are a genetic "train wreck" with an infinite number of mutations and epigenetic alterations in ~250 oncogenes and ~700 tumor suppressor genes. In contrast, cancer as a metabolic disease with only seven different "metabotypes" appears to be remarkably simple to deal with, since all the above mutations mainly affect three major metabolic pathways: aerobic glycolysis, glutaminolysis, and one-carbon metabolism [7].

Besides the traditional oncogenes and tumor suppressor genes [6], cell adhesion molecules (CAMs) also contribute directly to the tumor initiation and metastasis or orchestrate the tumor microenvironment to affect the tumor progression [8]. CAMs are involved in several biological functions, such as cellular social behaviors, tissue architecture, organ formation, blood vessel generation and angiogenesis, immune and inflammatory reactions, and wound healing [8]. An altered expression of CAMs has implications in tumor progression and metastasis, since most CAMs govern cellular social behaviors by directly contributing to cell adhesion, epithelial-to-mesenchymal transition (EMT), and cross talk with the intracellular signal transduction pathways affecting other tumor progression-related processes [8]. As a consequence, the aberrant expression of CAMs is capable of changing mobility and invasiveness, influencing outlasting ability and proliferation of tumor cells, and altering new blood vessel formation [8]. It also affects distant organ dissemination of carcinoma cells, because CAMs orchestrate complex interactions of tumor cells with various stromal cells in the tumor microenvironment, resulting in augmentation or reduction of the spreading potential of carcinoma cells [8].

Effects of the aberrant expression of the following CAMs on tumorigenesis and malignant progression are better studied, such as cadherin [9], integrins [10], CD44 [11], CEACAM [12], mucins [13], L1CAM [14], EpCAM [15], ALCAM [16], and METCAM/MUC18 [17]. Over the past 25 years, our team investigated the role of METCAM/MUC18 in several types of tumors, such as melanoma and breast, nasopharyngeal, ovarian, and prostate cancers [17–37].

2. METCAM/MUC18: an immunoglobulin-like (Ig-like) CAM

METCAM/MUC18 was first demonstrated to be abundantly expressed on the cellular membrane of most malignant human melanomas and hence was named as MUC18 [38] and MCAM [37]. It has been implicated to play a pivotal role in the malignant progression of human melanoma and hence was named as Mel-CAM [39]. However, subsequent studies showed that METCAM/MUC18 was not found to be exclusively expressed in melanoma, and furthermore, it did not initiate the transformation of normal cutaneous melanocytes to melanoma [39]. Instead METCAM/MUC18 was also expressed in endothelial cells and other epithelial tumors, and it could initiate or promote the transformation of other epithelial cells into carcinomas [40]. Thus METCAM/MUC18 also bears other names, such as S-endo1, CD146, A32, or METCAM [40, 41]. Later METCAM/MUC18 was also found to act as a suppressor in tumorigenesis and metastasis in some cancer cell lines [17, 37, 40].

The human METCAM/MUC18 (huMETCAM/MUC18) is a cell adhesion molecule (CAM) belonging to the Ig-like gene superfamily. The METCAM/MUC18 usually has an apparent molecular weight of 110–150,000 due to its high glycosylation in all cell types. The naked huMETCAM/MUC18 is a single-chain transmembrane protein of 65–72 kDa consisting of 646 amino acids with an extracellular

N-terminal domain of 558 amino acids, a transmembrane domain with 24 amino acids, and a cytoplasmic domain of 64 residues (**Figure 1**) [38, 42].

Figure 1 shows that the N-terminal extracellular domain of the protein is composed of a signal peptide sequence (SP) and five immunoglobulin-like domains and one X domain [37, 38, 40, 42]. The intracellular cytoplasmic domain has one, three, and one protein kinase consent sequences that are potentially to be phosphorylated by PKA, PKC, and CK2, respectively [37, 38, 40, 42]. The amino acid sequence of huMETCAM/MUC18 reveals nine potential N-glycosylation sites, of which six are conserved between human and mouse proteins, in the extracellular domain. METCAM/MUC18 is conserved in mouse, in which the amino acid sequences of mouse METCAM/MUC18 (moMETCAM/MUC18) are 72.6% identical to the huMETCAM/MUC18 [43]. Therefore, both huMETCAM/MUC18 and moMETCAM/MUC18 are capable of performing similar general functions of CAMs, such as controlling cellular social behaviors by impacting the adhesion status of cells and modulating signaling. Furthermore, overexpression of both human and mouse METCAM/MUC18s similarly affected tumor cells in in vitro motility and invasiveness, in vitro and in vivo tumorigenesis, and in vivo metastasis [42, 43].

The huMETCAM/MUC18 is expressed in at least ten normal tissues: hair follicular cells, smooth muscle cells, endothelial cells, cerebellum, basal cells of the lung, activated T cells, intermediate trophoblasts [44], breast epithelium [18–19], nasopharyngeal epithelium [23], and ovarian epithelium [27]. The protein is also expressed in several carcinomas, such as breast carcinoma, intermediate trophoblast tumors, melanoma, prostate adenocarcinoma, osteosarcoma, and others [17, 44]. Our studies also indicate that overexpression of METCAM/MUC18 augments tumorigenesis of breast carcinoma [18–20], nasopharyngeal carcinoma type III [24, 26], and prostate adenocarcinoma [34], but it does not have an obvious effect on tumorigenesis of most melanoma cell lines [21]. METCAM/MUC18 overexpression also initiates the distant organ dissemination of prostate cancer [32–33] and augments the distant organ dissemination of melanoma [21] and breast carcinoma [45].

In contrast, overexpression of METCAM/MUC18 represses tumorigenesis of a mouse melanoma cell line, K1735-9 [22], nasopharyngeal carcinoma type I [24–25], and perhaps hemangiomas [46]. METCAM/MUC18 overexpression also represses the distant organ dissemination of the mouse melanoma cell line, K1735-9 [22]. Thus, METCAM/MUC18 plays a dual role in some of these cancers [17, 37].

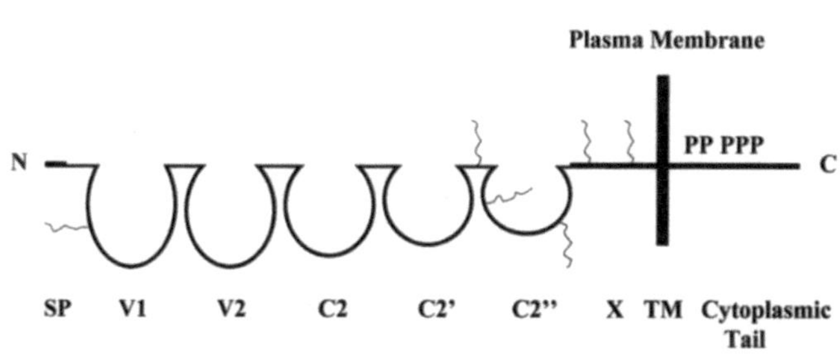

Figure 1.
The human METCAM/MUC18 (huMETCAM/MUC18). The figure represents the protein structure of huMETCAM/MUC18 with its three domains: (1) A large extracellular domain showing a signal peptide (SP), the five Ig-like variables (V1 and V2) and conserved (C1, C2, C2', and C2") domains, each of which held together by a disulfide bond, and one X domain; six conserved N-glycosylation sites indicated as wavy lines in V1, the interdomain C2'/C2", C2", and X domains. (2) A short transmembrane domain (TM). (3) A cytoplasmic domain containing five potential phosphorylation sites (P).

3. METCAM/MUC18: a promoter in tumor progression and metastasis of human cancers

The protein METCAM/MUC18 is expressed in breast cancer, melanoma, nasopharyngeal carcinoma, and prostate cancer and also expressed in others cancers, such as angiosarcoma, gestational trophoblastic tumors, Kaposi's sarcoma, leiomyosarcoma, some lung adenocarcinoma and squamous and small cell carcinomas, and some neuroblastomas [44]. However, its role in the progression of most of these cancers is not well known. Recent meta-analysis suggests that high METCAM/MUC18 expression in many solid tumors appears to be associated with poor prognosis and patient survival [47]. In addition, METCAM/MUC18 expression and its possible role in other solid tumors began to emerge, such as angiosarcoma, gastric cancer, hepatocellular carcinoma, glioma, non-small cell lung cancer (NSCLC), small cell lung cancer (SCLC), osteosarcoma, and pancreatic cancer, as described in the following.

3.1 Breast cancer

Breast carcinomas were heterogenous with three histological subtypes (ER+, PR+, and ERBB2 receptor (HER)) ([48] for a review), with at least five distinct molecular subtypes (luminal A (ER+ and PR+), luminal B (ER+ and PR±), basal-like (ER-, PR-, AR-), HER2-enriched (HER2+), and normal-like) [49], or with ten combined genomic/transcriptomic subtypes [50]. HuMETCAM/MUC18 was found to be expressed in breast cancer cell lines and tissues of basal-like and mesenchymal subtypes at much higher levels than in luminal subtypes, which poorly or very weakly expressed the protein [18, 51]. METCAM/MUC18 was suggested by two groups to play a tumor suppressor role [52, 53] but by two other groups as a tumor promoter in the progression of human breast cancer [51, 54]. To resolve this controversy, we started separate studies to explore the real role of METCAM/MUC18 in the tumor progression of human breast cancer. We demonstrated that ectopic expression of METCAM/MUC18 in two breast cancer cell lines (MCF-7 and SK-BR-3) augmented their ability in epithelial-to-mesenchymal transition (EMT) and formation of colony in vitro and increased tumor-take and tumorigenesis (in vivo tumorigenesis) in athymic nude mice [18–20].

Treatment with an anti-METCAM/MUC18 antibody decreased the motility and invasiveness of the two basal-like cell lines, MDA-MB-231 and MDA-MB-468, which endogenously express the protein [19]. Overexpression of huMETCAM/MUC18 could also induce metastasis of the MCF7 cells in SCID/beige mice with the supplement of estrogen [45]. Furthermore, enforced expression of METCAM/MUC18 increases the metastasis of both basal-like cell lines in athymic nude mice [45]. The tumor suppression role of huMETCAM/MUC18 in tumorigenesis of human breast cancer cells previously observed by one group [52] has not been supported by evidence published later [18, 45]. The most likely reason may be due to the artifact of including fetal bovine serum in their injection mixtures, as extensively discussed in our published paper [18]. The other discrepancy may be because only in vitro experiments were done, but no in vivo animal test [51, 53, 54]. Taken together, METCAM/MUC18 plays a positive role in the tumor progression of four human breast cancer cell lines. From the results of further preliminary mechanical study, we suggest that METCAM/MUC18 promotes the progression of human breast cancer cells by increasing proliferation, angiogenesis, epithelial-to-mesenchymal transition (EMT), and switching to aerobic glycolysis [18–20]. METCAM/MUC18's downstream signaling molecules may also be used as therapeutic targets for the treatment of breast cancer.

3.2 Melanoma

Most malignant human melanomas overly expressed huMETCAM/MUC18 on the cellular surface, suggesting that it may promote the malignant progression of human melanoma [38]. This notion is supported by the evidence that enforced expression of the huMETCAM/MUC18 increases the metastatic ability of three nonmetastatic human melanoma cell lines in the immune-incomplete mouse models [55, 56]. It is further corroborated by our results that enforced expression of moMETCAM/MUC18 also augments the lung nodule formation ability of two low-metastatic mouse melanoma cell lines, K1735-3 and K1735-10, in a syngeneic mouse model with the complete immunity [21]. However, overexpression of moMETCAM/MUC18 in K1735-3 and K1735-10 subline has a minimal effect on tumor formation.

METCAM/MUC18 enables melanoma cells to establish pulmonary metastasis only when the METCAM/MUC18-expressing melanoma cells are injected into the tail vein (experimental metastasis) [18–20, 55, 56], but not when the cells were injected subcutaneously (spontaneous metastasis) either in immune-deficient mouse models [55, 56] or in immune-competent syngeneic mouse models [21]. Thus, it bypassed the initial stages of metastasis, suggesting that METCAM/MUC18 may promote melanoma metastasis only in the later stage of metastasis. This result is consistent with a later observation in that huMETCAM/MUC18 does not confer melanocytes the ability to initiate the tumor progression into melanoma [39]. Surprisingly when another mouse melanoma cell line, K1735-9, was used for the similar test in the syngeneic brown mouse model, a totally opposite result was obtained [22], to be described in Section 4. The exact reason for the dual role of METCAM/MUC18 in the tumor progression and metastasis is not clear, but one possibility is suggested in Section 5.

Taken together, our syngeneic mouse system should be more useful than the immune-incomplete mouse system to comprehend the complex mechanisms played by METCAM/MUC18 in the malignant progression of melanoma cells. Furthermore, the knowledge learned from our syngeneic mouse systems should also be useful for testing the real efficacy of various therapeutic strategies before the treatment of clinical melanoma, because they should more closely mimic the clinical melanoma cases than the xenograft models.

3.3 Nasopharyngeal carcinoma

Most (90%) nasopharyngeal carcinoma (NPC) occurs in the non-lymphomatous, squamous epithelial lining of the posterior nasopharynx [23, 24]. Three histological subtypes of NPC are defined according to World Health Organization (WHO) classification: WHO type I (keratinizing squamous cell carcinomas), WHO type II (nonkeratinizing squamous cell carcinomas), and WHO type III (undifferentiated carcinomas) [23, 24]. Epidemiological studies suggested three major risk factors, such as genetic predisposition, dietary and environmental factors, and the Epstein-Barr virus (EBV) infection, that may induce the unusual incidence of NPC in endemic areas [23–26]. However, the biological mechanisms of their contribution to tumor initiation, development, and malignant progression remain elusive. Since aberrant expression of CAMs, such as CD44, connexin 43, E-cadherin, and ICAM, has been associated with the progression of NPC ([23] for a review), it is highly probable that these risk factors may alter cell adhesion molecule (CAM) expression and lead to tumorigenesis and malignant progression of NPC. In order to test this hypothesis, we initiated the studies on the possible role of altered METCAM/MUC18 expression in the malignant progression of nasopharyngeal carcinoma. First, we investigated if an aberrant expression of METCAM/MUC18 was associated with NPC

[23] and then the effect of METCAM/MUC18 overexpression on the tumorigenesis of two NPC cell lines in an athymic nude mouse model [24–26], as described next.

We used immunohistochemistry (IHC) method to determine the expression level of huMETCAM/MUC18 in 7 tissue specimens of normal nasopharynx and 97 specimens of three different types of NPC and also used immunoblot method to determine several cell lines established from type I to type III NPC [23]. The results showed a weak expression of the METCAM/MUC18 protein in only 27% of the NPC tissues (no expression in 73% of the NPC tissues), in contrast to all the normal nasopharynx tissues which exhibited a high expression of the protein, suggesting that METCAM/MUC18 may play a tumor suppressor role in the development of NPC during the progression of cancer [23]. Then, we further tested the hypothesis by examining the effect of ectopic METCAM/MUC18 expression on in vitro cellular behavior and in vivo tumorigenesis of the two NPC cell lines in athymic nude mice. Indeed, the predicted hypothesis was supported by the results when NPC-TW01 cells were used for the tests [24–26], as described in Section 4. Surprisingly, contrary to the hypothesis, when NPC-TW04 cell line was used for similar in vitro and in vivo tests, we observed that overexpression of METCAM/MUC18 actually promoted in vitro and in vivo tumor growth of NPC-TW04 cells [24, 26], which were established from type III NPC [57]. We thus conclude that METCAM/MUC18 plays a positive role in the tumor progression of the type III NPC [24, 26]. Overall, METCAM/MUC18 plays a dual role in the tumor progression of NPC.

3.4 Prostate cancer

For the past two decades, we have first demonstrated that METCAM/MUC18 expression in human tissues was associated with the progression of human prostate cancer [31] and also with that of mouse adenocarcinoma in a transgenic model, TRAMP [33]. We further showed that overexpression of METCAM/MUC18 promotes the progression of a human prostate cancer cell line, LNCaP, which was established from lymph node lesions [32, 34], as described next.

First, by using IHC and immunoblot assays to determine the expression of huMETCAM/MUC18 in the tissues of human normal prostate gland, patients with BPH, and patients with prostate cancer and metastatic lesions, we found that METCAM/MUC18 was highly expressed in all of the high-grade PINs and most of prostate carcinoma at advanced pathological stages and metastatic lesions, but it was not expressed in most normal prostate glands and in all BPH lesions. Thus, huMETCAM/MUC18 expression is associated with the progression of human prostate cancer [31].

Second, by using similar immunological methods to determine the expression of moMETCAM/MUC18 in the prostatic tissues of a transgenic mouse model, TRAMP, at different times of life span, we found that moMETCAM/MUC18 expression was increased with the progression of the mouse adenocarcinoma in this transgenic mouse model. Thus, moMETCAM/MUC18 overexpression is associated with the progression of mouse prostate adenocarcinoma in a transgenic mouse model, TRAMP [33].

Third, we tested the effect of overexpression of huMETCAM/MUC18 in a human prostate cancer cell line LNCaP on its tumorigenesis when the cells were injected at the non-orthotopic *SC* sites in nude mice. We observed that huMETCAM/MUC18 overexpression promoted the tumorigenesis of the cell line at the non-orthotopic sites [34]. Then, we tested the effect of overexpression of huMETCAM/MUC18 in the LNCaP cell line on its tumorigenesis and establishing metastatic lesions when the cells were injected at the orthotopic site (in the dorsal and lateral lobes of mouse prostate gland) in a male nude mouse model [32]. We found that huMETCAM/MUC18 overexpression promoted the tumorigenesis at the orthotopic prostate gland and also initiates metastatic lesions at periaortic lymph nodes and multiple distant sites (such as seminal vesicles, ureters, and the kidney). From the results, we conclude that ectopic overexpression of huMETCAM/MUC18 promotes in vivo tumorigenesis of the cells at either at non-orthotopic *SC* sites or at orthotopic prostate gland and also that it also initiates metastasis of the cells to multiple distant sites when cells were injected at the orthotopic mouse prostate gland. Taken together, we concluded that huMETCAM/MUC18 expression promotes the tumor progression of LNCaP cells in an athymic nude mouse model [31–36].

Fourth, to check if the above conclusion is also extended to another human prostate cancer cell line, DU145, we recently tested the effect of knocking down the endogenously expressed METCAM/MUC18 on tumorigenesis in a nude mouse system, since DU145 endogenously expresses a high level of METCAM/MUC18 [58]. We found that knocking down of the endogenously expressed METCAM/MUC18 with three shRNAs decreased the subcutaneous tumorigenesis in male nude mice in comparison to a control shRNA, as shown in **Figure 2**. We thus concluded that METCAM/MUC18 expression in DU145 cell line, which was established from brain lesions, plays a positive role in tumorigenesis (and perhaps metastasis) similar to in LNCaP cells.

In summary, we conclude that METCAM/MUC18 plays a positive role in the tumor progression and metastasis of two human prostate cancer cell lines, LNCaP and DU145. However, we recently observed an opposite result when the third human prostate cancer cell line PC-3 was used for the similar test, as described in Section 4, suggesting that METCAM/MUC18 also plays a dual role in the tumor progression of human prostate cancer.

3.5 Other solid tumors

3.5.1 Angiosarcoma

METCAM/MUC18 very likely promotes the formation of angiosarcoma, as supported by our preliminary results as described next. MoMETCAM/MUC18 was expressed at a higher level in one angiosarcoma clone, SVR, which was transfected with H-Ras, than in the control cell line, MS-1, an immortalized normal endothelial cell line [59]. Furthermore, the tumorigenicity of the SVR cell line was higher than the control cell line, thus in direct association with the higher expression level of

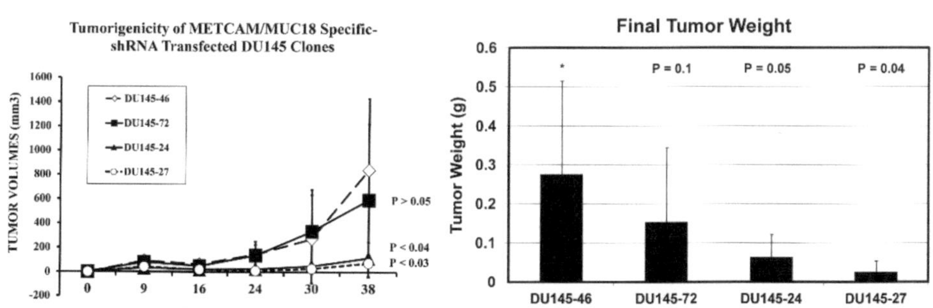

Figure 2.
Tumorigenicity of four shRNA knockdown clones of DU145. Effect of METCAM/MUC18 expression on in vivo tumorigenicity (left) and final tumor weight (right). (Left) Average tumor volumes from 5 mice S.C. injected with each of the 46 (control), 72, 24, and 27 clones/cells, which were transfected with 4 corresponding shRNAs in pGIPZ vector, were plotted against time. (Right) Average final tumor weights from five mice S.C. injected with the same clones/cells and standard deviations were plotted at the end point of experiment. P values are shown in the figure by comparing the data to the control clone [58].

moMETCAM/MUC18 [40, 59]. This suggests that METCAM/MUC18 very likely promotes the tumor progression of angiosarcoma [40, 59].

3.5.2 Gastric cancer

The expression of huMETCAM/MUC18 in gastric cancer was investigated to evaluate its clinical-pathological and prognostic significance [60]. The expression of huMETCAM/MUC18 and three EMT-related proteins (E-cadherin, β-catenin, and vimentin) was examined by IHC method in 144 gastric cancers. Forty-one percent of the gastric cancer specimens were positive for the huMETCAM/MUC18 expression. HuMETCAM/MUC18 was also correlated positively with lymph node involvement and a poor prognosis. Furthermore, the huMETCAM/MUC18 expression was directly correlated with the lost expression of the epithelial marker, E-cadherin, and the gained expression of the mesenchymal markers, nuclear β-catenin and vimentin, suggesting that huMETCAM/MUC18 promotes EMT and also tumor progression in gastric cancer. It is possibly used as an independent index for a poor prognosis in gastric cancer and as a potential therapeutic target for patients with gastric cancers [60].

3.5.3 Glioblastoma

Glioblastoma multiforme (GBM) is the most common brain malignancy, accounting for more than 45% of all primary malignant brain tumors. YY146, an anti-METCAM/MUC18 monoclonal antibody, was created and radiolabeled for the noninvasive positron-emission tomography (PET) imaging of orthotopic GBM models. ^{64}Cu-labeled YY146 was demonstrated to be preferentially accumulated in the U87MG xenografted tumors, which permitted the obtaining of high-contrast PET images of small tumor nodules (~2 mm). Furthermore, tumor-take of glioblastoma in an orthotopic xenograft mouse model correlates with the expression level of METCAM/MUC18 in a highly specific manner. Furthermore, YY146 can mitigate the EMT of these U87MG cells. Moreover, using YY146 as the primary antibody for histological studies of the World Health Organization, grades I through IV primary gliomas showed that there was a positive correlation between METCAM/MUC18-positive staining and high tumor grade, which concurred with the GBM data available in The Cancer Genome Atlas (TCGA). Taken together, METCAM/MUC18 appears to promote the aggressive phenotypes and hence the tumor progression of glioblastoma U87MG cells [61].

3.5.4 Hepatocellular carcinoma

Hepatocellular carcinoma (HCC) remains the fifth most common malignant cancer and as the third leading cause of cancer-related mortality [62]. High-throughput flow cytometry (HT-FC) profiling was used to characterize the expression of METCAM/MUC18 in the tumor cells from 30 human HCC samples. Increased expression of METCAM/MUC18 expression was significantly increased in hepatocellular carcinoma (HCC) tumor tissues as compared with the matched adjacent normal liver tissues. The METCAM/MUC18+ cells purified from HCC tumors have significantly increased colony-forming capacity, consistent with the characteristics of the cancer stem cells or the tumor-initiating cells, which are considered to contribute to the pathogenesis of HCC [63]. The high expression of METCAM/MUC18 in HCC samples and in HCC cell lines isolated from HCC samples was also confirmed by RT-PCR and Western blot analyses [64]. The HCC cell lines, which stably expressed METCAM/MUC18, had been shown to promote EMT, IL8 upregulation, and STAT1 downregulation, suggesting that METCAM/

MUC18 promotes tumor progression and metastasis and predicts poor prognosis of hepatocellular carcinoma [64].

3.5.5 Non-small cell lung cancer

Lung cancer is the cancer with the highest mortality rate in the world [62], and non-small cell lung cancer (NSCLC) is the cause for about 80% of all lung cancer. The frequency of occurrence of adenocarcinoma, which is one of the major histological subtypes of NSCLC, has recently increased [65]. Eighty-five specimens of NSCLC were immunohistochemically analyzed by using an anti-METCAM/MUC18 monoclonal antibody (clone N1238) on an NSCLC tissue microarray, and the staining was semiquantitatively scored. METCAM/MUC18 has been shown to express in 51% of NSCLC, preferentially squamous cell carcinomas. Positive expression of METCAM/MUC18 has also been associated with a shorter survival of patients with adenocarcinomas and used to predict the poor overall survival in patients with lung adenocarcinomas [65, 66]. Another group also used IHC to show that METCAM/MUC18 expression was more frequently detected in males than in females. The positive expression of METCAM/MUC18 was associated with a poorer 5-year overall survival rate according to the survival analysis, suggesting that METCAM/MUC18 may be a useful marker for predicting poor prognosis in patients with NSCLC following complete resection [65]. The third group reported that METCAM/MUC18 protein expression was found in 46.61% of squamous cell carcinomas and 37.47% of adenocarcinomas. METCAM/MUC18 expression positively correlated with vimentin but inversely with E-cadherin, indicating a positive correlation with EMT. METCAM/MUC18 expression in surgically treated primary tumor NSCLC is clearly associated with lymph node metastasis and is a statistically significant prognostic factor [67]. Consistent with the results and also supporting the conclusion described above, we also showed that METCAM/MUC18 is expressed in a lung type II alveolar epithelial cell carcinoma cell, A549, and highly expressed in an adenocarcinoma cell line, H838, in comparison with its no expression in an immortalized normal embryonic WI38 cell line [68], as shown in **Figure 3**.

Furthermore, the fourth group observed that METCAM/MUC18 expression mediates acquisition of cancer stemness and enhances tumor invasion and metastasis in a mouse model [69–70]. High expression of METCAM/MUC18 correlates with intrapulmonary metastasis of NSCLC cells in a mouse model [69–70]. Taken

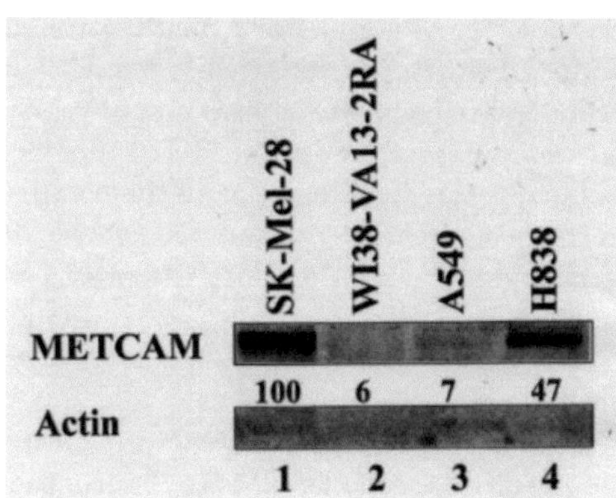

Figure 3.
Expression of METCAM/MUC18 in normal lung tissue (SV40-immortalized normal lung cells) (WI38, lane 2) and lung type II alveolar epithelial cell carcinoma cell (A549, lane 3) and lung primary adenocarcinoma (H838, lane 4) [From [68]].

together, METCAM/MUC18 plays a positive role in the tumor progression and metastasis of NSCLC.

3.5.6 Small cell lung cancer

Small cell lung cancer (SCLC), a lung cancer subtype with an aggressive and highly metastatic nature, is the cause for about 10–20% of lung cancer incidence. The 5-year survival rate is at 7%, still very gloomy because choices of systemic treatment for SCLC patients have not been much increased. SCLC is highly responsive to chemotherapy at the start of treatment. Despite favorable responses to initial therapy, SCLC relapse occurs within a year exhibiting a multidrug-resistant phenotype, which eventually contributes strongly to poor prognosis. Through in-depth proteomic profiling, METCAM/MUC18 was identified as a markedly upregulated surface receptor in chemoresistant SCLC cell lines that exhibited a mesenchymal phenotype as well as in chemoresistant patient-derived xenografts compared to matched treatment-naïve tumors. METCAM/MUC18 knockdown in chemoresistant cells reduced cell proliferation and decreased the IC50 inhibitory concentration of chemotherapeutic drugs. METCAM/MUC18 was found to modulate sensitivity of SCLC cells to chemotherapeutic drugs through upregulation of MRP1/ABCC1 expression and of the PI3/AKT pathway in a SOX2-dependent manner. Metabolomic profiling revealed that METCAM/MUC18 modulates lactate production in chemoresistant cells that exhibit a distinct metabolic phenotype characterized by low oxidative phosphorylation. METCAM/MUC18 may serve as a novel therapeutic target to overcome chemoresistance in SCLC [71]. In summary, the above results point to the positive role played by METCAM/MUC18 in the tumor progression and metastasis of SCLC.

3.5.7 Osteosarcoma

Osteosarcoma is the most common primary malignant bone tumor in children. Clinically evident metastatic disease is present in 10–20% of patients at diagnosis. Despite advancements in multimodality treatment, 5-year survival rates are ~40–50% [72]. METCAM/MUC18 was widely expressed on both osteosarcoma and Ewing's sarcoma cells. METCAM/MUC18 protein and RNA are highly expressed in osteosarcoma cell lines (SaOS, MG-63, U-2OS), but not in normal osteoblast cells [72–73]. ABX-MA1, an anti-METCAM/MUC18 antibody, did not appear to inhibit the in vitro proliferation of osteosarcoma cells, and neither did it significantly inhibit the in vivo growth of KRIB human osteosarcoma cells in the tibias of nude mice. Nevertheless, after 1½ months, a noticeably fewer number of ABX-MA1-treated mice spontaneously developed pulmonary metastatic lesions than the control antibody-treated mice. Furthermore, ABX-MA1 reduced the in vitro invasiveness of osteosarcoma cells in the Matrigel-coated trans-well assay and disturbed the homotypic adhesion among osteosarcoma cells and the heterotypic interaction of them with vascular endothelial cells. Osteosarcoma is effectively treated with anti-METCAM/MUC18 monoclonal antibodies [73–74]. Taken together, METCAM/MUC18 plays a positive role in the metastasis of osteosarcoma [72–74].

3.5.8 Human and mouse pancreatic cancer

Pancreatic ductal adenocarcinoma (PDAC) is the cancer that has the fourth highest mortality rate in the western countries [62]. The 5-year survival rate of all PDAC patients is 6%. Since this tumor is highly aggressive, cancer incidence is almost equivalent to its mortality rate [62]. Most pancreatic cancer deaths are due to metastasis. Especially, the events of tumor spreading are heterogeneous,

Tumor/cancer tissues or cell lines	Tumorigenesis	Metastasis	References
Angiosarcoma human cell lines MS1, SVR	Increasing	Not determined	[40, 59]
Human breast cancer cell line MCF-7	Promotion	Not determined	[18]
Human breast cancer cell line SK-BR-3	Promotion	Not determined	[19, 20]
Human breast cancer cell lines MDA-MB-231 and MDA-MB-468	Promotion	Promotion	[19, 45]
Gastric cancer human tissues	Promotion	Not determined	[60]
Glioma cell lines U87MG, U251	Promotion	Not Determined	[61]
Hepatocellular carcinoma human cell lines PLC/PRF/5, Huh7, MHCC97H and 97L HepG2, SMMC-7721, FOCUS, YY-8103, LM3, HLF, and primary HCC cell lines; normal liver cell line LO2	Promotion	Not determined	[63, 64]
Non-small cell lung cancer human cell lines A549, H23, H358, H460, H522, H838, HCC4006, H1650/ER, PC-9, and PC9GR and adenocarcinoma tissues	Promotion	Promotion	[65–70]
Small cell lung cancer human cell lines H69, H69AR, H82, H196, H209, DMS79	Promotion	Not determined	[71]
Clinical melanoma tissues and human melanoma cell lines SB-2, SK, XP-44	No effect	Increasing and affecting the late stage	[38, 55, 56]
Mouse melanoma cell lines K1735-3, K1735-10	No effect or slight suppression	Increasing and affecting the late stage	[21]
Nasopharyngeal carcinoma type III human cell line NPC-TW04	Promotion	Not determined	[24, 26]
Osteosarcoma human cell lines CR9, MNNG-HOS, OHS, KPDX, KRIB, MG-63, shYY1, SaOS, SaOS-2, TE85, U20S	Promotion	Augmentation	[72–74]
Pancreatic cancer human cell lines and mouse cell lines ptf1a, LSL-Kras, LSL-Trp53, Pdx1	Promotion	Possible augmentation	[75, 76]
Clinical prostate cancer human tissues	Increasing	Increasing and affecting initiation in the early stage (PIN)	[31]
Human prostate cancer cell line LNCaP	Increasing	Increasing and affecting initiation in the early stage	[32, 34–36]
Human prostate cancer cell line DU145	Increasing	Not determined	[58]
Prostate adenocarcinoma in TRAMP mice	Increasing	Increasing and affecting initiation in the early stage	[33]

Table 1.
The positive role of METCAM/MUC18 in the tumor progression of various solid tumors/cancers.

thus limiting the therapeutic choices for patients at late stages. METCAM/MUC18 expression in cancer cells is associated with a secretion of soluble METCAM/MUC18 (sMETCAM/MUC18) that plays an active role in tumor development. For example, sMETCAM/MUC18 causes the overproduction of its binding partner, angiomotin, in cancer cells and endothelial cells in the tumor micro-*milieu*, which augments angiogenesis and proliferation and survival of cancer cells. These are mediated in part by the promotion and activation of c-myc in cancer cells. Dispensation of a new specific monoclonal antibody pinpointing on sMETCAM/MUC18 represses tumor angiogenesis and growth of huMETCAM/MUC18+ pancreatic cancer cell xenografts in mice models. Taken together, sMETCAM/MUC18 secreted by METCAM/MUC18+ tumors exhibit promoting effects on tumor angiogenesis and growth. Thus, an antibody pinpointing on sMETCAM/MUC18 successfully represses vascularization, growth, and survival of METCAM/MUC18-positive pancreatic tumors [75].

The expression of a homeodomain transcription factor MEIS1 (myeloid ecotropic viral integration site) has been associated with a ductal phenotype in pancreatic tissue architecture. To investigate a possible role of MEIS1 in the malignant progression of PDAC, pancreatic cancer cell clones/lines, which overexpress MEIS1, were generated and tested for in vitro proliferation rate and motility. Overexpression of MEIS1 had no effect on in vitro proliferation rate but augmented motility. Furthermore, an upregulation of the MTCAM/MUC18 gene in the migrating cells has been found in the subsequent expression analysis. The interaction of MEIS1 with the enhancer DNA of METCAM/MUC18 is revealed by employing DNA pulldown and chromatin immunoprecipitation (ChIP) assay. Furthermore, the transcriptional activation of METCAM/MUC18 also facilitates migration of pancreatic cancer cells in vitro. Activation of METCAM/MUC18 through MEIS1 occurs in a cell type-dependent fashion, reflecting the different routes that lead to metastasis in vivo. Thus, the transcription factor MEIS1 activates METCAM/MUC18 expression to promote migration of mouse pancreatic tumor cell lines [76].

In summary, the positive role played by the METCAM/MUC18 in the progression of solid tumors has been extended from breast cancer, human and mouse melanoma, and prostate cancer to angiosarcoma [40, 59], gastric cancer [60], glioblastoma [61], hepatocellular carcinoma [63, 64], non-small cell lung adenocarcinoma [65–70], small cell lung cancer [71], osteosarcoma [72–74], human and mouse pancreatic cancer [75, 76], and prostate cancer [32–36, 58]. Taken together, METCAM/MCU18 appears to be more prevalently playing a positive role than a negative role in the tumor formation and/or cancer metastasis of various tumors/cancers. **Table 1** summarizes the positive role of METCAM/MUC18 in the tumor progression of many solid tumors/cancers.

4. METCAM/MUC18: a tumor suppressor and metastasis suppressor in some cancers

In contrast to the positive role played by METCAM/MUC18 in the above cancers, recent results of testing the effects of METCAM/MUC18 expression on tumorigenesis of other cancer types revealed that it also plays a negative role in the tumor progression and metastasis in some cancers, such as colorectal cancer, hemangioma, one mouse melanoma cell line K1735-9, NPC type I, ovarian cancer, human pancreatic cancer, and one human prostate cancer cell line PC-3, as described next.

4.1 Colorectal cancer

Colorectal cancer (CRC) is the third leading cause of cancer deaths in recent years [62]. Cancer stemness contributes to carcinogenesis, tumor relapse, and chemoresistance in traditional cancer therapeutics ([77] for a review). Stemness, which is the cell state with the properties of self-renewal, differentiation, and tumor-initiating potential, might be characterized by a set of more dynamic features influenced by the nature of the microenvironment. Various extrinsic cues and intrinsic signaling pathways, such as Wnt, Notch, and Hedgehog signals, are involved in the maintenance of stemness. Since METCAM/MUC18 has also been identified as a pluripotent marker for mesenchymal stem cells (MSCs), it was also hypothesized to exert potential effects on cancer cell stemness. One group of investigators has provided evidence to demonstrate that reduced expression of METCAM/MUC18 actually functions as a positive regulator of stem cell properties in colorectal cancer through augmenting the Wnt/β-catenin signaling pathway. METCAM/MUC18 may actually manifest multifaceted effects on tumor progression in a context-dependent manner. The above evidence suggests that METCAM/MUC18 expression suppresses the tumor progression and metastasis of colorectal cancer [77].

4.2 Hemangioma

The expression of METCAM/M/MUC18 in hemangioma is inversely proportional to the progression of hemangioma, suggesting that METCAM/MUC18 plays a negative role in the progression of hemangioma [46].

4.3 Mouse melanoma

As shown in the above section, moMETCAM/MUC18 does not have an obvious effect on the tumorigenesis of the two K1735 cell lines, such as K1735-3 and K1735-10 [21]. In contrast, moMETCAM/MUC18 definitely acts as a tumor suppressor for the K1735-9 cell line. Overexpression of moMETCAM/MUC18 in K1735-9 also completely suppressed lung nodule formation in immunocompetent syngeneic C3H brown mouse model [22]. Thus, METCAM/MUC18 expression suppresses the tumor progression and metastasis of the mouse melanoma K1735-9 cell line [22].

4.4 Nasopharyngeal carcinoma (NPC)

According to the IHC results as shown in the above section, we suggested a hypothesis that METCAM/MUC18 may play a tumor suppressor function in the development of NPC during the progression of the cancer [23]. Then, we further tested the hypothesis by examining the effect of METCAM/MUC18 overexpression on in vitro cellular behavior and in vivo tumorigenesis of the two NPC cell lines in athymic nude mice. When the METCAM/MUC18-overexpressing NPC-TW01 clones/cells, which were established from NPC type I, were used for the animal test, indeed tumor suppression was observed [24, 25]. However, the opposite results were obtained when the METCAM/MUC18-overexpressing NPC-TW04 clones/cells, which were established from NPC type III, were used for the similar tests. Thus, METCAM/MUC18 plays a dual role in the tumor progression of NPC [23, 24–26].

4.5 Ovarian cancer

Two independent groups showed that METCAM/MUC18 expression is correlated with the progression of ovarian cancer [27, 78] and it affects in vitro behaviors of ovarian carcinoma cells [79]; however, the role of METCAM/MUC18 in the progression of epithelial ovarian cancer has not been directly tested in animal models. For this purpose, we initiated testing the effect of METCAM/MUC18 overexpression on the in vitro cellular behaviors and in vivo tumorigenesis and malignant progression of human ovarian cancer cell lines in nude mice. First, we used a human ovarian cell line, SK-OV-3, for the in vitro and in vivo tests. We observed that overexpression of METCAM/MUC18 reduced in vitro motility and invasiveness [28] and suppressed in vivo tumorigenesis on subcutaneous (SC) sites and in intraperitoneal cavity as well as in vivo malignant progression of the human ovarian cancer cell line SK-OV-3 in intraperitoneal (IP) cavity in female athymic nude mice [28]. When the other human ovarian cancer cell line, BG-1, was similarly tested, similar results were also observed [80]. In summary, we supplied in vitro and in vivo evidence to definitely support the conclusion that METCAM/MUC18 plays a suppressor role in the tumorigenesis and malignant progression of two human ovarian cancer cell lines [28–30, 80], suggesting that METCAM/MUC18 is a strong candidate as a new tumor and metastasis suppressor in human ovarian cancer cells.

4.6 Human pancreatic cancer

In contrast to the above results of human and mouse pancreatic cancer that METCAM/MUC18 expression plays a positive role in the malignant progression of PDAC, a group has demonstrated that METCAM/MUC18 expression in cancer-associated fibroblasts (CAFs) has been correlated with the pre-pancreatic intraepithelial neoplasia (PIN) and the invasive ductal pancreatic cancer with a low histological grade. Furthermore, the prognosis for the patients with a low METCAM/MUC18 expression is poorer than those with a high METCAM/MUC18 expression. Suppressing METCAM/MUC18 expression in CAFs augmented tumor cell in vitro motility and invasiveness in a co-culture system that includes both tumor cells and CAFs. Knockdown of METCAM/MUC18 also augmented CAF activation, possibly via regulation of NF-kB activity, which in turn induces the yield of factors for tumorigenesis. In line with this notion, METCAM/MUC18 overexpression in CAFs decreased in vitro motility and invasiveness of the cancer cells co-cultured with CAFs. Moreover, METCAM/MUC18 expression in CAFs was decreased by interaction with cancer cells. Taken together, reduced METCAM/MUC18 expression in CAFs and reduction of METCAM/MUC18 augment tumor progression of pancreatic cancer [81]. Therefore, METCAM/MUC18 expression suppresses the tumor progression and metastasis of pancreatic cancer. In comparison with the results from Section 3.5.8, METCAM/MUC18 expression also plays a dual role in pancreatic cancer.

4.7 Prostate cancer

We recently used the knocking down strategy similar to that of DU145 cell line to test the effect of decreased endogenous METCAM/MUC18 expression on in vivo tumorigenesis of another human prostate cancer cell line, PC-3, which was established from bone lesions. Surprisingly we found that knocking down the endogenously expressed METCAM/MUC18 increased the tumor proliferation of PC-3 cells, suggesting that expression of METCAM/MUC18 suppressed the tumorigenesis of the human prostate cancer cell line PC-3 [82]. We thus conclude that METCAM/MUC18 serves as a tumor suppressor in the PC-3 cell line. Thus, similar to mouse melanoma, NPC, and pancreatic cancer, METCAM/MUC18 expression also plays a dual role in tumor progression and metastasis in human prostate cancer.

In summary, METCAM/MUC18 may also suppress tumor progression and metastasis of the following solid tumors, such as colorectal cancer [77], mouse melanoma K1735-9 subline [22], NPC type I [24, 25], ovarian cancer [28–30], human pancreatic cancer [81], one prostate cancer cell line PC-3 [82], and perhaps hemangioma [46]. Thus, METCAM/MUC18 appears to play a negative role in tumor progression and metastasis of some solid tumors but a dual role in some other solid tumors. It is not clear why METCAM/MUC18 plays a dual role. Since METCAM/MUC18 only plays a dual role in different cell lines from the same type of cancer or in different type of cancers, but never in the same cancer cell line, it is logical to suggest a possible explanation that the intrinsic properties of each cancer cell line may provide specific co-factors or heterophilic ligands that may positively or negatively modulate the METCAM/MUC18-mediated tumorigenesis and metastasis. This can be readily scrutinized by identifying these specific intrinsic cofactors or heterophilic ligands by using immunological coprecipitation method in the future studies, which is feasible as described in Section 5.5.

5. Preliminary and possible mechanisms

Since the huMETCAM/MUC18 was first discovered in the 1980s, three groups have worked on the role of huMETCAM/MUC18 in melanoma metastasis [38, 39, 55, 56], another group on the role of huMETCAM/MUC18 in the biology of endothelial cells [41, 83], and one group on breast cancer [45], and our group joined in the effort to study the role of huMETCAM/MUC18 in the progression of mouse melanoma [43] and prostate cancer [31–36] and later breast cancer [18–20], ovarian cancer [27–30], and NPC [23–26], as described above. Recently, more research groups have participated in further exploring the possible role of METCAM/MUC18 in other solid tumors in different organs, such as the colorectum [77], gastro-organ [60], glial cells [61], liver [63, 64], lung [65–71], bone [72–74], and pancreas [75, 76, 81]. Furthermore, preliminary work in leiomyosarcoma, esophagus squamous cell carcinoma, clear cell renal sarcoma, and gallbladder adenocarcinoma are also beginning to emerge [47]. Thus, after decades of group effort, we are beginning to understand the biology of METCAM/MUC18-mediated tumor progression.

However, we still know very little how METCAM/MUC18 mediates or regulates tumor progression and metastasis of cancer cells. Thus, the biological mechanisms describing the role of METCAM/MUC18 in tumorigenesis and malignant progression are still not well clarified. By deducing knowledge learned from the tumorigenesis of other tumors [6, 17, 37, 40] and angiogenesis [41, 83], we may be able to find some common clues to begin understanding its mechanisms. As such, the following five important aspects are much needed for immediate future studies, such as differential regulation at the transcription level in tumors of different organs; different signaling pathways involved; contributions of different domains of the protein; possible different extent of N-glycosylation in different cancer cell lines, which may critically modulate the function of METCAM/MUC18 in tumor progression; and different kinds or quantities of cofactors or heterophilic ligand(s) in different cancer cell lines.

5.1 Transcriptional regulation

The mechanism of transcriptional control of METCAM/MUC18 gene is minimally studied [17]. So far, only 900 bp of the core promoter region of the huMETCAM/MUC18 gene are sequenced [84]. The core promoter reflects a typical housekeeping gene, which is rich in GC sequences but does not contain a TATA box. Nevertheless, it includes many consensus sequences presumably as putative binding sites for various transcription regulatory factors, such as SP-1, CREB [85], AP-2 [86–87], c-Myb [88], N-Oct2 (Brn2) [89], Ets [90], CArG [91], and Egr-1 [92], and three insulin-responsive elements (one Ets and two E-box motifs) [93], suggesting that transcriptional control of the huMETCAM/MUC18 gene is regulated by various growth signals [37, 40]. For example, the huMETCAM/MUC18 gene is positively regulated by PKA/CREB (cAMP-responsive element binding protein) and negatively regulated by AP-2α [94]. Having a longer DNA containing sequences for tissue-specific expression of the gene is essential for further understanding the roles of other regulators [17]. In line with this hypothesis, recently, the Ets sequence in the 10 kilo-bp upstream region has been shown to regulate the expression of huMET-CAM/MUC18 gene [95]. We have also engaged in this task by screening in a phage library containing the human genomic sequences and obtained several phage clones which contain at least 4 kilo-bp of in the upstream region of the promoter region of the gene for future studies [96]. Thus, the regulatory mechanism of tissue-specific expression of the METCAMMUC18 gene may be forthcoming.

The epigenetic control of the expression of huMETCAM/MUC18 gene has been implicated in human cancers, because huMETCAM/MUC18 gene is located at the locus of human chromosome 11q23.3 [97] that has been shown to be hypermethylated in NPC [98], suggesting that the expression of this gene may be regulated by epigenetic controls. To support this notion, our preliminary results of treating NPC cell lines with 5-Aza-2′-deoxycytidine (Aza-C) showed that after the treatment with Aza-C, METCAM/MUC18 expression was somewhat elevated in the NPC-TW01 cell line, but not in the NPC-TW04 cell line [99]. METCAM/MUC18 has also been shown to be methylated in the early stage of most prostate cancer [100]. Thus, it is highly possible that the gene is epigenetically controlled in other cancers.

5.2 Signaling pathways

The cytoplasmic tail of huMETCAM/MUC18 contains consensus sequences potentially to be phosphorylated by PKA, PKC, and CK2, suggesting that its functions may be mediated by these protein kinases and regulated by cross talk with various signaling pathways [17, 37, 38, 40, 42]. First, it is necessary to biochemically prove how many sites are actually phosphorylated in the cytoplasmic tail of the METCAM/MUC18 protein purified from different cancer cell lines and which protein kinase is responsible for the phosphorylation. After this is answered, then we can further study how METCAM/MUC18 mediates cross talk and networking with different signal pathways and is to be compared with the cytoplasmic tails of other CAMs [6, 8, 41]. Knowledge learned from the impact of other CAMs on tumor progression suggests that METCAM/MUC18, as an integral membrane Ig-like CAM, should mediate inside-in, inside-out, and outside-in signals to participate in intercellular communication and interaction of cell with the extracellular matrix, which results in impacting EMT [6, 8, 41, 101]. Furthermore, huMETCAM/MUC18 has been shown to express in normal mesenchymal cells (smooth muscle, endothelium, and Schwann cells) in the tissue stroma and be a marker for the mesenchymal stem cells [102]; thus, expression of METCAM/MUC18 may augment the EMT of cancer cells and hence the progression of many cancers. Moreover, METCAM/MUC18 may affect cancer cell progression by cross talk with signaling pathways that affect apoptosis, survival and proliferation, angiogenesis, and energy metabolism of tumor cells [6, 8, 101]. This is indeed found in our preliminary mechanical studies in breast cancer [19, 20], melanoma [21, 22], NPC [24–26], ovarian cancer [28–30], and prostate cancer [34–37]. Further systematic studies by using specific RNAi's to knockdown the downstream effectors one by one in the METCAM/MUC18-expressing clones may be necessary to further understand this aspect of mechanism. Moreover, its interaction with cofactors or cognate heterophilic ligand(s) may alter these signals, which in turn should affect intrinsic tumor proliferation or impact tumor angiogenesis and/or mediate targeting to specific organs and promoting metastasis. Finally, METCAM/MUC18 may interact with various hormonal receptors, growth or anti-growth factors/receptors, various chemokines/receptors, and the Ca++-mediated signaling members and affect tumor progression [17].

HuMETCAM/MUC18 expression in melanoma cells is reciprocally regulated by AKT, in which AKT upregulates the level huMETCAM/MUC18 and overexpression of huMETCAM/MUC18 activates endogenous AKT, which in turn inhibits apoptosis and increases survival ability [103]. A similar mechanism is also likely to be used in other cancers; however, the detailed mechanism of how AKT upregulates the expression of METCAM/MUC18 in most cancers has not been reported. After the cytoplasmic tail is phosphorylated, then it may facilitate its interaction with FAK, thus promoting cytoskeleton remodeling, which in turn augments tumor cell motility and invasiveness [83]. Alternatively, after phosphorylation, huMETCAM/MUC18 may interact with the downstream effectors of Ras, activating ERK and JNK, which in turn may transcriptionally activate the expression of AKT or other genes that promote the proliferation and angiogenesis of tumor cells. Moreover, by predicting from the relatively less selectivity of CK2 for its substrate and many CAMs which are phosphorylated by CK2, such as CD44, E-cadherin, and L1-CAM, and one of the integrin receptors in the extracellular matrix protein, vitronectin [104], huMETCAM/MUC18 is very likely to be phosphorylated by CK2 and linked to AKT to affect the proliferation, survival, and other tumorigenesis-related functions [105]. Recent findings appear to support this mechanism in that METCAM/MUC18 may promote EMT of breast cancer cells via activation of RhoA and upregulation of slug [45]. HuMETCAM/MUC18 may play an important role in regulating tumor dormancy or awakening, driving or preventing cancer cells to pre-metastatic niche, and formatting a microenvironment for favorable or unfavorable tumor growth in secondary sites [17, 37].

HuMETCAM/MUC18 may mediate hematogenous spreading of melanoma cells, as implicated by its expression in endothelial cells and malignant melanoma cells [106] and presence in junctions of endothelial cells [107, 108], essential for tumor angiogenesis in three tumor cell lines [109] and human prostate cancer LNCaP cells [110], and it is highly likely for that in other cancers [111, 112]. HuMETCAM/MUC18 may also be implicated in promoting lymphatic metastasis of cancer cells, since it is one of the lymphatic metastasis-associated genes, which are upregulated in malignant mouse hepatocellular carcinoma [113]. However, the detailed mechanisms of huMETCAM/MUC18-mediated hematogenous and lymphatic spreading of cancer cells remain to be investigated. For this purpose, labeling cells with viable dyes and employing a newly developed non-intruding, but highly photo-penetrating imaging photoacoustic tomography (PAT) to monitor each step of the process in real time in hairless nude mice may be helpful to provide some answers [114].

HuMETCAM/MUC18 may interact with the host immune system and affect tumor progression, though the immune system may have a contradictory role in the process [115]. This notion is positively supported by a recent finding that a subset of host B lymphocytes may be implicated in regulating melanoma malignant progression via interaction with huMETCAM/MUC18 [116]. Our syngeneic mouse system for mouse melanoma should be useful for exploring the role of immune T and B cells in the progression of METCAM/MUC18-expressing melanoma cells. However, the role of B and T cells in the progression of most human cancer cells may not be explored in the athymic nude mouse models since most human cancer cells can only grow as xenografts in these immunodeficient mouse models. Nevertheless, to investigate the effect of huMETCAM/MUC18 expression on mediating NK cells in metastasis may be possible in these nude mouse models, which can be tested by pretreatment of nude mice with anti-NK surface marker antibodies to deplete the NK cells prior to injection of the huMETCAM/MUC18-expressing cancer cells. This possibility is supported by the finding that the surface huMETCAM/MUC18 expressed in cancer cells may have a homophilic interaction with the NK cells, which also express huMETCAM/MUC18 and enhance cytotoxic functions of NK cells [117].

5.3 Functional domain

To begin addressing the relation of the protein structure of huMETCAM/MUC18 to its functions in tumorigenesis and metastasis, we have generated mutant-deleted different domains of huMETCAM/MUC18 by using a special PCR method [118] and used them to determine their contribution to tumorigenesis. Surprisingly, our preliminary results showed that the ecto-domain and the intact copy of huMETCAM/MUC18 cDNA equally efficiently induced tumorigenesis in LNCaP cells in nude mice, suggesting the key role of the ecto-domain in inducing tumorigenesis of prostate cancer cells in vivo. However, this stirs up a puzzling question that the cytoplasmic domain was not essential for this process [119]. Nevertheless, critical direct test of using only the cytoplasmic domain for inducing tumor should be performed. It is essential that a systematic study has also to be performed in other cancer cell lines before a definitive conclusion can be drawn.

5.4 Glycosylation

Malignant progression of cancer cells has been shown to associate with an abnormal glycosylation, resulting in expression of altered carbohydrate determinants [120]. Thus, the glycosylated status of huMETCAM/MUC18 in different cancer types may be different from normal cells and may manifest either a positive or negative effect on the progression of different cancer types, which should be very intriguing since huMETCAM/MUC18 possesses six conserved N-glycosylation sites in the extracellular domain [17, 37, 40].

Glycosylation of a protein may affect the proper folding, stability, and/or activity of a protein [121]. Both huMETCAM/MUC18 and moMETCAM/MUC18 are very likely heavily glycosylated, sialylated, and/or posttranslationally modified, because both have an apparent molecular weight of about 110–150 kDa, in comparison with the naked protein with a molecular weight of about 65–70 kDa [122]. The possible roles of METCAM/MUC18 glycosylation in inducing/promoting or suppressing the metastasis of cancer cells should be explored [123]. To initiate the study, we subjected the huMETCAM/MUC18, which was isolated from one human cancer cell line, to the digestion with N-glycosidase F, neuraminidase (sialidase), O-glycosidase, or endoglycosidase H. We observed that the apparent molecular weight of the protein was decreased after digestion with N-glycosidase F and neuraminidase (sialidase), but not with O-glycosidase or endoglycosidase H [37, 40], suggesting that both sialic acid and N-glycans are probably the major carbohydrate side chains of huMETCAM/MUC18. It is also possible that glycosylation may differ depending on the type of cancers. Thus, we suggested that different N-glycans at the N-glycosylation sites of huMETCAM/MUC18 may differ in different cancer cell lines, which may have significant positive or negative impacts on their EMT abilities as well as tumorigenesis and metastasis. Our hypothesis is supported by a recent report that described GCNT3 as an upstream regulator of METCAM/MUC18 in that it glycosylates METCAM/MUC18 and extends its half-life which results in further elevation of S100A8/A9-mediated cellular motility in melanoma cells [124]. The role of glycosylation in the six N-glycosylation sites should be genetically altered to explore their effects on the functions of METCAM/MUC18 in tumor progression and metastasis.

5.5 Heterophilic ligands and cofactors that modulate the function of METCAM/MUC18

Since METCAM/MUC18 only plays a dual role in different cell lines from the same type of cancer or in different types of cancers, but never in the same cancer cell line, it is logical to suggest a possible explanation that the intrinsic properties of each cancer cell line may provide specific cofactors or heterophilic ligands that may positively or negatively modulate the METCAM/MUC18-mediated tumor progression and metastasis. This can be readily scrutinized by identifying these specific intrinsic cofactors or heterophilic ligands in different cancer cell lines by using immunological coprecipitation method. This approach appears to be feasible as shown in our preliminary result in that a putative heterophilic ligand, 72 kDa protein, is identified [17, 37, 40]. This protein is present at a higher concentration in PC-3 cells than in DU145 that may be responsible for an opposite role of METCAM/MUC18 in tumor progression of these two cell lines. Thus, it is possible that mechanisms of huMETCAM/MUC18-mediated cancer progression may be different in different cancer cell lines due to their different intrinsic properties, which possess different concentration or completely different heterophilic different ligands and/or cofactors. The heterophilic ligands and/or cofactors of METCAM/MUC18 may contribute to the cellular intrinsic properties, such as adhesion-associated signaling cascades and cytoskeleton rearrangement, leading to different EMT of these cells and modulating the huMETCAM/MUC18-mediated tumor progression and metastasis. Different intrinsic cofactors in different cancer cell lines may modulate METCAM/MUC18 and alter cell-to-cell and cell-extracellular matrix interactions in the tumor microenvironment, resulting in affecting tumor progression and metastasis in vivo. Finally, these cofactors/ligands may interact differently with METCAM/MUC18 in different cell lines and affect other host physiological factors, which may augment or suppress in vivo tumor progression and metastasis by affecting metabolic switch, pro-apoptosis/anti-apoptosis, tumor angiogenesis, and host immune system in the tumor micro-*milieu* and in various metastatic sites [17, 37, 40, 111, 112]. Thus, the identification of the cofactors and the huMETCAM/MUC18-cognate heterophilic ligand(s) is critical for understanding the mechanism.

6. Conclusions

METCAM/MUC18 also plays a key positive function in the progression of angiosarcoma, breast cancer, gastric cancer, glioblastoma, hepatocellular carcinoma, lung cancer, melanoma, NPC type III, osteosarcoma, pancreatic cancer, prostate cancer, and possibly other cancers. On the other hand, METCAM/MUC18 plays a key role in suppressing the progression of colorectal cancer, one mouse melanoma cell line, NPC type I, ovarian cancer, pancreatic cancer, prostate cancer PC-3 cell line, and perhaps hemangioma. To further understand its role in these processes, it is essential to further identify its cofactor regulators and cognate heterophilic ligands, define its functional domains, and study its cross talk with members of various signal transduction pathways, the regulation of its expression at the level of transcription, and effects of N-glycosylation on the functions of the protein.

7. Research perspectives and clinical applications

7.1 Research perspectives

The current studies have laid an important foundation for future intriguing investigation to further understand the detailed mechanism of METCAM/MUC18-mediated tumor progression and metastasis of various cancer cell lines. For this purpose besides those have been described above, other future endeavors may include (a) understanding the mechanisms in the METCAM/MUC18-mediated tumor progression and metastasis, such as intrinsic growth capability, key chemokines and cytokines participating in the evasion of immunological responses, and key pro-angiogenic and anti-angiogenic factors participating in the augmentation of angiogenesis, (b) identification of possible miRNAs and noncoding RNAs participating in the process upstream and downstream of METCAM/MUC18 [126], and (c) possible clinical applications that should be explored. Precaution should be taken that a thorough picture may be possibly revealed only after the comprehensive studies are successfully executed.

7.2 Clinical applications

Four major approaches may be taken to decrease or stop the progression and metastatic propensity of cancer cells and keep them staying at the primary site, stopping them in a dormant state or keeping the disseminating cancer cells at the state of micrometastases: (a) Dispense humanized anti-METCAM/MUC18 antibodies to the cancer patients [125]. (b) Knocking down the METCAM/MUC18 expression by siRNAs to silence the genes [35, 36]. For knocking down therapy, the METCAM/MUC18 gene-specific siRNAs may be delivered by liposomes or other delivery methods [126]. (c) Target at downstream key members in the signaling pathways which are activated by the promotion. (d) Target at the cofactors or the cognate heterophilic ligand(s) of METCAM/MUC18. The above strategies may be used in single or better in combination for treating the patients. However, the dual role of METCAM/MUC18 in cancer progression may limit the above clinical applications to only cancers exhibiting a positive METCAM/MUC18-mediated tumor progression and metastasis.

Acknowledgements

I thank the support of grants from the National Science Council, Taiwan.

Conflict of interest

The author has no conflict of interests.

Author details

Guang-Jer Wu[1,2]

1 Department of Bioscience Technology and Center for Biomedical Technology, Chung Yuan Christian University, Taoyuan, Taiwan

2 Department of Microbiology and Immunology, Emory University School of Medicine, Atlanta, GA, USA

*Address all correspondence to: guangj.wu@gmail.com

References

[1] Jackson M, Marks L, GHW M, Wilson JB. The genetic basis of disease. Essays in Biochemistry. 2018;**62**:643-723

[2] Klinsmith LJ. Principles of Cancer Biology. San Francisco: Pearson Education Press; 2006

[3] Weinberg RA. The Biology of Cancer. 1st ed. New York, USA and Abington, UK: Garland Science; 2007

[4] Baylin SB, Jones PA. Epigenetic determinants in cancer. Cold Spring Harbor Perspectives in Biology. 2016;**8**(a019505):1-35

[5] Yang H, Villani RM, Wang H, Simpson MJ, Roberts MS, Tang M, et al. The role of cellular reactive oxygen species in chemotherapy. Journal of Experimental & Clinical Cancer Research. 2018;**37**:266, 10 pages

[6] Hanahan D, Weinberg RA. Hallmarks of cancer: The next generation. Cell. 2011;**144**:646-674. DOI: 10.1016/j.cell.2011.02.013

[7] Wishart DS. Is cancer a genetic disease or metabolic disease? eBioMedicine. 2015;**2**:478-479

[8] Gkretsi V, Stylianopoulos T. Cell adhesion and matrix stiffness: Coordinating cancer cell invasion and metastasis. Frontiers in Oncology. 2018;**8**:145. DOI: 10.3389/fonc.2018.00145

[9] Mendonsa A, Na TY, Gumbiner BM. E-cadherin in contact inhibition and cancer. Oncogene. 2018;**37**(35): 4769-4780

[10] Hamidi H, Ivaska J. Every step of the way: Integrins in cancer progression and metastasis. Nature Reviews. Cancer. 2018;**18**(9):533-548. DOI: 10.1038/s41568-018-0038-z

[11] Wang Z, Zhao K, Hackert T, Zoller M. CD44/CD44v6 a reliable companion in cancer-initiating cell maintenance and tumor progression. Frontiers in Cell and Development Biology. 2018;**6**(97). DOI: 10.3389/fcell.2018.00097

[12] Calinescu A, Turcu G, Nedelcu RI, Brinzea A, Hodorogea A, Antohe M, et al. On the dual role of carcinoembryonic antigen-related cell adhesion molecule 1 (CEACAM1) in human malignancies. Journal of Immunology Research. 2018;**2018**:7169081, 8 pages. DOI: 10.1155/2018/7169081

[13] Bhatia P, Gautqm SK, Cannon A, Thompson C, Hall BR, Aithal A, et al. Cancer-associated mucins: Role in immune modulation and metastasis. Cancer Metastasis Reviews. 2019:1-14. DOI: 10.1007/s10555-018-09775-0

[14] Altevogt P, Doberstein K, Fogel M. L1CAM in human cancer. International Journal of Cancer. 2016;**138**:1565-1571

[15] Yahyazadeh Mashhadi SM, Kazemimanesh M, Arashkia A, Azadmanesh K, Meshkat Z, Golichenari B, et al. Shedding light on the EpCAM: An overview. Journal of Cellular Physiology. 2019;**234**(8):12569-12580

[16] Weidle UH, Eggle D, Klostermann S, GWM S. ALCAM/CD166: Cancer-related issues. Cancer Genomics & Proteomics. 2010;7(5):231-243

[17] Wu GJ. Chapter 13. Dual role of METCAM/MUC18 expression in the progression of cancer cells. In: Uchiumi F, editor. Gene Expression and Regulation in Mammalian Cells-Transcription from General Aspects. University Campus STeP Ri, Rijeka, Croatia: InTech Open Access Publisher; 2018. pp. 257-289. ISBN 978-953-51-3856-3, Print ISBN 978-953-51-3855-6

[18] Zeng GF, Cai SX, Wu GJ. Up-regulation of METCAM/MUC18 promotes motility, invasion, and tumorigenesis of human breast cancer cells. BMC Cancer. 2011;**11**:113. DOI: 10.1186/1471-2407-11-113

[19] Zeng GF, Cai SX, Liu Y, Wu GJ. METCAM/MUC18 augments migration, invasion, and tumorigenicity of human breast cancer SK-BR-3 cells. Gene. 2012;**492**:229-238

[20] Huang CY, Wu GJ. METCAM/MUC18 promoted tumorigenesis of human breast cancer SK-BR-3 cells in a dosage-specific manner. Taiwanese Journal of Obstetrics & Gynecology. 2016;**55**(2):202-212. DOI: 10.1016/j.tjog.2016.02.010

[21] Wu GJ, Fu P, Wang SW, MWH W. Enforced expression of MCAM/MUC18 increases in vitro motility and invasiveness and in vivo metastasis of two mouse melanoma K1735 sublines in a syngeneic mouse model. Molecular Cancer Research. 2008;**6**(11):1666-1677

[22] Wu GJ. Ectopic expression of MCAM/MUC18 increases in vitro motility and invasiveness, but decreases in vivo tumorigenesis and metastasis of a mouse melanoma K1735-9 subline in a syngeneic mouse model. Clinical & Experimental Metastasis. 2016;**33**(8):817-828. DOI: 10.1007/s10585-016-9812-z

[23] Lin JC, Chiang CF, Wang SW, Wang WY, Kwuan PC, Wu GJ. Significance and expression of human METCAM/MUC18 in nasopharyngeal carcinoma (NPC) and metastatic lesions. Asian Pacific Journal of Cancer Prevention. 2014;**15**(1):245-252

[24] Liu YC. Putative roles of huMETCAM in modulating the development and progression of nasopharyngeal carcinoma [thesis]. Chung Yuan Christian University; 2014. Available from: http://www.lib.cycu.edu.tw/thesis

[25] Liu YC, Chen, YR, Wu GJ. METCAM/MUC18 plays a tumor suppressor role in the development of nasopharyngeal carcinoma type I. 2019 (submitted)

[26] Liu YC, Ke CC, Chen YR, Wu GJ. METCAM/MUC18 plays a tumor pomoter role in the development of nasopharyngeal carcinoma type III. 2019 (submitted)

[27] Wu GJ, Dickerson EB. Frequent and increased expression of human METCAM/MUC18 in cancer tissues and metastatic lesions associates with the clinical progression of human ovarian carcinoma. Taiwanese Journal of Obstetrics & Gynecology. 2014;**53**:509-517

[28] Wu GJ, Zeng GF. METCAM/MUC18 is a novel tumor and metastasis suppressor for the human ovarian cancer SKOV3 cells. BMC Cancer. 2016;**16**:136. DOI: 10.1186/S12885-016-2181-9

[29] Wu GJ. METCAM/MUC18 plays a novel tumor and metastasis suppressor role in the progression of human ovarian cancer cells. Obstetrics & Gynecology International Journal. 2017;**6**(4):1-8

[30] Wu GJ. METCAM/MUC18 decreases the malignant propensity of human ovarian carcinoma cells. International Journal of Molecular Sciences. 2018;**19**:02976

[31] Wu GJ, Varma VA, MWH W, Yang H, SWC W, Liu Z, et al. Expression of a human cell adhesion molecule, MUC18, in prostate cancer cell lines and tissues. The Prostate. 2001;**48**:305-315

[32] Wu GJ, Peng Q, Fu P, Chiang CF, SWC W, Dillehay DL, et al. Ectopical expression of human MUC18 increases

metastasis of human prostate cancer LNCaP cells. Gene. 2004;**327**:201-213

[33] Wu GJ, Chiang CF, Fu P, Hess W, Greenberg N, MWH W. Increased expression of MUC18 correlates with the metastatic progression of mouse prostate adenocarcinoma in the (TRAMP) model. The Journal of Urology. 2005;**173**:1778-1783

[34] Wu GJ, MWH W, Liu Y. Enforced expression of human METCAM/MUC18 increases the tumorigenesis of human prostate cancer cells in nude mice. Journal of Urology. 2011;**185**:1504-1512

[35] Wu GJ. Human METCAM/MUC18 as a novel biomarker to drive and its specific SiRNAs to block the malignant progression of prostate cancer. Journal of Cell Science & Therapy. 2015;**6**:5.1000227

[36] Wu GJ. Human METCAM/MUC18 is a new diagnostic marker of and a driver for promoting and its specific siRNAs, derived oligopeptides and antibodies be used for decreasing the malignant progression of prostate cancer. Journal of Stem Cell Research & Therapeutics. 2016;**1**(5):00035

[37] Wu GJ. Dual role of METCAM in the progression of different cancers. Journal of Clinical Oncology. 2012;**2012**:853797. DOI: 10.1155/2012/853797

[38] Lehmann JM, Reithmuller G, Johnson JP. MUC18, a marker of tumor progression in human melanoma. Proceedings of the National Academy of Sciences of the United States of America. 1989;**86**:9891-9895

[39] Meier F, Caroli U, Satyamoorthy K, Schittek B, Bauer J, Berking C, et al. Fibroblast growth factor-2 but not Mel-CAM and/or β3 integrin promotes progression of melanocytes to melanoma. Experimental Dermatology. 2003;**12**:296-306

[40] Wu GJ. METCAM/MUC18 expression and cancer metastasis. Current Genomics. 2005;**6**:333-349

[41] Anfosso F, Bardin N, Frances V, Vivier E, Camoin-Jau L, Sampol J, et al. Activation of human endothelial cells via S-Endo-1 antigen (CD146) stimulates the tyrosine phosphorylation of focal adhesion kinase p125FAK. The Journal of Biological Chemistry. 1998;**273**:26852-26858

[42] Wu GJ, MWH W, Wang SW, Liu Z, Peng Q, Qu P, et al. Isolation and characterization of the major form of human MUC18 cDNA gene and correlation of MUC18 over-expression in prostate cancer cells and tissues with malignant progression. Gene. 2001;**279**:17-31

[43] Yang H, SWC W, Liu Z, MWH W, McAlpine B, Ansel J, et al. Isolation and characterization of murine MUC18 cDNA gene, and correlation of MUC18 expression in murine melanoma cell lines with metastatic ability. Gene. 2001;**265**:133-145

[44] Shih IM. The role of CD146 (Mel-CAM) in biology and pathology. The Journal of Pathology. 1999;**189**:4-11

[45] Zeng Q, Li W, Lu D, Wu Z, Duan H, Luo Y, et al. CD146, an epithelial-mesenchymal transition inducer, is associated with triple-negative breast cancer. Proceedings of the National Academy of Sciences of the United States of America. 2012;**109**(4):1127-1132

[46] Li Q, Yu Y, Bischoff J, Milliken JB, Olsen BR. Differential expression of CD146 in tissues and endothelial cells derived from infantile hemangioma and normal human skin. The Journal of Pathology. 2003;**201**:296-302

[47] Zeng P, Li H, Lu PH, Zhou LN, Tang M, Liu CY, et al. Prognostic value

of CD146 in solid tumor: A systematic review and meta-analysis. Scientific Reports. 2017;**7**(1):4223. DOI: 10.1038/s41598-017-01061-3

[48] Yeo SK, Guan J. Breast cancer: Multiple subtypes within a tumor. Trends Cancer. 2017;**3**(11):753-760

[49] Perou C, Sorlie T, Eisen MB, van de Rijn M, Jeffrey SS, Rees CA, et al. Molecular portraits of human breast tumors. Nature. 2000;**406**:747-752

[50] Curtis C, Shah SP, Chin S, Turashvili G, Rueda OM, Dunning MJ, et al. The genomic and transcriptomic architecture of 2000 breast tumors reveals novel subgroups. Nature. 2012;**486**:346-352

[51] Zabouo G, Imbert AM, Jacqemier J, Finetti P, Moreau T, Esterni B, et al. CD146 expression is associated with a poor prognosis in human breast tumors and with enhanced motility in breast cancer cell lines. Breast Cancer Research. 2009;**11**:R1. DOI: 10.1186/bcr2215

[52] Shih IM, Hsu MY, Palazzo JP, Herlyn M. The cell-cell adhesion receptor MEL-CAM acts as a tumor suppressor in breast carcinoma. The American Journal of Pathology. 1997;**151**:745-751

[53] Ouhtit A, Gaur RL, Abd Elmageed ZY, Fernando A, Thouta R, Trappey AK, et al. Towards understanding the mode of action of the multifaceted cell adhesion receptor CD146. Biochimica et Biophysica Acta. 2009;**1795**:130-136

[54] Garcia S, Dales JP, Charafe-Jauffret E, Carpentier-Meunier S, Andrac-Meyer L, Jacquemier J, et al. Poor prognosis in breast carcinomas correlates with increased expression of targetable CD146 and c-Met and with proteomic basal-like phenotype. Human Pathology. 2007;**38**:830-841

[55] Xie S, Luca M, Huang S, Gutman M, Reich R, Johnson JP, et al. Expression of MCAM/MCU18 by human melanoma cells leads to increased tumor growth and metastasis. Cancer Research. 1997;**57**:2295-2303

[56] Schlagbauer-Wadl H, Jansen B, Muller M, Polterauer P, Wolff K, Eichler HG, et al. Influence of MUC18/MCAM/CD146 expression on human melanoma growth and metastasis in SCID mice. International Journal of Cancer. 1999;**81**:951-955

[57] Lin CT, Wong CI, Chan WY, et al. Establishment and characterization of two nasopharyngeal carcinoma cell lines. Laboratory Investigation. 1990;**62**:713-724

[58] Wu G-J, Chang YR, Chu JT. METCAM/MUC18 plays a positive role in the tumorigenesis of human prostate cancer DU145 cells: Knockdown shRNAs decrease tumorigenicity in nude mice. 2019 (submitted)

[59] LaMontagne KR Jr, Moses MA, Wiederschain D, Mahajan S, Holden J, Ghazizadeh H, et al. Inhibition of MAP kinase causes morphological reversion and dissociation between soft agar growth and in vivo tumorigenesis in angiosarcoma cells. The American Journal of Pathology. 2000;**157**:1937-1945

[60] Liu WF, Ji SR, Sun JJ, Zhang Y, Liu ZY, Liang AB, et al. Gastric cancer CD146 expression correlates with epithelial-mesenchymal transition markers and a poor prognosis in gastric cancer. International Journal of Molecular Sciences. 2012;**13**:6399-6406

[61] Yang Y, Hernandez R, Rao J, Yin L, Qu Y, Wu J, et al. Targeting CD146 with a 64Cu-labeled antibody enables in vivo immunoPET imaging of high-grade gliomas. Proceedings

of the National Academy of Sciences of the United States of America. 2015;**112**(47):E6525-E6534

[62] Siegel RL, Miller KD, Jemal A. Cancer statistics 2019. CA: A Cancer Journal for Clinicians. 2019;**69**:7-34

[63] Jiang G, Zhang L, Zhu Q, Bai D, Zhang C, Wang X. CD146 promotes metastasis and predicts poor prognosis of hepatocellular carcinoma. Journal of Experimental & Clinical Cancer Research. 2016;**35**(38). DOI: 10.1186/s13046-016-0313-3

[64] Chen K, Ding A, Ding Y, Ghanekar A. High-throughput flow cytometry screening of human hepatocellular carcinoma reveals CD146 to be a novel marker of tumor-initiating cells. Biochemistry and Biophysics Reports. 2016;**8**:107-113

[65] Oka S, Uramoto H, Chikaishi Y, Tanaka F. The expression of CD146 predicts a poor over all survival in patients with adenocarcinoma of the lung. Anticancer Research. 2012;**32**:861-864

[66] Kristiansen G, Yu Y, Schlüns K, Sers C, Dietel M, Petersen I. Expression of the cell adhesion molecule CD146/MCAM in non-small cell lung cancer. Analytical Cellular Pathology. 2003;**25**:77-81

[67] Zhang X, Wang Z, Kang Y, Li X, Ma X, Ma L. MCAM expression is associated with poor prognosis in non-small cell lung cancer. Clinical and Translational Oncology. 2014;**16**:178-183

[68] Wu GJ et al. Effects of METCAM/MUC18 expression on the tumor progression of non-small cell lung cancer cells. (In press)

[69] Zhang F, Wang J, Wang X, Wei N, Liu H, Zhang X. CD146-mediated acquisition of stemness phenotype enhances tumor invasion and metastasis after EGFR-TKI resistance in lung cancer. The Clinical Respiratory Journal. 2019;**13**(1):23-33

[70] England CG, Jiang D, Hernandez R, Sun H, Valdovinos HF, Ehlerding EB, et al. ImmunoPET imaging of CD146 in murine models of intrapulmonary metastasis of non-small cell lung cancer. Molecular Pharmaceutics. 2017;**14**(10):3239-3247

[71] Tripathi SC, Fahrmann JF, Celiktas M, Aguilar M, Marini KD, Jolly MK, et al. A novel mechanism of chemoresistance in small cell lung cancer mediated by MCAM via PI3K/AKT/SOX2 signaling pathway. Cancer Research. 2017;**77**(16):4414-44252

[72] Schiano C, Grimaldi V, Casamassimi A, Infante T, Esposito A, Giovane A, et al. Different expression of CD146 in human normal and osteosarcoma cell lines. Medical Oncology. 2012;**29**(4):2998-3002

[73] EC MG, Heimberger A, Mills L, Weber K, Thomas GW, Shtivelband M, et al. A fully human anti-melanoma cellular adhesion molecule/MUC18 antibody inhibits spontaneous pulmonary metastasis of osteosarcoma cells in vivo. Clinical Cancer Research. 2003;**9**:6560-6566

[74] Westrøm S, Bønsdorff TB, Abbas N, Bruland ØS, Jonasdottir TJ, Mælandsmo GM, et al. Evaluation of CD146 as target for radioimmunotherapy against osteosarcoma. PLoS One. 2016;**11**(10):e0165382. DOI: 10.1371/journal.pone.0165382

[75] Stalin J, Nollet M, Garigue P, Fernandez S, Vivavancos L, Essaah A, et al. Targeting soluble CD146 with a neutralizing antibody inhibits vascularization, growth, and survival of CD146 positive tumors. Oncogene. 2016;**35**:5489-5500

[76] von Burstin J, Bachhuber F, Paul M, Schmid RM, Rustgi AK. The TALE homeodomain transcription factor MEIS1 activates the pro-metastatic melanoma cell adhesion molecule MCAM to promote migration of pancreatic cancer cells. Molecular Carcinogenesis. 2017;**56**(3):936-944

[77] Liu D, Du L, Chen D, Ye Z, Duan H, Tu T, et al. Reduced CD146 expression promotes tumorigenesis and cancer stemness in colorectal cancer through activating Wnt/β-catenin signaling. Oncotarget. 2016;**7**(26):40704-40718

[78] Aldovini D, Demichelis F, Doglioni C, Di Vizio D, Galligioni E, et al. M-CAM expression as marker of poor prognosis in epithelial ovarian cancer. International Journal of Cancer. 2006;**119**(8):1920-1926

[79] Wu Z, Wu ZY, Li J, Yang X, Wang Y, et al. MCAM is a novel metastasis marker and regulates spreading, apoptosis and invasion of ovarian cancer cells. Tumor Biology. 2012;**33**:1619-1628

[80] Wu GJ. Enforced expression of METCAM/MUC18 decreases in vitro motility and invasiveness and tumorigenesis and in vivo tumorigenesis of human ovarian cancer BG-1 cells. In: Schatten H, editor. Ovarian Cancer: Molecular & Diagnostic Imaging and Treatment Strategies, Advances in Experimental Medicine and Biology. Humana Press, (Springer Science+Business Media LLC); 2019 (in press)

[81] Zheng B, Ohuchida K, Chijiiwa Y, Zhao M, Mizuuchi Y, Cui L, et al. CD146 attenuation in cancer-associated fibroblasts promotes pancreatic cancer progression. Molecular Carcinogenesis. 2016;**55**(11):1560-1572

[82] Wu G-J, Chang YR, Chu JT. METCAM/MUC18 plays a negative role in the tumorigenesis of human prostate cancer PC-3 cells: Knockdown effects shRNAs increasing tumorigenicity in nude mice. 2019 (submitted)

[83] Anfosso F, Bardin N, Vivier E, Sabatier F, Sampol J, Dignat-George F. Outside-in signaling pathway linked to CD146 engagement in human endothelial cells. The Journal of Biological Chemistry. 2001;**276**:1564-1569

[84] Sers C, Kirsch K, Rothbacher U, Riethmuller G, Johnson JP. Genomic organization of the melanoma-associated glycoprotein MUC18: Implications for the evolution of the immunoglobulin domains. Proceedings of the National Academy of Sciences of the United States of America. 1993;**90**:8514-8518

[85] Rummel MM, Sers C, Johnson JP. Phorbol ester and cyclic AMP-mediated regulation of the melanoma-associated cell adhesion molecule MUC18/MCAM. Cancer Research. 1996;**56**:2218-2223

[86] Jean D, Gershenwald JE, Huang S, Luca M, Hudson MJ, Tainsky MA, et al. Loss of AP-2 results in up-regulation of CAM/MUC18 and an increase in tumor growth and metastasis of human melanoma cells. The Journal of Biological Chemistry. 1998;**273**:16501-16508

[87] Ruiz M, Pettaway C, Song R, Stoeltzing O, Ellis L, Bar-Eli M. Activator protein 2α inhibits tumorigenicity and represses vascular endothelial growth factor transcription in prostate cancer cells. Cancer Research. 2004;**64**:631-638

[88] Ness SA. The Myb oncoprotein: Regulating a regulator. Biochem Biophys Acta. 1996;**1299**:F123-F139

[89] JAF T, Murphy K, Baker E, Sutherland GR, Parsons PG, Sturm RA. The brn-2 gene regulates the melanocytic phenotype and tumorigenic

potential of human melanoma cells. Oncogene. 1995;**11**:691-700

[90] Yordy JS, Li R, Sementchenko VI, Pei H, Muise-Helmericks RC, Watson DK. S100 expression modulates ETS1 transcriptional activity and inhibits cell invasion. Oncogene. 2004;**23**:6654-6665

[91] L'honore A, Lamb NJ, Vandromme M, Turowski P, Carnac G, Fernandez A. MyoD distal regulatory region contains an SF binding CArG element required for MyoD expression in skeletal myoblasts and during muscle regeneration. Molecular Biology of the Cell. 2003;**14**:2151-2162

[92] Baron V, Duss S, Rhim J, Mercola D. Antisense to the early growth response-1 gene (Egr-1) inhibits prostate tumor development in TRAMP mice. Annals of the New York Academy of Sciences. 2003;**1002**:197-216

[93] O'Brien RM, Streeper RS, Ayala JE, Stadelmaier BT, Hornbuckle LA. Insulin-regulated gene expression. Biochemical Society Transactions. 2001;**29**:552-558

[94] Melnikova VO, Debroff AS, Zigler M, Villares GJ, Braeuer R, Wang H, et al. CREB inhibits AP-2α expression to regulate the malignant phenotype of melanoma. PLoS One. 2010;**5**:e12452

[95] Sechler M, Parrish JK, Birks DK, Jedlicka P. The histone demethylase KDM3A, and its downstream target MCAM, promote Ewing Sarcoma cell migration and metastasis. Oncogene. 2017;**36**(29):4150-4160

[96] Wu GJ et al. Transcriptional regulation of METCAM/MUC18 gene in the upstream region in cancer cells. (In press)

[97] Lung HL, Cheng Y, Kumaran MK, et al. Fine mapping of the 11Q22-23 tumor suppressive region and involvement of TSLC1 in nasopharyngeal carcinoma. International Journal of Cancer. 2004;**112**:628-635

[98] Wu GJ. MCAM (melanoma cell adhesion molecule). Atlas of Genetics and Cytogenetics in Oncology and Haematology. 2012. DOI: 10.4267/2042/47418. ID41314ch11q23. The manually annotated Biomax Human Genome Database Version 4.0, Biomax Informatics AG, www.biomax.com, the Biomax Solutions Inc., Falmouth, MA, USA

[99] Wu GJ et al. Epigenetic regulation of METCAM/MUC18 expression in nasopharyngeal carcinoma. (In press)

[100] Brait M, Banerjee M, Maldonado L, Ooki A, Loyo M, Guida E, et al. Promoter methylation of MCAM, ERα and ERβ in serum of early stage prostate cancer patients. Oncotarget. 2017;**8**(9):15431-15440. DOI: 10.18632/oncotarget.14873

[101] Wong CW, Dye DE, Coombe DR. The role of immunoglobulin superfamily cell adhesion molecules in cancer metastasis. International Journal of Cell Biology. 2012;**2012**: 9 p. Article ID 340296

[102] Sorrentino A, Ferracin M, Castelli G, Biffoni M, Tomaselli G, Baiocchi M, et al. Isolation and characterization of CD146+ multipotent mesenchymal stromal cells. Experimental Hematology. 2008;**36**:1035-1046

[103] Li G, Kalabis J, Xu X, Meier F, Oka M, Bogenrieder T, et al. Reciprocal regulation of MelCAM and AKT in human melanoma. Oncogene. 2003;**22**:6891-6899

[104] Maggio F, Pinna LA. One-thousand-and-one substrates of protein

kinase CK2? The FASEB Journal. 2003;**17**:349-368

[105] Datta SR, Brunet A, Greenberg ME. Cellular survival: A play in three AKTs. Genes & Development. 1999;**13**:2905-2927

[106] Sers C, Riethmuller G, Johnson JP. MUC18, a melanoma-progression associated molecule, and its potential role in tumor vascularization and hematogenous spread. Cancer Research. 1994;**54**:5689-5694

[107] Bardin N, Anfosso F, Masse J, Cramer E, Sabatier F, LeBivic A, et al. Identification of CD146 as a component of the endothelial junction involved in the control of cell-cell adhesion. Blood. 2001;**98**:3677-3684

[108] Kang Y, Wang F, Feng J, Yang D, Yang X, Yan X. Knockdown of CD146 reduces the migration and proliferation of human endothelial cells. Cell Research. 2006;**16**:313-318

[109] Yan X, Lin Y, Tang D, Shen Y, Yuan M, Zhang Z, et al. A novel anti-CD146 monoclonal antibody, AA98, inhibits angiogenesis and tumor growth. Blood. 2003;**102**:184-191

[110] Wu GJ, Son EL. Soluble METCAM/MUC18 blocks angiogenesis during tumor formation of human prostate cancer cells. In: Proceedings of the 97th Annual Meeting of American Association for the Cancer Research. Vol. 47. 2006. Abstract# 252

[111] Wu GJ. Chapter 7: The role of MUC18 in prostate carcinoma in Immunohistochemistry and in situ hybridization of human carcinoma. In: Hayat MA, editor. Molecular Pathology, Lung Carcinoma, Breast Carcinoma, and Prostate Carcinoma. Vol. 1. Maryland Heights, MO, USA: Elsevier Science/Academic Press; 2004. pp. 347-358

[112] Wu GJ. Chapter 11: Dual roles of the melanoma CAM (MelCAM/METCAM) in malignant progression of melanoma. In: Research on Melanoma: A glimpse into current directions and future trends. University Campus STeP Ri, Rijeka, Croatia: InTech Open Access Publisher; 2011. pp. 229-242

[113] Song B, Tang JW, Wang B, Cui XN, Zhou CH, Hou L. Screening for lymphatic metastasis-associated genes in mouse hepatocarcinoma cell lines Hca-F and Hca-P using gene chip. Chinese Journal of Cancer. 2005;**24**(7):774-780

[114] Wang LV. Prospects of photoacoustic tomography (PAT). Medical Physics. 2008;**35**(12):5758-5767

[115] deVisser KE, Eichten A, Coussens LM. Paradoxical roles of the immune system during cancer development. Nature Reviews. Cancer. 2006;**6**:24-37

[116] Staquicini F, Tandle A, Libutti SK, Sun J, Zigler M, Bar-Eli M, et al. A subset of host B lymphocytes controls melanoma metastasis through a melanoma cell adhesion molecule/MUC18-dependent interaction: Evidence from mice and humans. Cancer Research. 2008;**68**(20):8419-8428

[117] Despoix N, Walzer T, Jouve N, Blot-Chabaud M, Bardin N, Paul P, et al. Mouse CD146/MCAM is a marker of natural killer cell maturation. European Journal of Immunology. 2008;**38**:2855-2864

[118] Geiser M, Cebe R, Drewello D, Schmitz R. Integration of PCR fragments at any specific site within cloning vectors without the use of restriction enzyme and DNA ligase. BioTechniques. 2001;**31**:88-92

[119] Wu GJ et al. Functional domains of METCAM/MUC18 in the tumor progression. (In press)

[120] Kannagi R, Izawa M, Koike T, Miyazaki K, Kimura N. Carbohydrate-mediated cell adhesion in cancer metastasis and angiogenesis. Cancer Science. 2004;**95**(5):377-384

[121] Parodi A. Protein glycosylation and its role in protein folding. Annual Review of Biochemistry. 2000;**69**:69-93

[122] Lehmann JM, Holzmann B, Breitbart EW, Schmiegelow P, Riethmuller G, Johnson JP. Discrimination between benign and malignant cells of melanocytic lineage by two novel antigens, a glycoprotein with a molecular weight of 113,000 and a protein with a molecular weight of 76,000. Cancer Research. 1987;**47**:841-845

[123] Yamamoto H, Oviedo A, Sweeley C, Saito T, Moskal JR. α2,6-Sialylation of cell-surface N-glycans inhibits glioma formation in vivo. Cancer Research. 2001;**61**:6822-6829

[124] Sumardika IW, Youyi C, Kondo E, Inoue Y, Ruma MW, Murata H, et al. β-1,3-galactosyl-O-glycosyl-glycoprotein β-1,6-N-acetylglucosaminyltransferase 3 increases MCAM stability, which enhances S100A8/A9-mediated cancer motility. Oncology Research. 2018;**26**(3):431-444

[125] Leslie MC, Zhao YJ, Lachman LB, Hwu P, Wu GJ, Bar-Eli M. Immunization against MUC18/MCAM, a novel antigen that drives melanoma invasion and metastasis. Gene Therapy. 2007;**14**:316-323

[126] Kasinski AL, Slack FJ. MicroRNAs en route to the clinic: Progress in validating and targeting microRNAs for cancer therapy. Nature Reviews. Cancer. 2011;**11**:849-864

Chapter 2

Molecular Genetics of Metastatic Breast Cancer

Hülya Yazici and Beyza Akin

Abstract

Breast cancer is the most common form of cancer in women. Breast cancer has a heterogeneous etiology. Genetic and environmental factors contribute to the pathogenesis and progression of breast cancer. Various genes as proliferation and nuclear factors have been identified in breast cancer. Therefore, the genetic component of patients is important in determining disease behavior, response to anticancer therapeutics, and patient survival. Prognosis of breast cancer is associated with potential metastatic properties of primary breast tumors. Metastasis is the leading cause of death in patients with breast cancer. Therefore, it is important to understand the mechanisms underlying the development of distant metastases to specific regions and has clinical value. Metastasis shows an organ-specific spread pattern and occurs with a series of complex and multistep events associated with each other, such as angiogenesis, invasion, migration-motility, extravasation, and proliferation. Breast cancer often metastasizes to the bone, liver, brain, and lungs. Metastasis may develop years after successful primary treatment. The metastatic process will become clear, as information about molecules and genes associated with metastases increases, and this is extremely important for cancer treatment.

Keywords: breast cancer, metastasis, genes, pathways, organs

1. Introduction

Breast cancer, which is one of the most common malignant diseases of women worldwide, is a heterogeneous disease with unknown pathogenesis. Genetic and environmental factors contribute to the pathogenesis and progression of breast cancer. Although an improvement has recently been detected in the diagnosis and treatment of breast cancer compared with other cancers, its contribution to survival was inadequate.

Breast cancer-associated death or survival is associated with the potential metastatic features of the primary breast tumors. Metastatic disease is the leading cause of death in breast cancer patients. Distant metastasis develops in ~20–30% of the early-stage breast cancer patients. Approximately 90% of deaths result from the complications due to recurrent or metastatic diseases. Therefore, it is very important to understand the underlying mechanisms in the development of distant metastases to specific regions. Metastases may show an organ-specific dissemination pattern. Metastasis may develop years after successful primary treatment. Metastasis frequently develops in the bone, liver, brain, and lungs in breast cancer.

Identification of the molecules, and genes associated with metastasis, and clarification of the contribution of these molecules to metastatic process are important for the treatment of cancer. Metastasis is the dissemination of the cancer cells from their primary region to different tissues and organs in the body. Metastasis develops with a series of complex and multistep chains of events such as angiogenesis, invasion, migration-motility, extravasation, and proliferation.

The anomalies of different genes as *BRCA1*, *BRCA2*, *MYC*, *TP53*, *RB1*, *JUN*, and *CDK2A* which have roles in cell proliferation are detected in breast cancer [1]. Therefore, performing the genetic and molecular screenings of patients is important for the identification of the behavior of disease, the anticancer therapeutic response, and the survival.

Different breast cancer cellular subtypes in primary breast cancer tissue metastasize in relation to their target organ. The route of metastasis is generated with the interaction of this different subtype cells and microenvironment of the tumor and with the organ they will locate, and this is named as "organotrophic metastasis."

Understanding the molecular mechanism of organotrophic metastasis is very important for biological indicator prediction, developing the innovative therapeutic strategies, and for improving the survival. Development of metastasis in distant regions is associated with the interaction between the tumor cells and host microenvironment. Before the initiation of tumor dissemination, the host microenvironment is modified to support the tumoral growth, in other words to create a pre-metastatic niche (PMN). PMN is organized with the factors secreted from tumor cell with the changes in the host cell metabolism and microenvironment. In addition, tumor cells also interact with the extracellular matrix (ECM) of the host tissue to facilitate metastasis.

Generally, breast cancer is classified as in situ carcinoma and invasive carcinoma in a simple way, and most breast cancers are invasive. More than 80% of invasive breast cancers may be investigated in two different subgroups as invasive ductal carcinoma (IDC), and some breast cancers may be investigated as invasive lobular carcinoma (ILC). Organ preference of metastasis in ILC and IDC is significantly distinct. Invasive ductal carcinomas do metastasis to the lungs, distant lymphatic glands, and central nervous system (CNS); however, ILC is known to do threefold higher metastasis to the peritone, gastrointestinal system, and ovaries [2].

Breast cancer has a tendency to do metastasis on the bone, liver, lung, and distant lymphatic glands. The most common metastasis type is the bone metastases detected in 70% of metastatic breast cancer patients [1]. The second most common metastasis region was the liver with ~30%, and the brain was reported as the third most common metastasis region with a rate of 10–30% [1].

The most common metastatic region in all subtypes except basal-like tumors is the bone. Luminal B, HER2+/ER/PR+ and HER2+/ER/PR, tumors do more metastasis to the brain, liver, lungs, and bone than the luminal A tumors. Basal-like tumors do higher rates of the brain, lungs, and distant lymphatic node metastasis; however, the liver and bone metastases are less frequently detected in basal-like tumors [3]. Although triple negative breast cancer (TNBC) tumors show a metastatic ratio similar to non-basal tumors, TNBC tumors have less liver metastasis than the non-basal tumors [1].

Some molecules may have different roles in different metastasis regions in accordance with their content. Although transforming growth factor beta (*TGF-β*) promotes the lung metastasis of breast cancer, its interaction with Src signaling pathway may cause bone metastasis [4]. In cancer cells with insulin-like growth factor (*IGF1*) and *IGF1* receptor (*IGF1R*), bone metastasis shows higher expression than the cancer cells with brain metastasis [5]. EGFR ligands and cyclooxygenase 2 (*COX2*) were reported to be associated with lung metastasis and, however, were reported to be not associated with bone or liver metastasis [6].

Wnt-1-inducible-signaling pathway protein1 (*WISP-1*) and *CCN4* are heparin-binding glycoproteins of the CCN protein family that are rich in cysteine. These proteins are expressed in various inner organs such as the lung, kidney, and spleen. *WISP-1* binds to *BMP-2* and increases the mesenchymal cellular proliferation and osteoblastic differentiation. *WISP-1* was reported to be associated with the increased metastasis risk among early-stage ER-positive lymphatic node-negative breast cancer patients [7]. Therefore, future studies will demonstrate whether genetic factors associated with WISP-1 and EXT1 genes may show metastasis risk or may be used in identification of metastasis. In addition, the increase of WISP-1 expression was proven to be associated with the pathogenesis of the primary lung cancers. Although the possibility of *WISP-1* to be used as a prognostic indicator for lung metastasis of breast cancer was suggested, it was not clarified yet whether *WISP-1* was a tumor stimulant or a tumor suppressor.

Breast cancer cells are detected to highly express the chemokine receptors *CXCR4* and *CCR7* genes in the studies investigating the contribution of chemokine receptors to organ-specific metastases. Chemokine receptor-specific ligands *CXCL12* and *CCL21* were demonstrated to be highly expressed in the organs to which breast tumors do metastasis such as the lymph nodes, lungs, liver, and bone marrow [8]. In addition, the blockade of *CXCR4* gene in experimental animal models was demonstrated to inhibit the metastasis of breast cancer cells. The activation of the RAS/mitogen-activated protein kinase (MAPK) with chemokine signaling pathway causes changes in primary cancer cells such as changes in the intracellular actin molecule polymerization, development of pseudopodia, and increased cellular motility, cellular migration, and tissue invasion. Any of these changes contribute to the development of organ-specific metastasis by contributing to the survival, metastasis, and vitality ability of cancer cells.

2. Metastasis-associated signal transduction pathways and genes

2.1 p38/MAPK pathway

p38/MAPK signal transduction pathway increases the breast carcinoma vascularization and growth by promoting the expression and accumulation of pro-tumorigenic factors.

The inactivation of the p38/MAPK signaling pathway was provided by the expression of the kinase-inactive mutant (dn-p38) of p38/MAPK14 in metastatic breast cancer cells in the studies, and with the deterioration of the tumor p38/MAPK signal, the development of breast cancer and metastasis ability was shown to decrease in breast carcinoma xenografts [9]. The conducted kinase-inactive mutant significantly decreased the dn-p38, tumor blood vessel density, and lumen dimensions. p38 controls the expression of the pro-angiogenic extracellular factors such as matrix protein fibronectin, cytokine, vascular endothelial growth factor A (*VEGFA*), and *IL8*. p38/MAPK signal transduction was demonstrated to increase the tumoral growth, and vascularization in addition to increasing the expressions of tumor-associated fibroblasts, and pro-angiogenic factors. All these effects were suppressed by the dn-p38 kinase-inactive mutant. The data analyses showed that p38 had higher expression in breast cancers which was an indicator of recurrence and poor prognosis. The activation of the p38/MAPK signaling pathway in the tumor increased the development of breast cancer and metastasis. *p38* contributes to the vascularization of carcinoma by facilitating the expression and accumulation of the pro-angiogenic factors. In conclusion, all these results suggested that all the genes which have a role in p38/MAPK pathway might be a therapeutic target against tumor vascularization and metastasis.

Tumor microenvironment (TME) is an important factor in cancer progression, recurrence, and response to treatment. TME blood vessels consist of stromal cells (fibroblasts, adipocytes) and infiltrating immune cells. Myeloid cells stimulate the tumor vascularization and metastasis by secreting metalloproteinase *MMP9/gelatinase-B* cells which increase the gathering of endothelial cells and pericytes. In addition to myeloid cells, *MMP9* is also produced by the breast carcinoma cells, and the *MMP9* destruction in carcinoma cells significantly decreases tumor vascularization [10]. Therefore, all three cellular components of the TME of breast contribute to the tumor vascularization by interacting with *MMP9*. p38/MAPK signal contributes to the development of breast cancer and metastasis by increasing the tumor cell invasiveness and tumor vascularization.

MMP9 that has a role in tumor angiogenesis and intratumoral vascularization-associated *ICAM1* works correlated with p38/MAPK signal. *ICAM1* is also suggested as a target in triple negative breast cancer (TNBC) [11]. The inhibition of p38/MAPK signal affects the TNF-induced *ICAM1* expression or the induction of *MMP9* by the cytokines *TGF-β* and TNF.

The deterioration of p38/MAPK signal causes no decrease in the expression of *MMP9* and *ICAM1* that are secreted by tumor cells. p38/MAPK signal contributes to fibronectin expression by responding to cytokines and tumor-fibroblast interactions [9].

p38/MAPK induces the expression of pro-angiogenic cytokines that include *VEGFA*, *IL8*, and *HBEGF* in addition to inducing an extracellular matrix protein fibronectin. *TAK1* controls the expression of MMP9 which releases *VEGF* and activates the *IL8* (**Figure 1**). Pro-angiogenic cytokines increase the tumoral growth by stimulating the tumoral vascularization.

p38/MAPK affects the development and metastasis of breast cancer by changing the tumor microenvironment of p38/MAPK signal. The inactivation of p38/MAPK signal in breast cancer cells decreases the growth of tumor xenografts and metastasis. Tumoral and stromal cells in breast TME stimulate the cytokine-mediated p38/MAPK signal which increases the expression of the pro-angiogenic and pro-invasive factors such as *VEGFA*, *IL8*, *IL6*, *HBEGF*, and fibronectin. p38/MAPK which affects

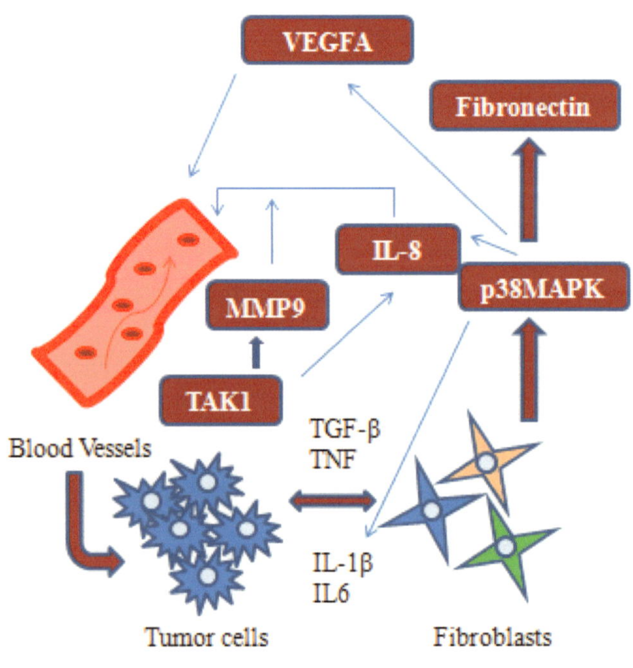

Figure 1.
The role of p38/MAPK in the regulation of tumor angiogenesis in breast cancer.

the vascular structure and stroma of tumor is detected to be definitely a potential target for anticancer treatment. Researchers suggested that anti-p38 drugs were a new therapeutic option in the treatment of breast cancer including metastatic disease [9].

2.2 Tumor endothelial marker 8 (TEM8)

Tumor endothelial marker (*TEM8*) was first discovered in the human tumor endothelial and was associated with tumor angiogenesis. TEM8 also known as Anthrax toxin receptor 1 (*ANTXR1*) is highly regulated in tumor endothelial and is expressed in breast cancer. *TEM8* was demonstrated to be required for tumoral growth and angiogenesis [12]. The role of *TEM8* in angiogenesis is organized with the regulation of downstream VEGF signal with its interaction with vascular endothelial growth factor receptor 2 (*VEGFR2*). Primary tumor development and metastasis are highly dependent on angiogenesis. Because the tumor cannot grow more than a few millimeters unless new blood vessels that will provide the oxygen and nutrients to tumor tissue are generated. The extravasation and dissemination of metastatic cells out of the vessel are facilitated and accelerated due to the leaky structure of the rapid developing tumor vessel network during tumor angiogenesis. Therefore, treatments targeting *TEM8* can differentiate the physiologic and pathological angiogenesis and can prevent the cancer progression without causing serious adverse effects. Due to this feature, *TEM8* is suggested to be a new possible therapeutic target in inhibiting the metastasis.

The destruction of *TEM8* in osteosarcoma cells causes the decrease of the cell proliferation [13]. *TEM8* interacts with the lipoprotein receptor associated protein 6 (*LRP6*) and regulates the downstream signaling of Wnt which is a protein that induces both the cellular proliferation and migration. *TEM8* was reported to regulate metastasis and a new molecule specific for metastasis by contributing the breast cancer stem cells (BCSC) and tumor growth with activating the Wnt signal with collagen VI [14]. *TEM8* is associated with invasive and aggressive phenotype in breast cancer. In addition, *TEM8* expression was demonstrated to be highly expressed in the tumor tissues of breast cancer patients compared to the normal tissues [14].

TEM8 expressed by cancer cells causes the development of angiogenesis by affecting the cancer cell proliferation and endothelial cell migration. *TEM8* knockout (KO) cells were generated using CRISPR/Cas9, *TEM8* expression was demonstrated to significantly disappear, and *TEM8* was inhibited in the studies investigating the association of *TEM8* with metastasis (**Figure 2**). Thus, angiogenesis decreased in tumor cells, and metastasis ability of *TEM8* significantly

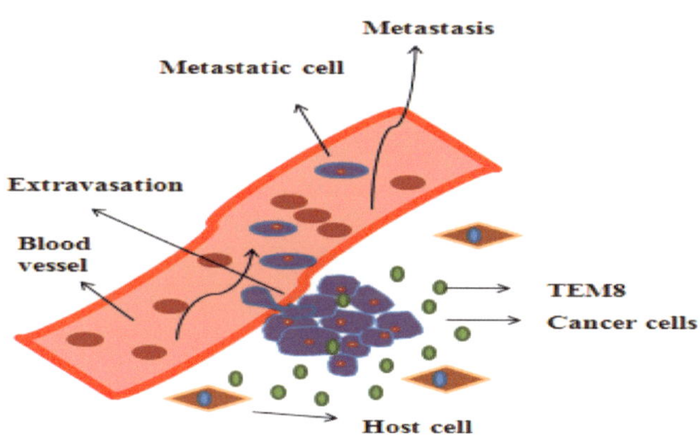

Figure 2.
The effect of TEM8 in breast cancer metastasis.

degraded with the deletion in cancer cells. Cancer cell proliferation, angiogenesis, and metastases are blocked with the prevention of cell cycle and the expression of the kinetochore-associated genes with the inhibition of *TEM* [15]. Cancer cells are known to secrete the pro-angiogenic signals such as *VEGFA* and open the angiogenic lock by affecting the tumor microenvironment. *TEM8* is known to work in cooperation with other factors such as *VEGF* for promoting endothelial cell migration and angiogenesis. In conclusion, *TEM8* expression is higher in tumor cells than in normal cells. Studies conducted using *TEM8* knockout metastatic breast cancer cell lines designed with CRISPR/Cas9 emphasize the role of *TEM8* in cancer development, tumor angiogenesis, and local metastasis. All these studies reveal the potential of *TEM8* as a therapeutic target for combating the disease; however, more clinical studies are required for developing the *TEM8*-targeted therapies [15].

2.3 APOBEC3B gene

Another important molecule in the development of metastatic potential of breast cancer is *APOBEC3B*. High level of *APOBEC3B* mRNA expression was demonstrated to be a significant prognostic biological indicator demonstrating the poor prognosis of breast cancer in ER-positive primary breast cancer cases. In addition, this molecule in distant metastasis regions was demonstrated to be highly expressed than the levels in regional lymph node metastases. This showed that *APOBEC3B* not only in the primary tumor stage has a role in the development of different metastatic stages of breast cancer. In conclusion, *APOBEC3B* causes the progression of metastatic breast cancer [16]. Therefore, the identification of different expression levels of *APOBEC3B* suggests that it carries a biological marker feature that may show a different metastatic stage and may be used in the identification of the metastasis stages in future.

3. Metastasis of breast cancer to different organs

3.1 Lymph node metastasis

Lymph node metastasis shows that distant metastasis risk is higher. The absence of lymph node metastases is associated with lower metastasis risk; however, the presence of more than four lymph node metastases is the precursor that distant metastasis risk is significantly higher. Distant tumor metastasis develops through axillary lymphoid nodes (ALD) and blood circulation. Therefore, lymph nodes are used as an indicator of the metastasis ability of tumor cells. There is an association between the tumor size and the rate of lymph node metastasis.

CCN proteins which have oncogenic functions in breast cancer mainly consist of *CCN1* and *CCN2*. *CCN1* protein is expressed in ~30% of breast cancers particularly in estrogen receptor (ER)-positive HER-2-negative tumors compared with the normal breast tissues. Higher *CCN1* expression is associated with lymph node metastasis and poor prognosis in breast cancer patients. *CCN1* increases the breast tumor vascularization and causes metastasis with Hg signaling [17]. In addition, *CCN1* has a regulatory role in fibroblast production by affecting MMP-1 for increasing the breast cancer cell migration and invasion. CCN4 expression is associated with lymph node metastasis and poor prognosis.

3.2 Bone metastasis

The common cause of morbidity and mortality in most advanced stage breast cancer patients is the development of osteolytic bone metastasis. The most frequently detected area of metastasis in metastatic breast cancer is the bone and constitutes 70% of the metastases. Most bone metastases detected in breast cancer are associated with osteolytic-type metastatic lesions owing to the osteoclast-mediated bone resorption. Although all subtypes of breast cancer have a tendency of bone metastases, luminal subtype tumors develop higher bone metastases (80.5%) than the basal-like (41.7%) and HER2+ tumors (55.6%) [18].

Tumor cells demonstrate different reactions in accordance with the environment in the new organ such as gene expression, growth ability, and response to treatment. Therefore, any of the breast cancer cell reaching to the bone may promote the excessive growth in molecular interaction with osteoblasts and osteoclasts. The molecules produced by cancer cells or with the parathyroid hormone-associated protein in the bone microenvironment and converting growth factor β (*TGF-β*) mediate this growth. The elimination of the tumor suppressor feature of *TGF-β* is suggested to stimulate the tumor invasion and metastasis [19]. Cytokines, chemokines, and other growth factors support the development of bone metastasis. Prometastatic cytokine *TGF-β*, osteolytic angiogenic factors interleukin-11 (*IL11*), and CTGF expression are accepted as the molecules that increase the osteolytic metastatic activity. Although *SMAD4* is a tumor suppressor which inhibits the tumor cell proliferation, it is an osteolytic metastasis promoter which binds the *TGF-β* signal to the following *IL11* induction [20]. *SMAD4* activates *VEGF* and *CXC* chemokine receptor 4 (*CXCR4*) to induce the bone metastasis in breast cancer through *HIF-lα* and *TGF-β* signal.

Some cancer cells in the primary tumor accumulate additional genetic changes which lead to bone metastasis. This causes invasion and colonization of tumor cells to the bone matrix. The destruction of the bone matrix with tumor cells facilitates the metastasis by the TGF and metastasis genes responding to TGF causing the increase of *CTGF* and *IL11* expression. *IL11*, *CTGF*, *CXCR4*, and *MMP-1* are the four most effective genes that are overexpressed in bone metastasis. Another effective gene is the protein osteopontin (OPN) which has various functions including the stimulating ability of the bone matrix to attach to the osteoclast. This protein is continuously overexpressed in metastatic cells. The genes effective in bone metastasis affect the tumor microenvironment toward metastasis. The overexpression of these genes develops the osteolytic bone metastasis. *IL11* is a strong osteoclast inducer which is synthesized by the progenitor cells in the bone marrow [17]. The in vivo testing of *IL11*-transfected MDA-MB-231 for metastatic activity of metastatic breast cancer cell line showed that the single expression of *IL11* did not significantly increase the metastasis. Therefore the presence of other genes in cooperation with IL11 in bone metastasis and their investigation were suggested [17]. *IL11* and *OPN* significantly increased the osteolytic bone metastasis by increasing the osteoclast function. *MMP-1* alone or in combination with *IL11* and *OPN* is another important molecule in the development of bone metastasis.

Because *TGF-β* is abundantly stored in the bone matrix, *TGF-β* that is secreted during osteolysis stimulates the metastatic breast cancer. *TGF-β* increases the *IL11* and *CTGF* expressions which are already higher in metastasis. The significantly overexpressed genes in bone metastasis encode the cell surface and secreting proteins which have functions that could possibly change the host tissue environment, each promoting the formation of osteolytic bone lesions.

Figure 3 demonstrates the functioning between the *CXCR4* gene responsible in bone marrow extravasation, *MMP-1* and *ADAMTS1* genes having roles of proteolysis and also *FGF5* and *CTGF* genes that are known to be expressed in angiogenesis, and IL11 genes which have a role in osteoclastogenesis.

Primary breast tumor develops with the accumulation of oncogenic mutations from normal breast epithelium. The increased expression of gene classes that facilitate metastasis to different organs among tumor cells enables the invasion of the bone matrix, colonization of metastatic tumor cell, and destruction of the bone matrix [21].

CCN protein family consists of six members as *CCN1* (*Cyr61*), *CCN2* (*CTGF*), *CCN3* (*Nov*), *CCN4* (*WISP-1*), *CCN5* (*WISP2*), and *CCN6* (*WISP3*) which have central roles in development, inflammation, and tissue repair [22]. In addition, CCN proteins have roles in various pathological cases by organizing the extracellular signals in the cellular environment. In MDA-MB-231 metastatic breast cancer cell line, *CCN3* reorganizes the actin cytoskeleton and increases the cell trafficking by activating the GTPase *Rac1* [23]. *CCN3* was demonstrated to increase the bone metastasis in the studies conducted in metastatic breast cancer cell line [23]. This significant effect of *CCN3* in metastasis was reported to deteriorate the osteoblast differentiation and provided a favorable environment for osteolytic breast cancer bone metastasis owing to supporting the osteoclastogenesis [23].

One of the overexpressed genes in bone-specific metastasis is the *NAT1* (N-acetyltransferase-1) and is a potential biological indicator for breast cancer.

3.3 Liver metastasis

The liver is the most common metastatic region for cancers and represents the second organ where breast cancer metastasis occurs. The development of liver metastasis in breast cancer patients is associated with Wnt signal and Ki67 signal independent of beta-catenin and an indicator of poor prognosis.

CXCR4 is the most common chemokine receptor that mediates the initiation of liver metastases. In addition, the dysregulation of cell adhesion molecules *N-cadherin* and *E-cadherin* was demonstrated to contribute to liver metastases in breast cancer (**Figure 4**). Breast cancer cells with higher *N-cadherin* level develop liver metastasis. *E-cadherin* which inhibits the metastasis was found lower in breast cancer cells with liver metastasis [24].

Although *N-cadherin* increases the liver metastasis, in normal conditions *E-cadherin* suppresses the development of liver metastasis. In addition, *IL-6*

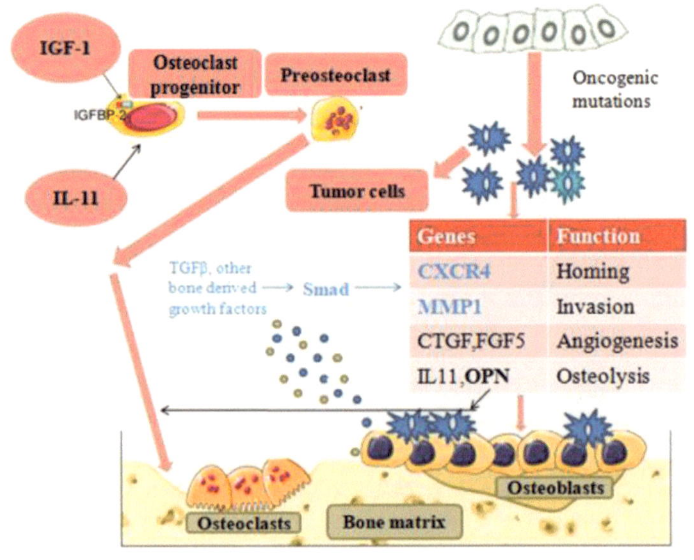

Figure 3.
The molecular mechanisms that are mediated by the genes effective in breast cancer-associated bone metastasis.

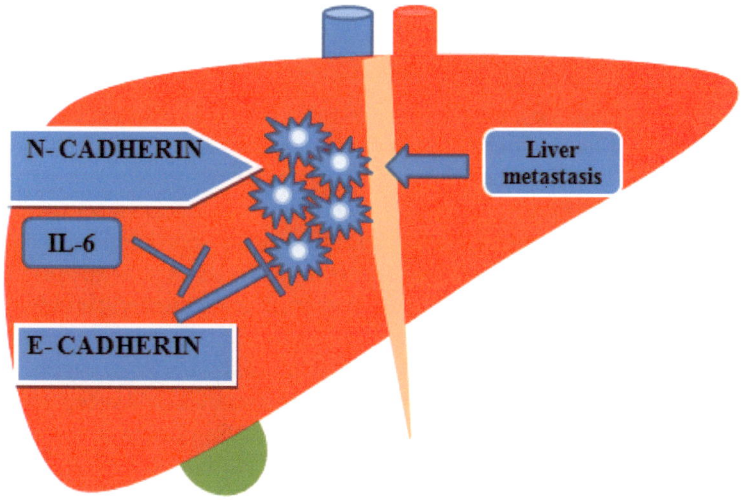

Figure 4.
Regulation of cell adhesion molecules in liver metastasis with N-cadherin and E-cadherin.

expression in liver metastasis of breast cancer facilitates the development of liver metastasis by inhibiting the *E-cadherin* expression [24].

Metastasis is a multistep procedure which is responsible for most cancer-associated deaths and is affected by both cell-cell or cell-matrix interactions and tumor microenvironment (vascularization, etc.).

Clinically, low oxygen level (hypoxia) is known to be associated with metastasis [17]. Lysyl oxidase (*LOX*) expression is both associated with tumor suppression and tumor progression, and its role in tumorigenesis changes in accordance with the cellular location, cell type, and transformation. *LOX* expression is regulated by the hypoxia-inducible factor (*HIF*). Mostly distant metastasis is detected, and overall survival is poor in patients who have tumors which highly express the *LOX*. The *LOX* inhibition eliminates metastasis in breast cancer patients. *LOX* is required in metastatic growth to form a niche. *LOX* is required for hypoxia-associated metastasis. Although LOX inhibition has no significant effect on primary tumor growth, *LOX* was associated to significantly decrease the lung metastases and inhibited the liver metastasis [25]. *LOX* molecule is suggested to be a good therapeutic target in prevention and elimination of metastasis [25].

3.4 Brain metastasis

Brain/CNS (central nervous system) metastasis develops in 10–30% of metastatic breast cancer patients. Brain metastasis (BM) is detected as a complication that generally develops in the late stages of disease. Brain metastases develop after systemic emergence of metastases in the lungs, liver, and bone [26]. Two main primary tumors that do metastasis to the brain are lung and breast adenocarcinomas [18]. Brain metastases are associated with neurological disorders by affecting both the cognitive and sensory functions in addition to their association with highly poor prognosis.

Breast cancer is the most common cancer type where brain metastasis develops after lung metastasis. Lung and breast cancer-associated brain metastasis is more frequently detected than the primary brain tumors. Brain metastasis incidence has gradually been increasing in breast cancer patients. Due to the development of systemic therapies, many breast cancer patients live longer, but still in a way brain metastases may develop. Various factors were described for increased brain metastasis risk in breast cancer patients. These factors may be reported as early age, poorly differentiated tumor histology (high grade), hormone receptor negativity, and metastasis in more than four lymph nodes. These factors were associated with the brain metastasis risk [26]. HER2-positive and TNBC patients have a higher risk of brain metastasis than the luminal-type breast cancer patients. Brain metastasis is detected in 30–40% of HER2-positive and triple negative breast cancer patients [26]. Brain metastasis in lung cancer generally develops within 2 years after the diagnosis of primary lung cancer, and brain metastasis in breast cancer is generally associated with the metastatic stage of the disease and develops 10 years after the primary diagnosis and after a successful treatment. However, brain metastasis in triple negative breast cancer patients develops in earlier periods. The development of brain metastasis in breast cancer was detected to be associated with Wnt, Notch, and EGFR pathways [27]. *CXCL12* that is expressed in the brain and *CXCR4* receptor located in the surface of the breast tumor cells block the cell signaling pathway together with *CXCR4* in brain metastasis. Breast cancer-associated brain metastasis generally develops in ~20–30% of breast cancer patients. Breast cancer-associated metastasis shows poor prognosis due to the lack of molecular therapeutic targets. The rate of detection of brain metastasis in HER2+ and triple negative breast cancer subtypes is 20–50%.

HER2 amplifications and mutations were frequently demonstrated in breast cancer and in breast cancers with brain metastasis [27]. There are no target-specific treatment options in the clinical practice generally in breast cancers that carry *BRCA1* and *BRCA2* gene mutation and triple negative brain metastasis. New molecular targets HER2, *EGFR*, *VEGFR*, *PARP*, *mTOR*, and *CDK-4/6* were discovered in the treatment of breast cancer with metastasis to the brain.

Brain metastasis is a multistep procedure with migration, intravasation, circulation, adhesion, extravasation, and brain microenvironment. Particularly the blood-brain barrier (BBB) is highly selective in the entrance of tumor cells and therapeutics to the brain microenvironment. In compliance with that, the cells to make a metastatic lesion in the brain have a specific clonal origin. This shows that a brain metastasis shared the common abnormalities with a metastasis ancestor cell, and the further abnormalities could only be present in only brain metastatic subclones. More frequent detection of *TP53* mutations in breast cancer with brain metastasis compared with the other breast cancers is an example. *COX2*, *EGFR*, and *HBEGF* were described as the extravasation stimulating factors through colonization in breast cancers with metastases to the brain and lung. The higher expression of the genes *CXCR4*, *PLLP*, *TNFSF4*, *VCAM1*, *SLC8A2*, and *SLC7A11* facilitates the development of brain metastases. In addition, the majority of snoRNAs and snRNAs have higher expression in breast cancer metastasizing to the brain [28].

3.5 Lung metastasis

Luminal breast tumors have the tendency to do metastasis to the bone; however, basal-like breast tumors mainly do metastasis to the lungs. The genes that are effective in the emergence of lung metastasis are generally associated with poor prognosis [29]. An epidermal growth factor receptor-ligand epiregulin (*EPR*) and the genes such as *COX2*, *MMP-1*, and *MMP-2* affect the tumor angiogenesis and facilitate the lung metastasis by reaching to the lung capillary vessels. The inhibition of *EGFR* and *COX2* minimizes the lung metastasis [30]. Protein deacetylase *SIRT7* was demonstrated to inhibit the development of lung metastasis of breast cancer cells by antagonizing the *TGF-β* signal [31]. An increased expression was reported in the genes *DSC2*, *TFCP2L1*, *UGT8*, *ITGB8*, *ANP32E*, and *FERMT1* that are associated with cell involvement and signal transduction in patients with lung metastasis of breast cancer [31].

Other genes except *PTEN* were detected to be overexpressed in the studies investigating the mechanism of lung metastasis. Although none of the described genes were found to be associated with previous metastasis, some of the encoded molecules were detected to have significant roles in the acquisition of proliferative and invasive characteristics to epithelial cells. The regulation of the epithelial-mesenchymal transition (EMT) is highly important in metastatic process. Integrins regulate the EMT by mediating the *TGF-β* signal activation [32]. *FERMT1* gene is known to be an effective gene in *TGF*-mediated epithelial-mesenchymal transition. Therefore, *FERMT1* gene is suggested to be associated with lung metastasis.

The decrease of the expression of a tumor suppressor gene *PTEN* was found to be associated with lung metastasis in a study [33]. *PTEN* is one of the main molecules which regulates the signaling pathways associated with reproduction, growth, cell viability, and cell migration and was detected to mutate in various different tumors. In addition, *PTEN* regulates the *EMT* in lung metastasis by affecting the cell viability and *CXCR4* chemotaxis. The biological indicators *EGFR* and *FOXC1* were demonstrated to be associated with each other and controlled the lung metastasis in breast cancer [33]. The survival rate of breast cancer patients with lung metastasis is very low despite the treatment options as chemotherapy, radiotherapy, and target-specific treatment against lung metastasis. Therefore, the development of new therapeutic strategies is significantly important for understanding the underlying mechanisms in lung metastasis.

A Notch signaling pathway receptor *Notch-1* was demonstrated to have a critical role in cell renewal, reproduction, and apoptosis of BCSC by regulating the epithelial-mesenchymal transition in breast cancer [34]. The abnormal activation of notch signaling pathway contributes to the breast cancer metastasis by primarily regulating the EMT and angiogenesis.

Wnt/β-catenin signaling has a significant role in the embryonic induction and tumorigenesis of the breast gland [35]. The nuclear localization and overexpression of β-catenin are an indicator of Wnt/β-catenin signal activation. Various clinical and laboratory studies showed that the abnormal activation of Wnt/β-catenin signaling was associated with poor prognosis in breast cancer patients and mainly increased in triple negative cancer subtype [36]. In addition, the Wnt-helper receptor *LRP6* was commonly overexpressed in highly aggressive triple negative breast cancer. Wnt/β-catenin signaling pathway contributes to the EMT and breast cancer metastases in addition to controlling the cell proliferation in breast cancer (**Table 1**).

Hedgehog (Hg) signaling pathway has a significant role in the development of ducts of the breast. In addition, Hg regulates the breast cancer stem cells and has a significant role in cancerogenesis [37]. Hg proteins regulate the breast cancer cell migration. Hg, Notch, and Wnt signaling pathways demonstrate joint behavior in tumor development and metastasis in cancer. These signaling pathways have significant roles in the development of breast cancer and lung metastasis.

Notch pathway	Wnt pathway	Hedgehog pathway
Uncontrolled growth	The self-renewal of breast cancer stem cells	*TGF-β*
The self-renewal of breast cancer stem cells	EMT	*CXCL12-CXC4*
Angiogenesis, EMT		
Formation of lung niches		
Development of lung metastasis		

Table 1.
The functioning of signaling pathways in breast cancer-associated lung metastasis.

Breast cancer is characterized with a separate metastatic pattern including the regional lymph nodes, bone marrow, lung, and liver. Chemokines are a group of small-molecular-weight protein which bind to chemokine receptors attached to G protein. Chemokines have a significant role in various pathological conditions such as cell migration, development, and inflammation. Binding of chemokines to receptors causes a structural change which activates the signaling pathways and promotes the migration. Chemokine and chemokine receptors have a critical role in identification of metastatic targets of tumor cells. Chemokines are divided into two groups in accordance with their functions as inflammatory chemokines and homeostatic chemokines. Inflammatory chemokines are induced by inflammation, and homeostatic chemokines are structurally expressed and have a role in homeostatic immune regulation [38].

Chemokines have a significant role in the progression of cancers [38] and have functions in tumoral growth, aging, angiogenesis epithelial-mesenchymal transition, and metastasis. The expression of chemokines and their receptors changes in malignity and then causes abnormal chemokine receptor signaling. This change stems from the inactivation of the tumor-suppressive genes or from the structural activation of oncogenes that have a role in the regulation of chemokines [38].

Chemokine receptors *CXCR4* and *CCR7* are highly expressed in human breast cancer cells, malignant breast tumors, and metastases [38]. In breast cancer cells, *CXCR4* or *CCR7* signaling mediates the actin polymerization and pseudopodia and then induces the chemotaxis and invasion.

The in vivo inactivation of *CXCL12/CXCR4* interactions significantly inhibits the metastasis of breast cancer cells to the regional lymph nodes and lungs [38]. *CXCL12/CXCR4* interactions also cause bone marrow metastasis of breast cancer cells.

Tumor cell migration and metastasis have various similarities with the leukocyte trafficking that are regulated by chemokines and their receptors. Cell trafficking-associated ligands *CXCL12/SDF-1α* and *CCL21/6Ckine* are highly expressed in the organs representing the first targets of metastatic breast cancer [38]. Malignant melanoma which has high skin metastasis and has a similar metastatic characteristic with breast cancer has high *CCR10* expression in addition to *CXCR4* and *CCR7* [38]. Therefore, both *CXCR4* and *CCR7* are highly critical molecules for cell trafficking and tissue homeostasis.

CXCL12 is the only ligand known for *CXCR4*. Metastatic breast cancers were demonstrated to selectively express CXCR4 and migrated to organs which highly express the ligand *CXCL12* that is also known as *SDF-1* [38]. *CXCR4* expression is known to be higher in malignant breast tumors than the levels in healthy breast tissues. *CXCL12* was highly expressed in organs such as the lung, bone, liver, and lymph nodes where the breast cancer cells preferred to do metastasis [38]. This showed that metastatic breast tumor cells selectively expressed *CXCR4*, and thus breast cancer cells which reached to organs have high *CXCL12* expression levels. In addition, the in vivo inhibition of *CXCR4-CXCL12* interactions was demonstrated to significantly decrease the metastasis of breast tumor cells to the lymph node and lungs [38]. Therefore, *CXCL12-CXCR4* signaling is suggested to be an important therapeutic target for metastatic breast cancer treatment.

CXCR4-CXCL12 receptor-ligand interactions in breast cancer allow the invading of tumor cells of neighboring tissues and for successful metastasis. The receptor-ligand interaction triggers the actin polymerization and facilitates the formation of pseudopodia. Thus, the invading of breast tumor cells of the neighboring tissues or distant tissue is induced or facilitated [39]. Chemokine *CXCL12* activates the chemokine receptor *CXCR4* in endothelial cell which supports the endothelial cell migration and growth [39]. The high expression of *CXCL12* in the lung, liver, and lymph nodes showed that these chemokines have a role in the metastasis of breast cancer cells for these anatomic regions.

CCL21 and its receptor *CCR7* have critical importance in the settlement of lymphocytes to secondary lymphoid organs. The primary breast cancer cells in lymph nodes and most metastatic cancer cells express *CCR7*, and there is an association between *CCR7* expression and lymph node metastasis. In addition, higher *CCR7* expression was demonstrated to be associated with poor prognosis and shorter survival [38].

Extracellular matrix (ECM) proteins tenascin-C (TNC), periostin (POSTN), and versican (VCAN) are highly important molecules in the formation of metastasis and have a critical role in the formation of breast cancer colonization in the lung tissue that has a tendency for metastasis. Tenascin-C, which is normally produced by fibroblasts, is also secreted by breast cancer stem cells. This abnormal expression of tenascin-C by breast cancer stem cells forms a niche in lung colonization and creates a metastasis-initiating effect. Periostin is a stromal factor that may bind to Wnt ligands and is effective in breast cancer metastasis [40].

Cancer-associated fibroblasts (*CAFs*) have a significant role in breast cancer metastasis by expressing the *Tiam1* and osteopontin in breast cancer tissue [40]. In addition, the expression of a *CAF*-associated protein thrombocyte-associated growth factor receptor (*PDGFRβ*) is highly associated with lung metastasis in breast cancer. In addition, CAFs increase the primary tumor growth through *TGF-β* and contribute to the development of lung metastasis-associated fibrous tissue in breast cancer [41]. Therefore, *CAF* is suggested to be a potential anti-cancer therapeutic target. The development of strategies targeting the micro-environment may be effective in the treatment or inhibition of breast cancer metastasis.

Because the lungs have a unique histological feature, cancer cell meets with high interstitial fluid pressure and thus supports the *PDGFRβ* expression when a cancer cell does metastasis to a small interstitial tissue between the alveoles. Lung metastasis is known to be associated with triple negative breast cancer.

As conclusion, the expression changes in these genes in breast cancer cells may be detected in bone, lung, brain, liver, and lymph node metastases. The studies revealed that there were important differences in metastatic behavior between breast cancer subtypes (**Table 2**). Therefore, the treatment of metastatic breast cancer must be performed by targeting the organ with metastasis, and the development of target molecules will form the future treatment protocols.

Luminal B, HER2+/ER/PR+ and HER2+/ER/PR, tumors do more metastasis to the brain, liver, lung, and bone than the luminal A tumors. Basal-like tumors do higher rates of brain and lung metastases. As demonstrated in **Table 2**, breast cancer cells do metastasis to the lung through triple negative breast cancer, basal, luminal B, HER2 molecular subtypes, the genes activated by growth factor receptors, matrix metalloproteinases, and the pathways of *COX2* and *LOX2* genes. Breast cancer cells with HER2+, luminal-HER2, triple negative breast cancer, and basal histologies primarily have a tendency to do metastasis to the brain. These molecular subtypes do metastasis to the brain with the effect of genes activated by growth factor receptors, matrix metalloproteinases, COX2, and chemokinesis. Clarifying the association of these signalings and genes with molecular subtypes suggests the significant new therapeutic targets for metastatic breast cancer treatment. The bone metastasis of luminal and HER2 breast cancer molecular subtypes is caused by growth factor genes and interleukins. Chemokine and integrin molecules that cause liver metastasis are more frequently detected in HER2+, ER+, luminal B, and luminal-HER2 molecular subtypes. BCR pathway proteins and CCN proteins, the genes responsible in Hg signaling pathway, cause lymph node metastasis in luminal type and HER2+ molecular subtypes [1].

Tissue	Lung	Brain	Bone	Liver	Lymph node
Molecular subtypes of breast cancer	TNBC Basal Luminal B HER2+	HER2+ Luminal-HER2 TNBC Basal	Luminal HER2	HER2+ ER+ Luminal B Luminal-HER2	Luminal HER2+
Molecular pathways and genes	**Growth factors** TGF-β EGFR VEGF **Matrix Metalloproteinases** MMP-1 MMP-2 **Chemokines** CXCL12 CXCR4 **BMP inhibitors** **Other factors** COX-2 LOX	**Growth factors** VEGF HBEGF **Matrix Metalloproteinases** MMP-9 MMP-1 **Chemokines** CXCR4 CXCL12 CCR7 CCL21 **Cytokines** CK5 **Notch pathways** **Wnt pathways** **Hg pathways** **Other factors** COX-2 LOX IL-8 COX-2 ICAM1 PTEN CAF	**Growth factors** IGF1 PGE2 TGF-β **Other factors** PDGF FGF2 IL11 IL-6 IL-1 OPN	**Chemokines** CXCR4 CXCL12 CCR7 CCL21 **Other factors** IL-6 N-cadherin E-cadherin LOX OPN VEGF TWIST WNT pathway ECM	**CCN proteins** **BCR pathways** **Hedgehog (Hg) pathway**

Table 2.
The organ-specific genes and signaling pathways effective in metastatic breast cancer.

Individualized target-specific appropriate treatment methods will be developed for metastatic breast cancer owing to the knowledge of the association of genes with each other that cause metastasis and the follow-up of the pathways where these genes gained function. There is an association between genomic differences and various gene expressions that cause poor prognosis in breast cancer. The gene expression profiles of primary tumors must be compared and associated with metastasis for describing and clarifying the tumor factors of metastatic breast cancer. The better understanding of the functioning of these genes will help to develop specific therapeutic approaches for metastatic breast cancer.

The molecules and genes on the pathways will be used in the diagnosis, prognosis and treatment response of metastatic breast cancer in the future. These effective molecules will be used as a tumor-specific indicator, and also detected in different biological materials like tissue, saliva, blood, serum, and urine in metastatic breast cancer. In addition, these genes may be used as therapeutic targets. The inactivation of these genes by inhibition or with biological antibodies through apoptosis is significantly important to resolve the tumor and metastasis. Different therapeutic strategies will be developed, and these molecules will be used in individualized treatment for inhibiting the tumor metastasis considering the associations between these genes, and chemokines, and integrins. The breast cancer molecular subtypes will be treated, and a progress will be enabled in the treatment of metastatic breast cancer with the development of molecular drugs which inhibit the active pathways or eliminate the pathway transition of the genes effective in metastatic breast cancer.

Acknowledgements

The authors thank Kadriye Yilmaz from the Department of Foreign Languages at the University of Istanbul for their language corrections.

Conflict of interest

The authors declare that they have no conflict of interests.

Author details

Hülya Yazici* and Beyza Akin
Division of Cancer Genetics, Istanbul University, Institute of Oncology, Istanbul, Turkey

*Address all correspondence to: hulyayazici67@gmail.com

References

[1] Kennecke H, Yerushalmi R, Woods R, Cheang MC, Voduc D, Speers CH. Metastatic behavior of breast Cancer subtypes. Journal of Clinical Oncology. 2010;**28**:3271-3277

[2] Antoine A, Khalil OI, Friedl P. Collective invasion in ductal and lobular breast cancer associates with distant metastasis. Clinical & Experimental Metastasis. Oct 2017;**34**(6-7):421-429

[3] Hess KR, Varadhachary GR, Taylor SH, Wei W, Raber MN, Lenzi R, et al. Metastatic patterns in adenocarcinoma. Cancer. 1 Apr 2006;**106**(7):1624-1633

[4] Zhang XH, Wang Q, Gerald W, Hudis CA, Norton L, Smid M, et al. Latent bone metastasis in breast cancer tied to Src-dependent survival signals. Cancer Cell. 7 Jul 2009;**16**(1):67-78

[5] Yoneda T, Williams PJ, Hiraga T, Niewolna M, Nishimura R. A bone-seeking clone exhibits different biological properties from the MDA-MB-231 parental human breast cancer cells and a brain-seeking clone in vivo and in vitro. Journal of Bone and Mineral Research. Aug 2001;**16**(8):1486-1495

[6] Bos PD, Zhang XH, Nadal C, Shu W, Gomis RR, Nguyen DX, et al. Genes that mediate breast cancer metastasis to lung. Nature. 18 Jun 2009;**459**(7249):1005-1009

[7] Ono M, Inkson CA, Kilts TM, Young MF. WISP-1/CCN4 regulates osteogenesis by enhancing BMP-2 activity. Journal of Bone and Mineral Research. Jan 2011;**26**(1):193-208

[8] Haghshenas MR, Haghshenas MR, Ashraf MJ, Khademi B, Ghaderi A, Erfani N, et al. Chemokine and chemokine receptor patterns in patients with benign and malignant salivary gland tumors: A distinct role for CCR7. European Cytokine Network. 1 Mar 2017;**28**(1):27-35

[9] Limoge M, Safina A, Truskinovsky AM, Aljahdali I, Zonneville J, Gruevski A, et al. Tumor p38MAPK signaling enhances breast carcinoma vascularization and growth by promoting expression and deposition of pro-tumorigenic factors. Oncotarget. 2017;**8**(37):61969-61981

[10] Safina A, Vandette E, Bakin A. ALK5 promotes tumor angiogenesis by upregulating matrix metalloproteinase-9 in tumor cells. Oncogene. 2007;**26**(17):2407-2422

[11] Ahmadiankia N, Bagheri M, Fazli M. Gene expression changes in pomegranate Peel extract-treated triple-negative breast Cancer cells. Reports of Biochemistry & Molecular Biology. Oct 2018;**7**(1):102-109

[12] Chaudhary A, Hilton MB, Seaman S, Haines DC, Stevenson S, Lemotte PK. TEM8/ANTXR1 blockade inhibits pathological angiogenesis and potentiates tumoricidal responses against multiple Cancer types. Cancer Cell. 14 Feb 2012;**21**(2):212-226

[13] Cao C, Wang Z, Huang L, Bai L, Wang Y, Liang Y, et al. Down-regulation of tumor endothelial marker 8 suppresses cell proliferation mediated by ERK1/2 activity. Scientific Reports. 2016;**6**:23419

[14] Chen D, Bhat-Nakshatri P, Goswami C, Badve S, Nakshatri H. ANTXR1, a stem cell enriched functional biomarker, connects collagen signaling to cancer stem-like cells and metastasis in breast cancer. Cancer Research. 2014;**73**(18):5821-5833

[15] Høye AM, Tolstrup SD, Horton ER. Tumor endothelial marker 8 promotes cancer progression and

metastasis. Oncotarget. 10 Jul 2018;**9**(53):30173-30188

[16] Sieuwerts AM, Schrijver WA, Dalm SU, Weerd VD, Moelans CB, Hoeve NT, et al. Progressive APOBEC3B mRNA expression in distant breast cancer metastases. PLoS ONE. 2017;**12**(1):e0171343

[17] Awolaran O, Brooks SA, Lavender V. Breast cancer osteomimicry and its role in bone specific metastasis; an integrative, systematic review of preclinical evidence. The Breast. Dec 2016;**30**:156-171

[18] Savci-Heijink CD, Halfwerk H, Koster J, van de Vijver MJ. A novel gene expression signature for bone metastasis in breast carcinomas. Breast Cancer Research and Treatment. Apr 2016;**156**(2):249-259

[19] Khoshakhlagha M, Soleimaniab A, Moradi MB, Avan A, Fernse GA, et al. Therapeutic potential of pharmacological TGF-β signaling pathway inhibitors in the pathogenesis of breast cancer. Science Direct. Jun 2019;**164**:17-22

[20] Kang Y, He W, Tulley S, Gupta GP, Serganova I, Chen CR, et al. Breast cancer bone metastasis mediated by the Smad tumor suppressor pathway. Proceedings of the National Academy of Sciences of the United States of America. 27 Sep 2005;**102**(39):13909-13914

[21] YibinKang M, Siegel P, WeipingShu, MariaDrobnjak M, Kakonen S, Cordón-Cardo C. A multigenic program mediating breast cancer metastasis to bone. Cancer Cell. 2003;**3**(6):537-549

[22] Soon LL, Yie TA, Shvarts A, Levine AJ, Su F, Tchou-Wong KM. Overexpression of WISP-1 Down-regulated motility and invasion of lung Cancer cells through inhibition of Rac activation. The Journal of Biological Chemistry. 2003;**278**:11465-11470

[23] Ouellet V, Tiedemann K, Mourskaia A, Fong JE, Tran-Thanh D, Amir E, et al. CCN3 impairs osteoblast and stimulates osteoclast differentiation to favor breast Cancer metastasis to bone. The American Journal of Pathology. May 2011;**178**(5):2377-2388

[24] Hazan RB, Phillips GR, Qiao RF, Norton L, Aaronson SA. Exogenous expression of N-cadherin in breast Cancer cells induces cell migration, invasion, and metastasis. The Journal of Cell Biology. 21 Feb 2000;**148**(4):779-790

[25] Erler JT, Bennewith KL, Nicolau M, Dornhöfer N, Kong C, Le QT, et al. Lysyl oxidase is essential for hypoxia-induced metastasis. Nature. 27 Apr 2006;**440**(7088):1222-1226

[26] Witze I, Oliveira-Ferrer L, Pantel K, Müller V, Wikman H. Breast cancer brain metastases: Biology and new clinical perspectives. Breast Cancer Research. 2016;**18**:8

[27] SR S, RL C. EGFR and HER2 signaling in breast cancer brain metastasis. Frontiers in Bioscience (Elite Edition). 2016;**8**:245-263

[28] Schulten H-J, Bangash M, Karim S. Comprehensive molecular biomarker identification in breast cancer brain metastases. Journal of Translational Medicine. 2017;**15**:269

[29] Blanco MA, Kang Y. Signaling pathways in breast cancer metastasis: Novel insights from functional genomics. Breast Cancer Research. 2011;**206**

[30] Eltarhouny SA, Elsawy WH, Radpour R, Hahn S, Holzgreve W, Zhong XY. Genes controlling spread of breast cancer to lung "gang of 4".

Experimental Oncology. Jun 2008;**30**(2):91-95

[31] Tang X, Shi L, Xie N, Liu Z, Qian M, Fanbiao Meng QX-G. SIRT7 antagonizes TGF-β signaling and inhibits breast cancer metastasis. Nature Communications. 2017;**318**

[32] Margadant C, Sonnenberg A. Integrin–TGF-β crosstalk in fibrosis, cancer and wound healing. EMBO Reports. Feb 2010;**11**(2):97-105

[33] Y J, Han B, Chen J, Wiedemeyer R, Orsulic S, Bose S, et al. FOXC1 is a critical mediator of EGFR function in human basal-like breast cancer. Annals of Surgical Oncology. Dec 2014;**21**(Suppl 4):S758-S766

[34] Damodaran DP, Kolluru V, Chandrasekaran B, Baby BV, Aman M, Suman S, et al. Targeting aberrant expression of Notch-1 in ALDH+ cancer stem cells in breast cancer. Molecular Carcinogenesis. Mar 2017;**56**(3):1127-1136

[35] MacDonald BT, Tamai K. Wnt/β-catenin signaling: Components, mechanisms, and diseases. Developmental Cell. Jul 2009;**17**(1):9-26

[36] Khramtsov AI, Khramtsova GF, Tretiakova M, Huo D, Olopade OI, Goss KH. Wnt/β-catenin pathway activation is enriched in basal-like breast cancers and predicts poor outcome. The American Journal of Pathology. Jun 2010;**176**(6):2911-2920

[37] Flemban A, Qualtrough D. The potential role of hedgehog Signaling in the luminal/basal phenotype of breast epithelia and in breast Cancer invasion and metastasis. Cancers (Basel). 16 Sep 2015;**7**(3):1863-1884

[38] Müller A, Homey B, Soto H, Ge N, Catron D, Buchanan ME, et al. Involvement of chemokine receptors in breast cancer metastasis. Nature. 1 Mar 2001;**410**(6824):50-56

[39] Baetselier HV, Verschueren H, Van der Taelen I, Dewit J, De Braekeleer J, De Baetselier P. Metastatic competence of BW5147 T-lymphoma cell lines is correlated with in vitro invasiveness, motility and F-actin content. Journal of Leukocyte Biology. Apr 1994;**55**(4):552-556

[40] Xu K, Tian X, Oh SY, Movassaghi M, Naber SP, Kuperwasser C, et al. The fibroblast Tiam1-osteopontin pathway modulates breast cancer invasion and metastasis. Breast Cancer Research. 2016;**14**

[41] Kim HM, Jung WH, Koo JS. Expression of cancer-associated fibroblast related proteins in metastatic breast cancer: An immunohistochemical analysis. Journal of Translational Medicine. 2015;**13**:222

Chapter 3

Protein Tyrosine Phosphatases in Tumor Progression and Metastasis: Promoter or Protection?

Carmen V. Ferreira-Halder, Stefano Piatto Clerici, Alessandra V. Sousa Faria, Patrícia Fernandes de Souza Oliveira, Helon Guimarães Cordeiro and Erica Akagi

Abstract

Reversible phosphorylation of proteins, executed by kinases and phosphatases, is the major posttranslational protein modification in eukaryotic cells, causing them to become activated or deactivated. This intracellular event represents a critical regulatory mechanism of several signaling pathways and can be related to a broad number of diseases, including cancer. Few decades ago, protein tyrosine phosphatases (PTPs) were considered as tumor suppressors. However, nowadays, accumulating evidence demonstrates that a misregulation of PTP activities plays a crucial and decisive role in cancer progression and metastasis. In this chapter, we will focus on the molecular aspects that support the crucial role of PTPs in cancer and in turn make them promising for prediction, monitoring, and rational appropriate therapy selection of individual patients.

Keywords: protein tyrosine phosphatases, cancer hallmarks, tumor suppressor, metabolism, epithelial-mesenchymal transition

1. Introduction

Protein tyrosine phosphorylation plays a key role in cellular biology, once it can create a new recognition site for protein-protein interactions, control protein stability, and specify the protein location, and, more importantly, regulates enzymatic activity. Therefore, this intracellular event represents a critical regulatory mechanism of several signaling pathways and, once it is dysregulated, can be related to a broad number of diseases, including tumor development. Reversible phosphorylation of proteins is controlled reciprocally by both protein tyrosine kinases (PTKs) and protein tyrosine phosphatases (PTPs). These phosphatases are hydrolases that preferentially act on phosphotyrosine residue of a wide range of proteins, having as products dephosphorylated protein at tyrosine residue and inorganic phosphate. PTPs consist of a large protein superfamily with 107 members that can be divided into four families (class I, II, III, and IV) according to differences in the amino acid sequence at their catalytic domains and the amino acid used in the catalytic reaction, cysteine-based PTPs (class 1, 2, and 3) and aspartate-based PTPs (class 4) [1, 2]. So far, most of PTPs have been reported to act as tumor suppressors;

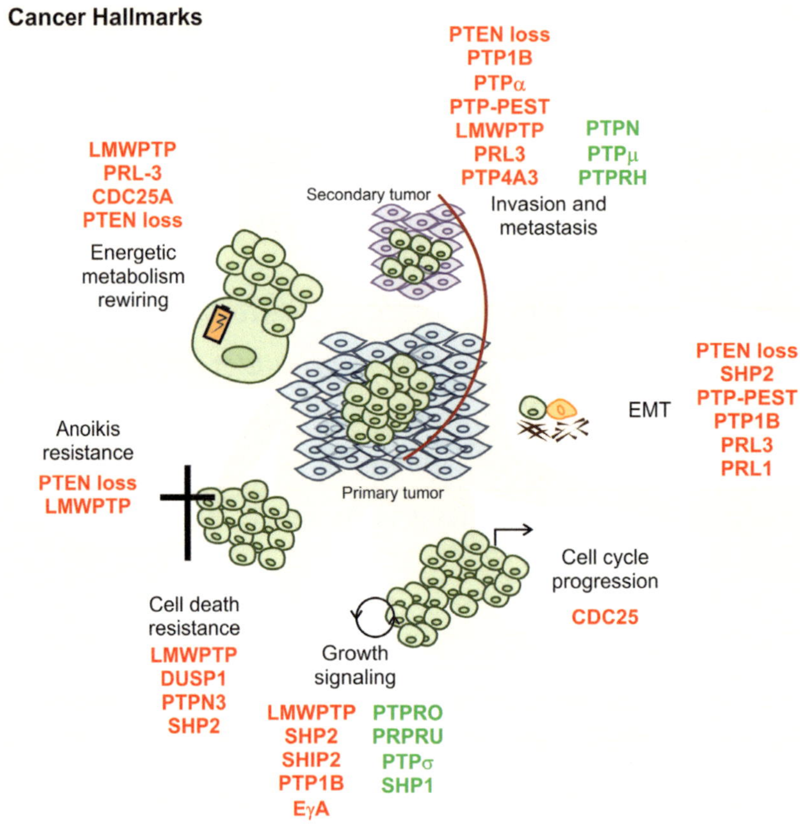

Figure 1.
Schematic overview of the role of PTPs in tumor plasticity. During tumor progression, cells acquire extra mutations and reprogram their metabolism in order to sustain proliferation, migration, and survival. These capacities are in part sustained by key signaling pathways in which PI3K, AKT, MAPK, and mTOR have central roles. In this context, hyperactivation and loss of specific PTPs are crucial for keeping these kinases active.

however, some PTPs can also act as oncogenes depending on the tumor stages or the expression of their interacting partners.

Along human tumor development, cells acquired biological plasticities that were firstly defined by Hanahan and Weinberg, as hallmarks of cancer. These authors proposed some capabilities of cancer cells that contribute for the disease complexity, aggressiveness, and invasiveness: sustaining proliferative signaling, evading growth suppressors, resisting cell death, enabling replicative immortality, inducing angiogenesis, deregulating cellular energetics, avoiding immune destruction, and activating invasion and metastasis [3]. Surprisingly, in the last decade, some reports have shown the relevance of PTPs for tumor cell plasticities. In this chapter we aim to draw an organized picture of the molecular mechanisms by which PTPs take part on tumor biological plasticity acquisition (**Figure 1**).

2. PTPs modulate energetic metabolism in tumors

Under normal conditions, cell metabolism depends on a tightly coordinated regulation of key regulatory enzymes and, consequently, metabolic pathways responsible for converting nutrients into building blocks for synthetic macromolecules, energy production, and biomass. However, cancer cells display efficiency capacity in reprogramming their metabolism through genetic or epigenetic changes in order to get survival, proliferation, migration, invasiveness, and resistance to death stimuli [5]. In recent years, it has been demonstrated that PTPs display a key role in favoring cancer cell metabolic plasticity.

2.1 PTPs and Warburg effect

Otto Warburg showed that tumor cells substantially metabolize glucose to lactate, even with the availability of oxygen. Under normal conditions, glucose is metabolized to pyruvate by a series of enzymatic steps in the glycolytic pathway, which is subsequently oxidized by the TCA and respiratory chain, generating CO_2, H_2O, and 32 or 34 molecules of ATP per glucose molecule, while in glycolysis, 2 ATPs/glucose are produced. This alteration in glucose metabolism depends on increased transcription of GLUTs, glycolytic enzymes, and oncogenes and increased demand of mitochondrial metabolism for biosynthetic processes [4–6].

Until a few years ago, the importance of protein kinases for the Warburg effect had been focused on several studies. However, recently, in the discovery that PTPs also have relevance in tumor onset and progression, attention has been given to the role of these phosphatases in tumor metabolism, as it is the case of Cdc25A, LMWPTP, PRL-3, and PTEN.

Cdc25A—Until 2016 it was believed that the relevance of Cdc25A in cancer was due to its positive effect on CDK. However, Liang and collaborators [7] performed an elegant study showing the Cdc25A as a positive regulator of PKM2 in human glioblastoma specimens. PKM2 catalyzes the conversion of phosphoenolpyruvate to pyruvate, the last step of glycolysis pathway. These authors described that the EGFR activation triggers the phosphorylation of Cdc25A at Y59 residue, mediated by Src. Consequently, the interaction between Cdc25A and PKM2 is favored at a nuclear compartment, leading to PKM2 dephosphorylation at S37, and in turn induces PKM2-dependent β-catenin transactivation and c-Myc-upregulated expression of the glycolytic genes *GLUT1*, *PKM2*, and *LDHA* [7].

LMWPTP—Our group demonstrated that, in chemoresistant chronic myeloid leukemia cells, the LMWPTP was overactivated and cooperated to Warburg effect. A downregulation of mitochondrial proteins—PDH1, SDHA, and VDAC— was also observed, while GLUT 1 expression and production of lactate were increased [8]. Later on, Lori and colleagues performed a phosphoproteomic analysis of A375 melanoma cells with silenced LMWPTP. These authors identified six possible substrates, of which four, PKM2, GAPDH, α-enolase, and triose phosphate isomerase, take part in the glycolytic pathway. In contrast to the findings reported by Faria and coworkers, it was observed that the inhibition of LMWPTP leads to an inactivation of PKM2, which causes a decrease in glycolytic flux and increase of GLUT1 and hexokinase 2 [8, 9].

PRL-3—It was reported that when colorectal cancer cells (LoVo cell line) overexpress, this phosphatase had an increase of glucose consumption and lactate production in comparison to LoVo cell line wild type. Accordingly, high amount of HK2, PKM2, and LDH were detected when PRL-3 is overexpressed [10]. Importantly, these authors also reported similar results when patient colorectal carcinoma samples were screened. PRL-3 displays a lower expression level in adjacent normal tissue but was overexpressed in colorectal carcinoma lesions. Furthermore, there was a positive correlation between the expression of glycolytic enzymes (GLUT1, HK2, PKM2, LDHA) and PRL-3.

PTEN—In different models (MEFs, prostate cancer cell lines, xenografts, genetically modified mouse and patient prostate cancer samples), the loss of PTEN specifically increases the expression of HK2 [11]. More recently, it was reported that the knockdown of PTEN in prostate cancer cells (DU145 cell line) leads to an increase of lactate, pyruvic acid, succinic acid, citric acid, fumaric acid, malic acid, and 2-ketoglutarate, in comparison to DU145 wild type [12]. These findings indicate that glycolysis and glutaminolysis pathways are active in prostate cancer DU-145 cells when PTEN is not functional. Accordingly, it was demonstrated that the PTEN higher expression compromises the proliferation and Warburg effect, in melanoma and breast tumor, by dropping the expression of HIF1 and increasing the mitochondrial function, which are, at least in part, caused by decreasing glucose uptake and inhibiting PI3K/mTOR pathway [13–16].

2.2 PTPs and glutamine/lipid metabolism

Some tumor cells become "addicted" to glutamine, once this amino acid can provide energy and substrates necessary for cell division. As a consequence, the tumor increases the mass of tumor cells and controls the potential redox through the synthesis of NADPH [17]. PTEN knockdown, in prostate cancer, reduces the protein level of GLS, enzyme involved in the glutaminolysis pathway, and increases the FASN expression [12]. Tumor cells also exhibit substantial alterations in lipid metabolism. During fast growth and aggressive progression, tumor cells required many metabolic intermediates and coordinate the activation of lipid synthesis leading to membrane formation, energy storage, and second messenger production [17, 18].

3. PTPs favor tumor growth through survival positive regulation, and cell death resistance

While normal cells tightly control the synthesis, secretion of growth factors, and proliferative signaling pathways, in order to ensure cellular homeostasis, cancer cells carry one or more defects along the signaling pathways from extracellular compartment, for example, growth ligands and their receptors, to intracellular mediators, such as PI3K, MAPK, and Akt, which give them survival advantages [19, 20]. In this context, PTPs' overexpression through gene amplification, loss, or inhibition contributes for aberrant signaling and, in turn, promoting tumor cell survival as exemplified below:

CDC25A, CDC25B, and CDC25C—CDC25A regulates cell cycle transition, from G1 to S phase, where it activates the cyclin E/CDK2 complex, whereas the phosphatases CDC25B and CDC25C act in the G2/M phase progression [21, 22]. Deregulations of these enzymes are correlated with imbalance in the cell cycle, genetic instability, and uncontrolled proliferation. In addition, the high expression level of these proteins is related to tumorigenesis [23, 24]. For instance, the overexpression of CDC25A was related to proliferation of breast, colon, hepatocellular, ovarian, lung, and nonmelanoma cancers [25]. Besides propitiating cancer cell proliferation, it was reported that CDC25A modulates Foxo1, consequently activating the expression of matrix metalloproteinase (MMP)-1, key mediator of cell dissemination. Moreover, the CDC25B overexpression was associated with gastric cancer, and its knockdown reduces the proliferation rate of gastric cells [26].

EYA—EYA dephosphorylates tyrosine residues of H2AX, a protein involved with DNA repair that prevents cell death caused by damage to the DNA molecule. Chemical inhibition of EYA phosphatase diminished angiogenesis and tumor growth [27]. WD-repeat-containing protein 1 (WDR1) is a specific substrate of EYA3; thus, this PTP can modulate cytoskeletal reorganization [28]. Another identified substrate of EYA is ERβ, which its dephosphorylation decreases the antitumor potential [29].

LMWPTP—In normal cells, the increase of LMWPTP expression was associated with a reduction of PDGFR phosphorylation, consequently dropping in the mitogenic capacity [30]. However, later on, LMWPTP was described as a positive modulator of Ras-MAPK, FGF, and Eph receptors [31, 32]. It was also reported that the overexpression of LMWPTP contributes for invasive profile and primary sarcoma formation in nude mice [33]. In this context, higher LMWPTP amount (mRNA and protein) in primary human prostate cancer in relation to normal adjacent tissue was found. Interestingly, the high level of mRNA of LMWPTP was detected in lymph nodes, an indication that this phosphatase takes part in the metastasis process [34]. In the same study, 147 patients out of 481 with prostate cancer presented higher expression of LMWPTP and worse clinical outcome [34]. Accordingly, the LMWPTP has been categorized as a potential biomarker for recurrence prediction for prostate cancer [35]. The importance of the LMWPTP in cancer progression was also reported in colorectal cancer. It was demonstrated that the LMWPTP overexpression in colorectal cancer correlated to a higher potential to liver metastasis [36]. Importantly, it was also demonstrated that the LMWPTP knockdown decreases CRC cell survival and sensitizes them to chemotherapy [36].

PTP1B—PTP1B is overexpressed in several cancers, such prostate, ovarian, stomach, and colorectal [37–40]. For instance, in esophagus squamous cell carcinoma, this phosphatase overexpression is directly related to invasion and metastasis [38]. Similar effect was described in lung cancer, which was due to Src and Erk activation. Interestingly, the PTP1B knockdown in colorectal cancer cells decreases proliferation rate by blocking β-catenin signaling, a pathway responsible for supporting the cancer secondary site colonization [39, 41].

SHIP2—SHIP2 positively affects tumor cell proliferation and migration. For instance, it was observed that the overexpression of SHIP2 in colorectal cancer was associated with migration and invasive profile through AKT activation [42].

SHP2 (PTPN11)—SHP2 (PTPN11) propiciates activation of Ras and MAPK triggered by mitogens (insulin, EGF, and lysophosphatidic acid) and cell adhesion. Notably, it has been shown that this phosphatase controls cell shape by contributing to cytoskeletal organization. In addition, SHP2 also regulates integrin-mediated cell adhesion, spreading, and migration. Also, inhibition of SHP2 is accompanied by expressive increase in the numbers of actin stress fibers and focal adhesion contacts. In contrast, overexpression of the SHP2 mutant also increased the strength of cell-substratum adhesion [43]. SHP2 has been considered as a proto-oncogene in several human cancers such as leukemia, glioblastoma, gastric carcinoma, lung cancer, and breast cancer. This phosphatase improves cancer progression and poor prognostic by activation of Ras/Raf/ERK and PI3K/Akt/mTOR pathways [44]. In hepatocellular carcinoma, the overexpression of SHP2 correlates with malignant cancer profile. Accordingly, it was reported that the inhibition of SHP2 diminishes metastasis by inhibition of cell adhesion and migration [45].

During cell transformation to malignancy, tumor cells became expert in overcoming a broad diversity of stresses, such as uncontrolled signaling regulation, starvation, DNA damage, hypoxia, and also anticancer therapy. In this aspect, different researchers have shown that PTPs are involved in tumor cells resistant to chemotherapeutic agents.

DUSP1 or PTPN10—It was shown that DUSP1 inhibits the MAPK (JNK) by dephosphorylation and in turn blocks apoptosis process. This effect might be one of the explanations in which DUSP1 promotes cancer cells escaping from apoptosis. Indeed, it has been reported that DUSP1 is involved in many cancers: gastric intestinal, lung, breast, squamous cell carcinoma, and head and neck [46].

LMWPTP—Our group has reported that in chemoresistant human chronic myeloid leukemia cells (Lucena-1), LMWPTP is around 20-fold more active than in their sensitive counterpart (K562). Importantly, the knockdown of LMWPTP in Lucena-1 cells reverted chemoresistance to vincristine and imatinib mesylate and culminated in inactivation of Src kinase and Bcr-Abl. Both kinases are well known to have a relevant contribution in leukemogenesis [47].

PTPN3—Wang and collaborators [40] performed a very elegant study, in which they found somatic mutations in six PTPs, including PTPN3, in colorectal, lung, breast, and gastric cancers. Later on, it was reported that PTPN3 induces drug resistance (cisplatin and doxorubicin) in ovarian cancer [48].

SHP2—A study using a RNA interference-based genetic screen in BRAF-mutant colon cancer cells identified the SHP2 as one of the key mediators of intrinsic and acquired resistance. Once this phosphatase maintains the receptor tyrosine kinases activated, even in the presence of BRAF inhibitor, it is still possible to have activation of cell proliferation and survival through involvement of ERK [49].

4. PTPs contribute for metastasis through extracellular matrix remodeling and epithelial-mesenchymal transition

In this chapter subtitle, we will focus on strategies for migration and invasion as part of the metastasis process.

PTPs activate the extracellular matrix remodeling and epithelial-mesenchymal transition. ECM is a three-dimensional noncellular scaffold crucial for life in multicellular organisms which is dynamically and continuously remodeled. ECM is mainly composed of water and almost 300 proteins, for example, collagens (fibrillar forms such as I–III, V, XI and non-fibrillar forms), proteoglycan (aggrecan and glycosaminoglycan such as heparin sulfate and hyaluronic acid), and glycoproteins (especially elastin, laminins, and fibronectin) [50, 51]. This essential component is considered an extremely organized meshwork in a strict contact with cells providing both biochemical and biomechanical support. It is well known that despite the physical support to cells, ECM also modulates cell differentiation, migration, and proliferation [50, 52]. Therefore, abnormal ECM remodeling (exacerbate deposition or degradation) can be observed during pathological conditions such as fibrosis and cancer [50, 52]. In tumor microenvironment, much of the ECM proteins are produced not only by stroma cells, e.g., cancer-associated fibroblasts [52], but also tumor cells can produce ECM proteins [53]. Malignant transformation is characterized by changes in the organization of cytoskeleton resulting in abnormal cell signaling related to cell-cell and to cell-ECM adhesion, a phenomenon termed epithelial-mesenchymal transition (EMT). EMT consists of the loss of epithelial cell characteristics to possess properties of mesenchymal cells. Several studies have shown that the EMT contributes to tumor progression, invasion, metastasis, and acquisition of therapeutic resistance. During the EMT process, the cancer cells acquire a fibroblastic morphology with a positive regulation of mesenchymal markers (N-cadherin, vimentin, and α-actin) and a negative regulation of epithelial cell markers (E-cadherin, ZO-1, claudins, occludins, and cytokeratin) as well as a regulation of transcription factors that are associated with increased migratory capacity (Slug, ZEB1/ZEB2, Twist1/Twist2). These factors bind to the E-cadherin gene promoter and repress it [54–56]. EMT requires a rupture of basement membrane permitting invasion and migration of cancer cells through the ECM, then causing remodeling, and creating a tumor-permissive environment [57].

Characteristic loss of E-cadherin-mediated cell-cell adhesion is commonly found during malignant transformation [58] in which process kinases and phosphatases have key roles [59, 60]. Several PTKs, including SRC and EGFR, phosphorylate the cadherin-catenin complex on different residues, resulting in a loss of cell adhesion [60]. For instance, PTP1B regulates cadherin-based adhesion by dephosphorylating β-catenin at Tyr654 [61]. In addition to β-catenin, p120-catenin phosphorylation increases binding and affinity to E-cadherin, and PTPμ appears to be a regulator of p120-catenin phosphorylation status, also acts as a scaffold, and recruits similar and regulatory molecules to sites of cell adhesion [61, 62]. SHP2 is also able to bind to cadherin-catenin complex and integrin molecules [62].

Cell migration through ECM requires integrin-mediated adhesion as well as turnover of focal adhesions [63]. A decrease in tyrosine phosphorylation by PTPs is involved in the formation and disassembly of focal adhesions. For instance, PTPα is required for the activation of Src kinase following integrin interaction [64], and the dephosphorylation of p130 CRK-associated substrate, by PTP-PEST, is necessary for disassembly of focal adhesions, enabling cell migration [64]. The relation between PTPs and upstream regulators of cell matrix adhesion and Rho family of small GTPases has also been shown [65]. Most Rho proteins have intrinsic GTPase activity which is stimulated by GTPase-activating proteins (GAPs), and these GAPs are modulated by phosphorylation at tyrosine sites. Consequently, PTPs can influence Rho protein activation through regulating the phosphorylation state of GAPs. Sastry and colleagues showed that PTP-PEST overexpression reduces Rac1 (a kind of G protein) activity resulting in protrusion and retraction during cell migration [66]. On the other hand, SHP2 seems to have some contradictory action, while some literatures reported a RhoA activity inhibition by SHP2 [67] and others suggested a stimulation [43]. In addition, p190RhoGAP, a GAP for RhoA, is a target for SHP-2 and LMWPTP and, in turn, regulating cytoskeletal rearrangement [68].

Metalloproteinases (MMPs) are one of the most important ECM-remodeling enzymes produced by tumoral cells, which are linked to tumorigenesis and metastasis [69]. More recently, it was reported that MMPs promote cell survival, angiogenesis [69], and induction of EMT [70]. Hwang and coworkers [71] observed that the treatment of MCF-7 breast cancer cells with BVT948 (a PTP inhibitor) decreases invasion through suppression of NF-κB-mediated MMP-9 expression. On the converse side, PTPμ knockdowns resulted in elevated adhesion, invasion, and proliferation of breast cancer cells due to activation of ERK and JNK signaling pathway and consequent elevated MMP-9 activity [72]. It was demonstrated that the overexpression of PRL-3 increased the migration and invasion capacity of DLD-1 colorectal cancer cells, which was dependent on the expression of MMP-7 [73]. Maacha and coworkers demonstrated that the contribution of the PTP4A3 for malignancy of uveal melanoma is related to MMP-14 [74]. Yuan and colleagues found that overexpression of PTPN9 reduces invasion and decreases MMP-2 gene expression in MDA-MB-231 cells through inhibition of STAT3 downregulation [75]. Interestingly, still in the context of breast cancer, William Du and his team [76] analyzed the levels of microRNA-24 in patients with breast carcinoma and found higher content of this microRNA in breast carcinoma samples than in benign breast tissue. They also generated constructs expressing miRNA-24 and studied their functions in vivo and in vitro. In vivo experiments in mice indicated that the expression of miRNA-24 enhanced tumor growth, invasion, and metastasis to the lung and decreased survival. Molecularly, in vitro and in vivo experiments showed high EGFR phosphorylation but repressed expression of PTPN9 and PTPRF due to direct target of these phosphatases by miRNA-24. Consistently, they found in patients with metastatic breast carcinoma a higher phosphorylation of EGFR but lower levels of PTPN9 and PTPRF. Another confirmation was the upregulation of MMP-2 and MMP-11 but downregulation of MMP inhibitor (TIMP-2) which supports the roles of miRNA-24 in tumor invasion and metastasis in breast cancer suggesting miRNA-24 as a potential target for cancer intervention. In another study, Liu and collaborators [41] observed that PTP1B promotes the aggressiveness of brain cancer through decreasing PTEN levels and, consequently, promoting AKT activation and increasing of MMP-2 and MMP-7. Previously, it was reported that PTP1B promotes gastric cancer cell invasiveness through modulating the expression of MMP-2, MMP-9, and MMP-14 [77]. Another interesting study shows the relationship of PTP1B and interruption of cell adhesion and induction of the *anoikis* effect in cancer cells. Inhibition of PTP1B in breast cancer cells leads to cell death and loss of extracellular matrix fixation, leading to negative regulation of cell adhesion proteins and interrupted actin polymerization. They saw that with the inhibition of PTP1B the activity of Src is consequently decreased by the adhesion pathway and motility is impaired [78].

Besides being involved in ECM remodeling by modulating MMP activities, PTPs (PTEN, SHP2, PTP1B, PRL3, PTP1B, PTRB, and PTPN9) have a key role in signaling cascades that promote expression of EMT markers.

DUSP1—It has been reported that the knockdown of DUSP1 culminates in low migratory and invasive efficiency of non-small cell lung cancer (NSCLC). Similar effect was also observed in in vivo model [79].

PTEN—It has been reported that the loss of PTEN or its negative modulation by phosphorylation or microRNA propiciates EMT. For instance, in lung cancer cells, the inactivation of PTEN stimulated the nuclear translocation of β-catenin and transcription factors snail and slug [80]. The authors also observed that the PI3K/AKT/GSK-3β pathway is essential for inducing EMT in PTEN-knocked-down cells. The relation between PTEN and negative regulation of AKT/β-catenin pathway was also described by Li and colleagues in squamous cell carcinoma of the esophagus [81]. It was observed that the glycan-1, a cell surface proteoglycan, promotes cell proliferation by regulating the PTEN/AKT/β-catenin pathway, which culminates in a positive regulation of N-cadherin and β-catenin and a negative regulation of E-cadherin. In colorectal cancer cells, the loss of PTEN is associated with a change in E-cadherin protein expression which was linked to EMT [82]. Wang and co-authors [83] reported that tetraspanin 1 induced liver cancer cell EMT via the PI3K/AKT/GSK-3β pathway. These authors also show that the PTEN repression was fundamental for this process. In addition to the effects reported above, one event that is associated with PTEN induction of EMT is the dysregulation of microRNAs. Studies have shown that PTEN is a target of some microRNAs. Wu and collaborators [84] showed that MiR-616-3p is upregulated in metastatic gastric cancer cells during angiogenesis process, and PTEN was one of the targets of this microRNA. Li [85] also showed that MiR-181-a is associated with lung cancer cell EMT through inhibition of PTEN protein expression. Another strategy to inhibit PTEN is via TGF-β cascade. The phosphorylation of the PTEN C-terminus leads to a conformational change, consequently provoking the loss of membrane binding and downregulation of PTEN phosphatase activity [86].TGF-β derived from the tumor microenvironment induces malignant phenotypes such as EMT and aberrant cell motility in lung cancers, by at least in part, due to inhibition of PTEN by phosphorylation [87].

SHP2—Sun and coworkers reported that IL-6 induces SHP2 activation by phosphorylation, which was required for breast cancer cell EMT stimulation in response to IL-6 [88]. This phosphatase also has a positive connection in lung cancer cell EMT triggered by TGF-β1 [89]. In addition, these authors identified the protein Hook1 as an interactor of SHP2 and classified this protein as an endogenous negative regulator of SHP2. The expression of Snail and Twist1, key mediators of EMT process, has been positively modulated by SHP2 in oral cancer, via its interaction with ERK1/ERK2 [89].

PTP1B—Hiraga and colleagues reported that PTP1B is one of the mediators of pancreatic cancer cell EMT induced by TGF-β [90].

PRL-1—This phosphatase causes activation of AKT, and inhibition of GSK3β, consequently, contributes for elevated levels of Snail expression and decreased E-cadherin expression. In agreement, the high level of this enzyme was associated with more aggressive phenotype and poorer prognosis in hepatocellular carcinoma patients [46].

PRL-3—**PRL-3** activates the PI3K/PKB pathway and promotes EMT by decreasing PTEN protein expression [23]. In addition, it was demonstrated that expression of PRL-3 in hepatocellular carcinoma patients was positively correlated with the expression of MMPs 1, 9, 10, and 12 [46].

PTRB—Overexpression of PTRB has an opposite effect on EMT markers: decreased the expression of E-cadherin and increased the amount of vimentin [91].

5. PTPs that act as tumor suppressors

Tumor suppressors operate in different ways and compartments to limit cell growth and proliferation. Besides the important contribution of PTPs in cancer progression, some PTPs that act as tumor suppressors are described below:

PTEN—Is a central tumor suppressor, mainly due to its negative effect on key pathways related to cell proliferation, survival, and metastasis: PI3K-Akt–mTOR, NF-κB, and HIF [92, 93]. Therefore, the loss of PTEN, which occurs in the major of the tumors, is correlated with tumor aggressiveness and low response to therapy. In prostate cancer studies, PTEN has been shown to ameliorate the malignant phenotype by dephosphorylating the activator residue of PTK6 (Tyr 342), a kinase related to a cancer aggressive phenotype [94]. In addition, other oncogenic kinases, such as PDGFR and FAK, have been reported as a substrate of PTEN [95, 96]. Although the molecular mechanisms by which PTEN acts as a tumor suppressor are well known, until few years ago, there were not a lot of information about the posttranslational regulation of PTEN. Recently, Park and collaborators [97] have reported two mechanisms of PTEN regulation that directly are connected to its tumor suppressor property: (a) deubiquitination by ubiquitin-specific protease 11 (USP11), responsible for increasing the stability of nuclear and cytosolic PTEN; (b) the level and activity of PTEN are also autoregulated by this phosphatase via PI3K-forkhead transcription factor (FOXO)-USP11 cascade [97].

SHP1 (PTPN6)—Has been described as a major negative regulator of MAPK, JAK/STAT, and NF-κB signaling pathways [98, 99]. Therefore, SHP1 activity is inversely related to cancer development. Indeed, the SHP1 expression in stomach cancer is very weak. Accordingly, the overexpression of SHP1 in stomach cancer cell lines induces a decrease of proliferation, migration, and invasion [100]. In addition, Chen and colleagues showed that SHP1 dephosphorylates and inhibits PKM2, a kinase that stimulates proliferation in hepatocellular carcinoma [46].

SHIP1—Is expressed only in hematopoietic-derived cells and acts as a negative modulator of PI3K pathway [101]. It was described that the PTEN and SHIP1 loss is deeply related to lymphoma survival [102].

PTPN9 (PTP-MEG2)—Low expression of this phosphatase predicted poor survival in patients with hepatocellular carcinoma. It was observed that PTPN9 indirectly inhibits activity of STAT3 and STAT5 through direct dephosphorylation of EGFR and HER2, in breast cancer [46]. In addition, the overexpression of PTPN9 decreases the phosphorylation of AKT protein at its activatory residue, which culminated in diminishing the EMT process efficiency [103].

PTPN12 (PTP-PEST)—Regulates oncogenic tyrosine kinases such as HER2 and EGFR and has a role in modulating EMT. Not surprisingly, it has been decreased or lost in human hepatocellular carcinoma tissues, and by using this carcinoma cell lines as models, it was demonstrated that PTPN12 downregulation stimulated cell migration [46].

FAP-1 (PTPN13)—Downregulates Src-ERK pathway by inhibiting EphrinB1 [104]. FAP-1 can also interact and dephosphorylate Her2, thus reducing the aggressive potential of tumors that have high expression of this receptor [105]. It was also demonstrated that overexpression of this phosphatase caused an upregulation of the epithelial marker, E-cadherin, and downregulated mesenchymal markers such as Snail, Slug, and MMP-9, which are a strong indication that FAP-1 inhibits EMT in hepatocellular carcinoma progression [46].

DUSP2—It has been shown that DUSP2 is involved in P53-induced cell apoptosis; however, this phosphatase is dramatically reduced in different solid tumors compared to their normal counterparts. Accordingly, it was reported that the diminished DUSP2 leads to prolonged ERK phosphorylation, increased drug resistance, as well as an inflammatory response due to overproduction of prostaglandin in colorectal cancer [106]. It was also reported that DUSP2 knockdown in xenograft tumors promotes higher vessel density and metastasis events from colorectal cancer to the liver [107].

PTPRT (PTPρ)—Is commonly mutated in several types of cancer, including colorectal cancer [40]. Many studies have reported the tumor suppressor potential of this PTP, and among the possible substrates of this phosphatase are paxilin and STAT3 [108, 109].

PTPRH—This phosphatase interacts with Grb2 and then modulates Ras pathway activity. Studies have reported that PTPRH blocks cell growth and migration by dephosphorylating proteins associated with focal adhesion, such as p130 [110].

PTPRD—It has been shown that patients with the high level of PTPRD display better long-term survival rate and low chance of liver cancer recurrence. However, the mechanisms underlying this action are not elucidated.

PTP receptor type F (PTPRF)—Is involved in Src kinase inactivation; therefore, it is not surprising that this enzyme is frequently downmodulated in hepatocellular carcinoma patients and upregulation of PTPRF is associated with better prognosis [46].

PTP receptor type O (PTPRO)—Plays as a chronic lymphocytic leukemia, lung, and breast tumor suppressor by inhibiting proliferation and stimulating apoptosis, at least in part, due to STAT3 dephosphorylation [46].

PTP receptor S (PTPσ)—Is an important negative modulator of EGFR. Therefore, the downregulation of this phosphatase has been connected to decreased overall survival and high risk of postoperative recurrence in HCC patients [46].

6. Conclusions

Over the past two decades of research on PTPs, the field has achieved a great progress in understanding the immense role of these phosphatases in cancer progression. Here, we presented an organized picture that clearly shows the participation/contribution of PTPs as key mediators of cancer plasticity, due to their loss of function or overexpression. In summary the above compendium highlights the importance of PTPs not only in cancer progression but also as potential targets for therapeutic interventions. Indeed, during the transition from good to poor outcome of different cancer subtypes, PTPs are extremely plastic, with the capacity to readjust themselves across a wide spectrum of stimuli. This plasticity of PTPs together with the loss of function of PTP suppressors provides tumor cells with all conditions for growth, proliferation, and survival. Illustrative examples are PTEN (loss), LMWPTP, PRL-3, and PTP1B serving as "signaling hubs" that connect different hallmarks (such as sustaining proliferative signaling, evading growth suppressors, resisting cell death, deregulating cellular energetics, and activating invasion and metastasis). This connection might explain, at least in part, the great capacity of tumor cells' plasticity.

Acknowledgements

Our research on this field has been supported by Fundação de Amparo à Pesquisa do Estado de São Paulo (FAPESP) (grant 2015/20412-7) and Conselho Nacional de Desenvolvimento Científico e Tecnológico (CNPq) (grant 303900/2017-2).

Conflict of interest

The authors declare no conflict of interest.

Appendices and nomenclature

130 CRK	p130 Crk-associated substrate (member of an adapter protein family that binds to several tyrosine-phosphorylated proteins)
AKT	also known as *protein kinase B (PKB)*, is a serine/threonine-specific protein kinase
Bcr-Abl	tyrosine-protein kinase
Cdc25	dual-specificity phosphatase
CDK2	*cyclin-dependent kinases*
DUSP1 (PTPN10)	dual-specificity protein *phosphatase* 1
DUSP	dual-specificity protein *phosphatase*
ECM	extracellular matrix
EGFR	epidermal growth factor receptor
EMT	epithelial-mesenchymal transition
Eph	ephrin
ERbeta	estrogen receptor beta
ERK	extracellular signal-regulated kinase
Eya	eyes absent
FAK	focal adhesion kinase
FGF	fibroblast growth *factor*
FOXO-1	forkhead box protein O1
GAPDH	glyceraldehyde 3-phosphate dehydrogenase
GAPs	GTPase-activating proteins or GTPase-accelerating proteins
GLS	glutamine synthetase
GLUT	glucose transporter 1
GSK-3beta	glycogen synthase kinase 3 beta
H2AX	H2A histone family member X
HIF	*hypoxia-inducible factor*
HK	hexokinase
JAK	Janus kinase 2
LDHA	lactate dehydrogenase A
LMWPTP	low-molecular-weight protein tyrosine phosphatase, also known as ACP1
MAPK	mitogen-activated protein kinase

MEF	mouse embryonic fibroblast
MMP-1	matrix metalloproteinase-1
mTOR	mammalian target of rapamycin
NFKB	nuclear factor kappa-light-chain-enhancer of activated B cells
PI3K	phosphatidyl inositol-3-kinase
PKM2	pyruvate kinase isozymes M2
PRL-3	phosphatase of regenerating the liver-3, also recognized as PTP4A3
PTEN	phosphatase and tensin homologue
PTKs	protein tyrosine kinases
PTP σ	protein tyrosine phosphatase sigma
PTP μ	protein tyrosine phosphatase
PTP-PEST (PTPN12)	PTP-PEST (PTP—proline, glutamic acid, serine, and threonine rich)
PTP1B	tyrosine-protein phosphatase non-receptor type 1
PTPN3	protein tyrosine phosphatase non-receptor type 3
PTPN11	protein tyrosine phosphatase non-receptor type 11
PTPN13	PTP also referred to as FAP1
PTPN9	tyrosine-protein phosphatase non-receptor type 9
PTPRδ	protein tyrosine phosphatase receptor delta
PTPRF	protein tyrosine phosphatase receptor type F
PTPRH	receptor-type protein tyrosine phosphatase H, also referred to as stomach cancer-associated protein tyrosine phosphatase-1 (SAP-1)
PTPRO	protein tyrosine phosphatase receptor type O
PTPρ	protein tyrosine phosphatase receptor T
PTPs	protein tyrosine phosphatases
Raf	serine/threonine-specific *protein* kinase
Ras	class of protein called small GTPase
Rho	Ras homologue of small *GTPase*
RhoA	Ras homologue of small *GTPase* member A
SHIP1	Src homology 2 (SH2) domain-containing inositol polyphosphate 5-phosphatase 1
SHIP2	Src homology 2 (SH2) domain-containing inositol polyphosphate 5-phosphatase 2
SHP1	Src homology 2 (SH2) domain-containing phosphotyrosine phosphatase, also known as PTPN6
SHP2	Src homology 2 (SH2) domain-containing phosphotyrosine phosphatase 2, also known as PTPN11
Slug	*SNAI2,* a zinc finger transcription factor
Src	proto-oncogene tyrosine-protein *kinase*
STAT3	signal transducer and activator of transcription type 3
TCA	tricarboxylic acid cycle
TGFbeta	transforming growth factor beta
Twist	*Twist*-related *protein*
WDR1	WD-repeat-containing protein 1
ZEB 1/2	zinc finger E-box-binding homeobox ½

Author details

Carmen V. Ferreira-Halder*, Stefano Piatto Clerici, Alessandra V. Sousa Faria, Patrícia Fernandes de Souza Oliveira, Helon Guimarães Cordeiro and Erica Akagi
Laboratory of Oncobiomarkers, Department of Biochemistry and Tissue Biology, Biology Institute, University of Campinas, São Paulo, Brazil

*Address all correspondence to: carmenv@unicamp.br

References

[1] Hunter T. The genesis of tyrosine phosphorylation. Cold Spring Harbor Perspectives in Biology. 2014;**6**(5): a020644. DOI: 10.1101/cshperspect.a020644

[2] Alonso A, Sasin J, Bottini N, Friedberg I, Friedberg I, Osterman A, et al. Protein tyrosine phosphatases in the human genome. Cell. 2004;**117**: 699-711. DOI: 10.1016/j.cell.2004.05.018

[3] Hanahan D, Weinberg RA. Hallmarks of cancer: The next generation. Cell. 2011;**144**(5):646-674. DOI: 10.1016/j.cell.2011.02.013

[4] Warburg O. On the origin of cancer cells. Science. 1956;**123**(3191):309-314

[5] Le A. The Heterogeneity of Cancer Metabolism. 1st ed. Vol. 1063. Cham: Springer; 2018. 183 pp. DOI: 10.1007/978-3-319-77736-8

[6] White MA, Lin C, Rajapakshe K, Dong J, Shi Y, Tsouko E, et al. Glutamine transporters are targets of multiple oncogenic signaling pathways in prostate cancer. Molecular Cancer Research. 2017;**15**(8):1017-1028. DOI: 10.1158/1541-7786.MCR-16-0480

[7] Liang J, Cao R, Zhang Y, Xia Y, Zheng Y, Li X, et al. PKM2 dephosphorylation by Cdc25A promotes the Warburg effect and tumorigenesis. Nature Communications. 2016;7:12431. DOI: 10.1038/ncomms12431

[8] Faria AVS, Tornatore TF, Milani R, Queiroz KCS, Sampaio IH, Fonseca EMB, et al. Oncophosphosignaling favors a glycolytic phenotype in human drug resistant leukemia. Journal of Cellular Biochemistry. 2017;**118**(11): 3846-3854. DOI: 10.1002/jcb.26034

[9] Lori G, Gamberi T, Paoli P, Caselli A, Pranzini E, Marzocchini R, et al. LMW-PTP modulates glucose metabolism in cancer cells. Biochimica et Biophysica Acta: General Subjects. 2018;**1862**(12):2533-2544. DOI: 10.1016/j.bbagen.2018.08.003

[10] Xu H, Zeng Y, Liu L, Gao Q, Jin S, Lan Q, et al. PRL-3 improves colorectal cancer cell proliferation and invasion through IL-8 mediated glycolysis metabolism. International Journal of Oncology. 2017;**51**(4):1271-1279. DOI: 10.3892/ijo.2017.4090

[11] Wang L, Xiong H, Wu F, Zhang Y, Wang J, Zhao L, et al. Hexokinase 2 mediated Warburg effect is required for PTEN- and p53-deficiency-driven prostate cancer growth. Cell Reports. 2014;**8**(5):1461-1474. DOI: 10.1016/j.celrep.2014.07.053

[12] Zhou X, Yang X, Sun X, Xu X, Li X, Guo Y, et al. Effect of PTEN loss on metabolic reprogramming in prostate cancer cells. Oncology Letters. 2019; **17**(3):2856-2866. DOI: 10.3892/ol.2019.9932

[13] Garcia-Cao I, Song MS, Hobbs RM, Laurent G, Giorgi C, de Boer VC, et al. Systemic elevation of PTEN induces a tumor-suppressive metabolic state. Cell. 2012;**149**(1):49-62. DOI: 10.1016/j.cell.2012.02.030

[14] Li AG, Murphy EC, Culhane AC, Powell E, Wang H, Bronson RT, et al. BRCA1-IRIS promotes human tumor progression through PTEN blockade and HIF-1α activation. Proceedings of the National Academy of Sciences of the United States of America. 2018;**115**(41): E9600-E9609. DOI: 10.1073/pnas.1807112115

[15] Bagati A, Moparthy S, Fink EE, Bianchi-Smiraglia A, Yun DH, Kolesnikova M, et al. KLF9-dependent ROS regulate melanoma progression in

stage-specific manner. Oncogene. 2019; **38**(19):3585-3597. DOI: 10.1038/ s41388-019-0689-6

[16] Pavlova NN, Thompson CB. The emerging hallmarks of cancer metabolism. Cell Metabolism. 2016; **23**(1):27-47. DOI: 10.1016/j. cmet.2015.12.006

[17] DeBerardinis RJ, Chandel NS. Fundamentals of cancer metabolism. Science Advances. 2016;**2**(5):e1600200. DOI: 10.1126/sciadv.1600200

[18] Martinez-Outschoorn EU, Peiris-Pages M, Pestell RG, Sotgia F, Lisanti MP. Cancer metabolism: A therapeutic perspective. Nature Review Clinical Oncology. 2017;**14**(1):11-31. DOI: 10.1038/nrclinonc.2016.60. Erratum in: Nat Rev Clin Oncol. 2017;14(2):113, 10.1038/nrclinonc.2017.1

[19] Verma A, Warner SL, Vankayalapati H, Bearss DJ, Sharma S. Targeting Axl and Mer kinases in cancer. Molecular Cancer Therapeutics. 2011;**10**(10):1763-1773. DOI: 10.1158/ 1535-7163.MCT-11-0116

[20] Linger RM, Cohen RA, Cummings CT, Sather S, Migdall-Wilson J, Middleton DH, et al. Mer or Axl receptor tyrosine kinase inhibition promotes apoptosis, blocks growth and enhances chemosensitivity of human non-small cell lung cancer. Oncogene. 2013;**32**(29):3420-3431. DOI: 10.1038/ onc.2012.355

[21] He RJ, Yu ZH, Zhang ZY. Protein tyrosine phosphatases as potential therapeutic targets. Acta Pharmacologica Sinica. 2014;**35**(10): 1227-1246. DOI: 10.1038/aps.2014.80

[22] Lyon MA, Ducruet AP, Wipf P, Lazo JS. Dual-specificity phosphatases as targets for antineoplastic agents. Nature Reviews. Drug Discovery. 2002; **1**(12):961-976. DOI: 10.1038/nrd963

[23] Jiang Y, Liu XQ, Rajput A, Geng L, Ongchin M, Zeng Q, et al. Phosphatase PRL-3 is a direct regulatory target of TGFbeta in colon cancer metastasis. Cancer Research. 2011;**71**(1):234-244. DOI: 10.1158/0008-5472.CAN-10-1487

[24] Zhang YX, Knyazev PG, Cheburkin YV, Sharma K, Knyazev YP, Orfi L, et al. AXL is a potential target for therapeutic intervention in breast cancer progression. Cancer Research. 2008;**68**(6):1905-1915. DOI: 10.1158/ 0008-5472.CAN-07-2661

[25] Al-Matouq J, Holmes T, Hammiller B, Tran N, Holmes M, Freeman SC, et al. Accumulation of cytoplasmic CDC25A in cutaneous squamous cell carcinoma leads to a dependency on CDC25A for cancer cell survival and tumor growth. Cancer Letters. 2017;**410**:41-49. DOI: 10.1016/j.canlet.2017.09.023

[26] Feng X, Wu Z, Wu Y, Hankey W, Prior TW, Li L, et al. Cdc25A regulates matrix metalloprotease 1 through Foxo1 and mediates metastasis of breast cancer cells. Molecular and Cellular Biology. 2011;**31**(16):3457-3471. DOI: 10.1128/ MCB.05523-11

[27] Wang Y, Pandey RN, Riffle S, Chintala H, Wikenheiser-Brokamp KA, Hegde RS. The protein tyrosine phosphatase activity of eyes absent contributes to tumor angiogenesis and tumor growth. Molecular Cancer Therapeutics. 2018;**17**(8):1659-1669. DOI: 10.1158/1535-7163.MCT-18-0057

[28] Mentel M, Ionescu AE, Puscalau-Girtu I, Helm MS, Badea RA, Rizzoli SO, et al. WDR1 is a novel EYA3 substrate and its dephosphorylation induces modifications of the cellular actin cytoskeleton. Scientific Reports. 2018; **8**(1):2910. DOI: 10.1038/s41598-018- 21155-w

[29] Yuan B, Cheng L, Chiang HC, et al. A phosphotyrosine switch determines the antitumor activity of ERbeta. The

Journal of Clinical Investigation. 2014; **124**(8):3378-3390. DOI: 10.1172/ JCI74085

[30] Ramponi G, Stefani M. Structure and function of the low Mr phosphotyrosine protein phosphatases. Biochimica et Biophysica Acta. 1997; **1341**(2):137-156. DOI: 10.1016/ S0167-4838(97)00087-3

[31] Stein E, Lane AA, Cerretti DP, Schoecklmann HO, Schroff AD, Van Etten RL, et al. Eph receptors discriminate specific ligand oligomers to determine alternative signaling complexes, attachment, and assembly responses. Genes & Development. 1998; **12**(5):667-678. DOI: 10.1101/ gad.12.5.667

[32] Park EK, Warner N, Mood K, Pawson T, Daar IO. Low-molecular-weight protein tyrosine phosphatase is a positive component of the fibroblast growth factor receptor signaling pathway. Molecular and Cellular Biology. 2002;**22**(10):3404-3414. DOI: 10.1128/mcb.22.10.3404-3414.2002

[33] Chiarugi P, Taddei ML, Schiavone N, Papucci L, Giannoni E, Fiaschi T, et al. LMW-PTP is a positive regulator of tumor onset and growth. Oncogene. 2004;**23**(22):3905-3914. DOI: 10.1038/ sj.onc.1207508

[34] Ruela-de-Sousa RR, Hoekstra E, Hoogland AM, Souza Queiroz KC, Peppelenbosch MP, Stubbs AP, et al. Low-molecular-weight protein tyrosine phosphatase predicts prostate cancer outcome by increasing the metastatic potential. European Urology. 2016; **69**(4):710-719. DOI: 10.1016/j. eururo.2015.06.040

[35] Kurose H, Ueda K, Kondo R, Ogasawara S, Kusano H, Sanada S, et al. Low-molecular-weight protein tyrosine phosphatase is a possible biomarker for predicting postoperative biochemical recurrence in prostate cancer with negative surgical margins. Anticancer Research. 2019;**39**(2):957-964. DOI: 10.21873/anticanres.13199

[36] Hoekstra E, Kodach LL, Das AM, Ruela-de-Sousa RR, Ferreira CV, Hardwick JC, et al. Low molecular weight protein tyrosine phosphatase (LMWPTP) upregulation mediates malignant potential in colorectal cancer. Oncotarget. 2015;**6**(10):8300-8312. DOI: 10.18632/oncotarget.3224

[37] Lessard L, Labbe DP, Deblois G, et al. PTP1B is an androgen receptor-regulated phosphatase that promotes the progression of prostate cancer. Cancer Research. 2012;**72**:1529-1537. DOI: 10.1158/0008-5472.CAN-11-2602

[38] Wang J, Liu B, Chen X, Su L, Wu P, Wu J, et al. PTP1B expression contributes to gastric cancer progression. Medical Oncology. 2012; **29**(2):948-956. DOI: 10.1007/ s12032-011-9911-2

[39] Hoekstra E, Das AM, Swets M, Cao W, van der Woude CJ, Bruno MJ, et al. Increased PTP1B expression and phosphatase activity in colorectal cancer results in a more invasive phenotype and worse patient outcome. Oncotarget. 2016;**7**(16):21922-21938. DOI: 10.18632/ oncotarget.7829

[40] Wang Z, Shen D, Parsons DW, et al. Mutational analysis of the tyrosine phosphatome in colorectal cancers. Science. 2004;**304**(5674):1164-1166. DOI: 10.1126/science.1096096

[41] Liu X, Chen Q, Hu XG, Zhang XC, Fu TW, Liu Q, et al. PTP1B promotes aggressiveness of breast cancer cells by regulating PTEN but not EMT. Tumour Biology. 2016;**37**(10):13479-13487. DOI: 10.1007/s13277-016-5245-1

[42] Hoekstra E, Das AM, Willemsen M, Swets M, Kuppen PJ, van der Woude CJ, et al. Lipid phosphatase SHIP2 functions as oncogene in colorectal cancer by

regulating PKB activation. Oncotarget. 2016;**7**(45):73525-73540. DOI: 10.18632/oncotarget.12321

[43] Inagaki K, Noguchi T, Matozaki T, Horikawa T, Fukunaga K, Tsuda M, et al. Roles for the protein tyrosine phosphatase SHP-2 in cytoskeletal organization, cell adhesion and cell migration revealed by overexpression of a dominant negative mutant. Oncogene. 2000;**19**(1):75-84. DOI: 10.1038/sj.onc.1203204

[44] Chen YN, LaMarche MJ, Chan HM, Fekkes P, Garcia-Fortanet J, Acker MG, et al. Allosteric inhibition of SHP2 phosphatase inhibits cancers driven by receptor tyrosine kinases. Nature. 2016;**535**(7610):148-152. DOI: 10.1038/nature18621

[45] Han T, Xiang DM, Sun W, Liu N, Sun HL, Wen W, et al. PTPN11/Shp2 overexpression enhances liver cancer progression and predicts poor prognosis of patients. Journal of Hepatology. 2015;**63**(3):651-660. DOI: 10.1016/j.jhep.2015.03.036

[46] Huang Y, Zhang Y, Ge L, Lin Y, Kwok HF. The roles of protein tyrosine phosphatases in hepatocellular carcinoma. Cancers (Basel). 2018;**10**(3). DOI: 10.3390/cancers10030082

[47] Ferreira PA, Ruela-de-Sousa RR, Queiroz KC, Souza AC, Milani R, Pilli RA, et al. Knocking down low molecular weight protein tyrosine phosphatase (LMW-PTP) reverts chemoresistance through inactivation of Src and Bcr-Abl proteins. PLoS One. 2012;**7**(9):e44312. DOI: 10.1371/journal.pone.0044312

[48] Li S, Cao J, Zhang W, Zhang F, Ni G, Luo Q, et al. Protein tyrosine phosphatase PTPN3 promotes drug resistance and stem cell-like characteristics in ovarian cancer. Scientific Reports. 2016;**6**:36873. DOI: 10.1038/srep36873

[49] Prahallad A, Heynen GJ, Germano G, Willems SM, Evers B, Vecchione L, et al. PTPN11 is a central node in intrinsic and acquired resistance to targeted cancer drugs. Cell Reports. 2015;**12**(12):1978-1985. DOI: 10.1016/j.celrep.2015.08.037

[50] Bonnans C, Chou J, Werb Z. Remodelling the extracellular matrix in development and disease. Nature Reviews. Molecular Cell Biology. 2014;**15**:786-801. DOI: 10.1038/nrm3904

[51] Yue B. Biology of the extracellular matrix: An overview. Journal of Glaucoma. 2014;**23**(8 Suppl. 1):S20-S23. DOI: 10.1097/IJG.0000000000000108

[52] Poltavets V, Kochetkova M, Pitson SM, Samuel MS. The role of the extracellular matrix and its molecular and cellular regulators in cancer cell plasticity. Frontiers in Oncology. 2018;**8**:431. DOI: 10.3389/fonc.2018.00431

[53] Hynes RO, Naba A. Overview of the matrisome—An inventory of extracellular matrix constituents and functions. Cold Spring Harbor Perspectives in Biology. 2012;**4**(1):a004903. DOI: 10.1101/cshperspect.a004903

[54] Pei D, Shu X, Gassama-Diagne A, Thiery JP. Mesenchymal–epithelial transition in development and reprogramming. Nature Cell Biology. 2019;**21**(1):44-53. DOI: 10.1038/s41556-018-0195-z

[55] Singh A, Settleman J. EMT, cancer stem cells and drug resistance: An emerging axis of evil in the war on cancer. Oncogene. 2010;**29**(34):4741-4751. DOI: 10.1038/onc.2010.215

[56] Yang Y, Mani AS, Donaher JL, Ramaswamy S, Itzykson RA, Come C, et al. Twist, a master regulator of morphogenesis, plays an essential role in tumor metastasis. Cell;**117**(7):927-939. DOI: 10.1016/j.cell.2004.06.006

[57] Quail D, Joyce J. Microenvironmental regulation of tumor progression and metastasis. Nature Medicine. 2013;**19**(11): 1423-1437. DOI: 10.1038/nm.3394

[58] Elisha Y, Kalchenko V, Kuznetsov Y, Geiger B. Dual role of E-cadherin in the regulation of invasive collective migration of mammary carcinoma cells. Scientific Reports. 2018;**8**(1):4986. DOI: 10.1038/s41598-018-22940-3

[59] Lilien J, Balsamo J. The regulation of cadherin-mediated adhesion by tyrosine phosphorylation/dephosphorylation of β-catenin. Current Opinion in Cell Biology. 2005;**17**(5):459-465. DOI: 10.1016/j.ceb.2005.08.009

[60] Nelson WJ. Regulation of cell-cell adhesion by the cadherin-catenin complex. Biochemical Society Transactions. 2008;**36**:149-155. DOI: 10.1042/BST0360149

[61] Sallee JL, Wittchen ES, Burridge K. Regulation of cell adhesion by protein-tyrosine phosphatases. II. Cell-cell adhesion. Journal of Biological Chemistry. 2006;**281**(24):16189-16192. DOI: 10.1074/jbc.R600003200

[62] Hale JS, Li M, Lathia JD. The malignant social network: Cell-cell adhesion and communication in cancer stem cells. Cell Adhesion & Migration. 2012;**6**(4): 346-355. DOI: 10.4161/cam.21294

[63] Burridge K, Sastry SK, Sallee JL. Regulation of cell adhesion by protein-tyrosine phosphatases: I. Cell-matrix adhesion. Journal of Biological Chemistry. 2006;**281**(23):15593-15596. DOI: 10.1074/jbc.R500030200

[64] Ostman A, Hellberg C, Böhmer FD. Protein-tyrosine phosphatases and cancer. Nature Reviews. Cancer. 2006; **6**(4):307-320. DOI: 10.1038/nrc1837

[65] Lawson CD, Ridley AJ. Rho GTPase signaling complexes in cell migration and invasion. The Journal of Cell Biology. 2018;**217**(2):447-457. DOI: 10.1083/jcb.201612069

[66] Sastry SK, Rajfur Z, Liu BP, Cote JF, Tremblay ML, Burridge K. PTP-PEST couples membrane protrusion and tail retraction via VAV2 and p190RhoGAP. The Journal of Biological Chemistry. 2006;**281**(17):11627-11636. DOI: 10.1074/jbc.M600897200

[67] Kodama A, Matozaki T, Fukuhara A, Kikyo M, Ichihashi M, Takai Y. Involvement of an SHP-2-rho small G protein pathway in hepatocyte growth factor/scatter factor-induced cell scattering. Molecular Biology of the Cell. 2000;**11**(8):2565-2575. DOI: 10.1091/mbc.11.8.2565

[68] Chiarugi P, Cirri P, Taddei L, Giannoni E, Camici G, Manao G, et al. The low M(r) protein-tyrosine phosphatase is involved in rho-mediated cytoskeleton rearrangement after integrin and platelet-derived growth factor stimulation. The Journal of Biological Chemistry. 2000;**275**(7): 4640-4646. DOI: 10.1074/jbc.275.7.4640

[69] Shay G, Lynch CC, Fingleton B. Moving targets: Emerging roles for MMPs in cancer progression and metastasis. Matrix Biology. 2015;**44–46**: 200-206. DOI: 10.1016/j.matbio.2015.01.019

[70] Radisky ES, Radisky DC. Matrix metalloproteinase-induced epithelial–mesenchymal transition in breast cancer. Journal of Mammary Gland Biology and Neoplasia. 2010;**15**(2):201-212. DOI: 10.1007/s10911-010-9177-x

[71] Hwang BM, Chae HS, Jeong YJ, Lee YR, Noh EM, Youn HZ, et al. Protein tyrosine phosphatase controls breast cancer invasion through the expression of matrix metalloproteinase-9. BMB Reports. 2013;**46**(11):533-538. DOI: 10.5483/BMBRep.2013.46.11.053

[72] Sun PH, Ye L, Mason MD, Jiang WG. Protein tyrosine phosphatase µ (PTP µ or PTPRM), a negative regulator of proliferation and invasion of breast cancer cells, is associated with disease prognosis. PLoS One. 2012;**7**(11). DOI: 10.1371/journal.pone.0050183

[73] Lee SK, Han YM, Yun J, Lee CW, Shin DS, Ha YR, et al. Phosphatase of regenerating liver-3 promotes migration and invasion by upregulating matrix metalloproteinases-7 in human colorectal cancer cells. International Journal of Cancer. 2012;**131**(3). DOI: 10.1002/ijc.27381

[74] Maacha S, Anezo O, Foy M, Liot G, Mery L, Laurent C, et al. Protein tyrosine phosphatase 4A3 (PTP4A3) promotes human uveal melanoma aggressiveness through membrane accumulation of matrix metalloproteinase 14 (MMP14). Investigative Ophthalmology and Visual Science. 2016;**57**(4):1982-1990. DOI: 10.1167/iovs.15-18780

[75] Yuan T, Wang Y, Zhao ZJ, Gu H. Protein-tyrosine phosphatase PTPN9 negatively regulates ErbB2 and epidermal growth factor receptor signaling in breast cancer cells. The Journal of Biological Chemistry. 2010;**285**(20):14861-14870. DOI: 10.1074/jbc.M109.099879

[76] Du WW, Fang L, Li M, Yang X, Liang Y, Peng C, et al. MicroRNA miR-24 enhances tumor invasion and metastasis by targeting PTPN9 and PTPRF to promote EGF signaling. Journal of Cell Science. 2013;**126**(6): 1440-1453. DOI: 10.1242/jcs.118299

[77] Wang N, She J, Liu W, Shi J, Yang Q, Shi B, et al. Frequent amplification of PTP1B is associated with poor survival of gastric cancer patients. Cell Cycle. 2015;**14**:732-743. DOI: 10.1080/15384101.2014.998047

[78] Hilmarsdottir B, Briem E, Halldorsson S, Kricker J, Ingthorsson S, Gustafsdottir S, et al. Inhibition of PTP1B disrupts cell-cell adhesion and induces anoikis in breast epithelial cells. Cell Death & Disease. 2017;**8**:e2769. DOI: 10.1038/cddis.2017.177

[79] Moncho-Amor V, Ibañez de Cáceres I, Bandres E, Martínez-Poveda B, Orgaz JL, Sánchez-Pérez I, et al. DUSP1/MKP1 promotes angiogenesis, invasion and metastasis in non-small-cell lung cancer. Oncogene. 2011;**30**(6):668-678. DOI: 10.1038/onc.2010.449

[80] Perumal E, So Youn K, Sun S, et al. PTEN inactivation induces epithelial-mesenchymal transition and metastasis by intranuclear translocation of β-catenin and snail/slug in non-small cell lung carcinoma cells. Lung Cancer. 2019;**130**:25-34. DOI: 10.1016/j.lungcan.2019.01.013

[81] Li JY, Huang WX, Zhou X, et al. Numb inhibits epithelial-mesenchymal transition via RBP-Jκ-dependent Notch1/PTEN/FAK signaling pathway in tongue cancer. BMC Cancer. 2019;**25**: 391. DOI: 10.1186/s12885-019-5605-5

[82] Bowen KA, Doan HQ, Zhou BP, et al. PTEN loss induces epithelial-mesenchymal transition in human colon cancer cells. Anticancer Research. 2009; **29**(11):4439-4449

[83] Wang Y, Liang Y, Yang G, et al. Tetraspanin 1 promotes epithelial-to-mesenchymal transition and metastasis of cholangiocarcinoma via PI3K/AKT signaling. The Journal of Experimental & Clinical Cancer Research. 2018;**37**(1): 300. DOI: 10.1186/s13046-018-0969-y

[84] Wu ZH, Lin C, Liu CC, et al. MiR-616-3p promotes angiogenesis and EMT in gastric cancer via the PTEN/AKT/mTOR pathway. Biochemical and Biophysical Research Communications. 2018;**501**:1068-1073. DOI: 10.1016/j.bbrc.2018.05.109

[85] Li H, Zhang P, Sun X, et al. MicroRNA-181a regulates epithelial-mesenchymal transition by targeting

PTEN in drug-resistant lung adenocarcinoma cells. International Journal of Oncology. 2015;**47**:1379-1392. DOI: 10.3892/ijo.2015.3144

[86] Rahdar M, Inoue T, Meyer T, et al. A phosphorylation-dependent intramolecular interaction regulates the membrane association and activity of the tumor suppressor PTEN. Proceedings of the National Academy of Sciences of the United States of America. 2009;**106**(2):480-485. DOI: 10.1073/pnas.0811212106

[87] Aoyama D, Hashimoto N, Sakamoto K, et al. Involvement of TGFβ-induced phosphorylation of the PTEN C-terminus on TGFβ-induced acquisition of malignant phenotypes in lung cancer cells. PLoS One. 2013;**8**(11):e81133. DOI: 10.1371/journal.pone.0081133

[88] Sun X, Zhang J, Wang Z, et al. Shp2 plays a critical role in IL-6-induced EMT in breast cancer cells. International Journal of Molecular Sciences. 2017; **18**(2):395. DOI: 10.3390/ijms18020395

[89] Li S, Wang L, Zhao Q, et al. SHP2 positively regulates TGFβ1-induced epithelial-mesenchymal transition modulated by its novel interacting protein Hook1. The Journal of Biological Chemistry. 2014;**289**(49):34152-34160. DOI: 10.1074/jbc.M113.546077

[90] Hiraga R, Kato M, Miyangawa S, et al. Nox4-derived ROS Signaling contributes to TGF-β-induced epithelial-mesenchymal transition in pancreatic cancer cells. Anticancer Research. 2013;**33**:4431-4438

[91] Weng X, Chen W, Hu W, et al. PTPRB promotes metastasis of colorectal carcinoma via inducing epithelial-mesenchymal transition. Cell Death & Disease. 2019;**10**(5):352. DOI: 10.1038/s41419-019-1554-9

[92] Fruman DA, Rommel C. PI3K and cancer: Lessons, challenges and opportunities. Nature Reviews. Drug Discovery. 2014;**13**(2):140-156. DOI: 10.1038/nrd4204

[93] Maynard MA, Ohh M. The role of hypoxia-inducible factors in cancer. Cellular and Molecular Life Sciences. 2007;**64**(16):2170-2180. DOI: 10.1007/s00018-007-7082-2

[94] Wozniak DJ, Kajdacsy-Balla A, Macias V, et al. PTEN is a protein phosphatase that targets active PTK6 and inhibits PTK6 oncogenic signaling in prostate cancer. Nature Communications. 2017;**8**(1):1508. DOI: 10.1038/s41467-017-01574-5

[95] Mahimainathan L, Choudhury GG. Inactivation of platelet-derived growth factor receptor by the tumor suppressor PTEN provides a novel mechanism of action of the phosphatase. The Journal of Biological Chemistry. 2004;**279**: 15258-15268. DOI: 10.1074/jbc.M314328200

[96] Tamura M, Gu J, Matsumoto K, et al. Inhibition of cell migration, spreading, and focal adhesions by tumor suppressor PTEN. Science. 1998;**280**: 1614-1617. DOI: 10.1126/science.280.5369.1614

[97] Park MK, Yao Y, Xia W, et al. PTEN self-regulates through USP11 via the PI3K-FOXO pathway to stabilize tumor suppression. Nature Communications. 2019;**10**(1):636. DOI: 10.1038/s41467-019-08481-x

[98] López-Ruiz P, Rodriguez-Ubreva J, Cariaga AE, et al. SHP-1 in cell-cycle regulation. Anti-Cancer Agents in Medicinal Chemistry. 2011;**11**(1):89-98. DOI: 10.2174/187152011794941154

[99] Liu J, Wang Y, Sun X, et al. Promoter methylation attenuates SHP1 expression and function in patients with primary central nervous system lymphoma. Oncology Reports. 2017;**37**(2):887-894. DOI: 10.3892/or.2016.5308

[100] Joo MK, Park JJ, Yoo HS, et al. Epigenetic regulation and anti-tumorigenic effects of SH2-containing protein tyrosine phosphatase 1 (SHP1) in human gastric cancer cells. Tumour Biology. 2016;**37**(4):4603-4612. DOI: 10.1007/s13277-015-4228-y

[101] Dempke WCM, Uciechowski P, Fenchel K, Chevassut T. Targeting SHP-1, 2 and SHIP pathways: A novel strategy for cancer treatment? Oncology. 2018;**95**(5):257-269. DOI: 10.1159/000490106

[102] Miletic AV, Anzelon-Mills AN, Mills DM, Omori SA, Pedersen IM, Shin DM, et al. Coordinate suppression of B cell lymphoma by PTEN and SHIP phosphatases. The Journal of Experimental Medicine. 2010;**207**(11): 2407-2420. DOI: 10.1084/jem.20091962

[103] Ying D, Ruan Y, Zhou X. MEG2 inhibits the growth and metastasis of hepatocellular carcinoma by inhibiting AKT pathway. Gene. 2019;**687**:1-8. DOI: 10.1016/j.gene.2018.11.003

[104] Vermeer PD, Bell M, Lee K, et al. ErbB2, EphrinB1, Src kinase and PTPN13 signaling complex regulates MAP kinase signaling in human cancers. PLoS One. 2012;**7**(1):E30447. DOI: 10.1371/journal.pone.0030447

[105] Zhu JH et al. Protein tyrosine phosphatase PTPN13 negatively regulates Her2/ErB2 malignant signaling. Oncogene. 2008;**27**(18): 2525-2531. DOI: 10.1038/sj.onc.1210922

[106] Hou PC, Li YH, Lin SC, Lin SC, Lee JC, Lin BW, et al. Hypoxia-induced downregulation of DUSP-2 phosphatase drives colon cancer stemness. Cancer Research. 2017;**77**(16):4305-4316. DOI: 10.1158/0008-5472.CAN-16-2990

[107] Lin SC, Hsiao KY, Chang N, Hou PC, Tsai SJ. Loss of dual-specificity phosphatase-2 promotes angiogenesis and metastasis via up-regulation of interleukin-8 in colon cancer. The Journal of Pathology. 2017;**241**(5): 638-648. DOI: 10.1002/path.4868

[108] Zhao Y, Zhang X, Guda K, et al. Identification and functional characterization of paxillin as a target of protein tyrosine phophatase receptor T. Proceedings of the National Academy of Sciences of the United States of America. 2010;**107**(6):2592-2597. DOI: 10.1073/pnas.0914884107

[109] Kim M, Morales LD, Jang IS, Cho YY, Kim DJ. Protein tyrosine phosphatases as potential regulators of STAT3 signaling. International Journal of Molecular Sciences. 2018;**19**(9). DOI: 10.3390/ijms19092708

[110] Noguchi T, Tsuda M, Takeda T, Inagaki K, Yamao T, Fukunaga K, et al. Inhibition of cell growth and spreading by stomach cancer-associated protein-tyrosine phosphatase-1(SAP-1) through dephosphorylation of p130cas. The Journal of Biological Chemistry. 2001; **276**(18):15216-15224. DOI: 10.1074/jbc.M007208200

Section 2

Tumorigenesis Risk Factors and Role of Neuroimmune Regulations

Chapter 4

Risk Factors for Ovarian Cancer

Marliyya S. Zayyan

Abstract

Ovarian cancers remain a perplexing group of diseases that continue to raise questions over their etiology and clinical behavior. They are the most fatal of gynecological cancers. Despite a global lifetime risk of only 1–2%, they contribute the highest mortality and the lowest 5-year (overall) survival rate of just 35%. The three broad histological groups: epithelial, sex cord-stromal and germ cell cancers have different biologic behavior and may constitute different clinical disease entities. Of the eight subtypes in the epithelial group, high-grade serous are universally the most common and have the worst prognosis. Globally making 65–85% of all ovarian cancers, most of the focus on risk factors has been directed on the epithelial group but the importance of other primary malignancies cannot be overemphasized as a step towards understanding their etiology and clinical behavior. The normal ovary has none of the epithelia that produce the range of epithelial ovarian cancers or there is an obvious premalignant stage, symptoms are very vague, screening and early diagnosis are difficult and indeed unrewarding. No specific etiology is known for any of the histologic groups. However, commonly mentioned risk factors like increasing age, genetics, nulliparity, prolonged infertility, use of fertility drugs, high animal fat, obesity, endometriosis, polycystic ovary syndrome, previous history of cancer, use of hormone replacement therapy, pelvic inflammatory disease and smoking may not apply to all the subtypes, while factors like increasing parity, breast feeding, use of oral contraceptive pills, hysterectomy, tubal ligation and use of antioxidants may differ in the degree of protection they provide. There may also be geographical and probably racial variations in the relevance of some of the risk factors. Thorough understanding of the predisposing and protective factors of the various histologic subtypes is an important step understanding the disease and therefore improving treatment outcome or providing effective prevention.

Keywords: risk factors, ovarian cancers, histologic subtypes, variation

1. Introduction

Ovarian cancer (OC) is an important public health problem with a lifetime risk of 1–2%. Recent estimates indicate that 295,414 cases are expected in 2018 with about 184,000 of victims dying from the disease [1]. This reflects an increase of over 54,000 cases in incidence and 32,000 cases in mortality compared with earlier figures [2, 3]. Public screening for ovarian cancer has been neither feasible nor beneficial due to a lack of most appropriate screening test for the range of malignancies produced by the ovary. Use of tumor markers is largely unreliable since different tumor markers are secreted by different histological varieties and up to 50% of early disease may be associated with insignificant rise of tumor markers [4, 5]. Besides tumor markers could be raised by non-malignant conditions as well as other malignancies [6–8]. Cancers of the lung, pancreas, colorectal, breast and non-Hodgkin's lymphomas are associated with a rise in CA125 [9, 10] which is also raised in benign conditions such as endometriosis, ovarian cyst, leiomyoma uteri and pelvic inflammatory disease [4, 8, 11]. Only 50% of early OC is associated with raised CA125 making it unreliable for early diagnosis. More than 75% of OC are diagnosed in late stages of disease [12–14] when prognosis is very poor. Screening did not reduce mortality in two large trials [12, 15].

The ovaries are totipotential in their ability to form wide histologic varieties of cancers with different biology, natural history and possibly mechanism of onset [16–18]. These heterogeneous tumors differ in their clinical behavior including response to treatment and prognosis. Knowledge of the cause or genesis of OCs is very scant and the available hypotheses do not explain observed disease phenomena [19, 20]. The uniqueness of OC in having no known premalignant stage, no reliable screening tool, very vague symptoms in early and advanced stages make identification of at risk group important for prevention, early diagnosis and possibly as a step towards defining its etiology.

The World Health Organization classifies ovarian cancers based on histologic origins of the cells, as epithelial, sex cord-stromal and germ cell tumors [16, 21] (**Table 1**). The epithelial ovarian cancers are made up of eight histologic subtypes with different cellular origin, pathogenesis, gene expression and response to treatment [13, 16, 17]. The most common type, serous cyst adenocarcinoma with two distinct subtypes may be arising from the fallopian tube epithelium. The high grade serous accounts for 85% of the epithelial ovarian cancers and up to 80% of

Histological
I. Epithelial tumors A. Serous cyst adenocarcinoma B. Mucinous Cyst adenocarcinoma C. Endometrioid D. Clear cell (mesonephroid) E. Brenner's F. Mixed epithelial G. Undifferentiated H. Unclassified
II. Sex cord-stromal tumors A. Granulosa B. Androblastoma C. Gynandroblastoma D. Unclassified
III. Lipid cell tumors
IV. Germ cell tumors A. Dysgerminoma B. Endodermal sinus tumors C. Polyembroyoma D. Choriocarcinoma E. Teratoma F. Mixed tumors
V. Gonadoblastoma
VI. Soft tissues not specific to the ovary
VII. Unclassified
VIII. Metastatic

Table 1.
WHO histological classification for ovarian cancers.

ovarian cancers generally [22]. It is the most challenging in terms of treatment outcome. Mucinous adenocarcinomas have cells similar to the cervical epithelium, endometrioid cancer cells resemble the endometrium, while Brenners tumors have transitional epithelium akin to that of the bladder [19].

The fimbriated end of the fallopian tube has morphologic and molecular similarities with high grade serous ovarian cancers which also expresses TP53 signature suggesting that neoplastic process may be originating from tubal epithelium and shed into the ovary where aggressive neoplastic process proceeds [14, 19]. Low-grade serous ovarian cancers share similar histiogenesis but progress through a separate pathway and has different prognosis [18, 23, 24]. It represents less than 5% of the epithelial cancer [25].

The sex cord-stromal tumors are a heterogeneous group, which include several histologic subtypes (**Table 1**). Apart from adult granulosa tumor that affects women in their fifth decade, sex cord-stromal tumors mainly affect women in the second or third decade of life and account for about 5% of malignancies in women 15–24 years [26]. Several subtypes are associated with genetic predisposition, including in patients with Peutz-Jeghers syndrome [27].

The germ cell tumors, which include dysgerminomas, immature teratoma, embryonal tumors and endodermal sinus tumors form only 1.5–5% of OC. Approximately one-third are dysgerminomas, another third immature teratomas and a further one-third include the rest three (embryonal tumors, endodermal sinus tumors, choriocarcinoma and mixed cell types) [19, 28]. Malignant germ cell tumors of the ovary may be developing through similar pathways with testicular germ cell tumors but the ovarian have greater histological complexity than most solid somatic tumors.

This diversity in genesis may partly explain the observed differences in clinical behavior.

2. Hypothesis for ovarian carcinogenesis

Development of OC has remained a mystery since hypotheses advanced do not convincingly explain the observed phenomena. It is important to explain how other surface epithelia form aggressive primary neoplasm in a separate organ.

The 'incessant ovulation' theory explains that repetitive ovulatory micro trauma to the ovarian surface in association with the tubal epithelium results in carcinogenesis through mistakes in repair of the damaged surface epithelium [29, 30]. While this hypothesis partly explain serous cystadenocarcinoma, it fails to explain other subtypes in the epithelial group and does not offer plausible explanation for the germ cell tumors and the sex cord-stromal tumors.

The pituitary "gonadotropin hypothesis" indicates that high levels of estrogens and gonadotropins such as luteinizing hormone and follicle-stimulating hormone would over stimulate the ovarian epithelium causing increased proliferation and subsequent malignant transformation [31, 32].

The "inflammation hypothesis" proposes that factors such as endometriosis, pelvic inflammatory disease and other inflammatory conditions may stimulate cancer formation [31, 33].

These theories have failed to provide plausible genesis for ovarian cancer therefore new hypothesis have been proposed [19, 34].

Understanding a clear etiology is far from site, a thorough global analysis of the risk factors of the disease may be a good starting point to unraveling the etiology and therefore an effective strategy towards disease control and prevention. It is however expected that the range of tumors may very well differ in risk factors and epidemiology.

3. Predisposing factors

Predisposing and protective factors for ovarian cancers vary according to histologic type [13, 18]. Although most studies concentrate on epithelial ovarian cancers, particularly serous cystadenocarcinoma, which tends to form the major global disease burden, risk factors to other histologic types are important prerequisite to their genesis and will be considered in this review.

4. Racial and geographical risk

Ovarian cancer is a cosmopolitan disease as it occurs in every geographical location and in every race [1, 30]. Epithelial ovarian cancer is the commonest subtype all around the world with high-grade serous accounting for 60–85% of cases [22, 35–38].

Highest incidence of OC is found among white females in Northern and Western Europe and in North America with age adjusted incidence exceeding 8.4/100,000 [1, 30]. Recent statistics from the US show a decline in incidence from 16.6/100,000 in 1985 to 11.8/100,000 in 2018 [39]. Incidence is also high in New Zealand and among Jewish women in Israel but low in Africa and Asia with estimated rates of <3/100,000 [37]. Japan, though reported to have low incidence is experiencing a rising trend in the disease of recent [40].

All regions of North America show higher incidence of invasive ovarian cancer among white women [41].

Within Europe too, there is difference in incidence and mortality across the region. Using WHO data base of 28 European countries from 1953 to 2000, Bray et al. reported Nordic countries, Austria, Germany and the United Kingdom to have the highest trend in the 1960s but the trend tended to decline over the recent years while Southern European countries showed an upward trend. Similarly, central and eastern European countries with hitherto low incidence are experiencing a rising over time [12, 35] . In the most recent 5-year period (2003–2007), the incidence of ovarian cancer was highest in Eastern/Southern Europe, followed by Northern Europe, and Western Europe [22] Asian sub region reports lower rates than Europe and America [2, 3].

South Eastern Asia have highest rate in the subcontinent and Eastern Asia has the lowest rate.

Migration to areas of high risk increases the risk of disease therefore cultural and dietary factors may be responsible for the observed difference. Japanese immigrants to the US have equivalent risk as natives [42].Racial variations in the incidence of ovarian cancer are best observed in the USA. Age adjusted incidence rate are higher in whites than in non-whites and Indians in the USA have lowest mortality from ovarian cancer. While Caucasian Americans have higher disease incidence, African-Americans have 1.3 times higher disease mortality and lower survival rates even with equal access to care [43]. They also experienced poorer 5-year survival rates irrespective of stage of diagnosis [44, 45].

From the Surveillance Epidemiology and End Result (SEER)database (1992–1998), AA experienced a fall in 5-year survival rates from 47.9 to 40.3%, while their Caucasian counterparts witnessed an improved survival from 40.7 to 45% in the same period. The observed disparities have been linked to interplay of socioeconomic, environmental, genetic and epigenetic factors [43].

Determining the incidence of ovarian cancer in four US populations of heterogeneous racial-ethnic composition, Weiss and Paterson found 19–42% lower incidence among Japanese, Chinese, Hispano and black women compared with white women [44]. The observed difference is primarily due to lower rates of serous and papillary tumors. Chinese women also had decreased incidence of mucinous tumors, while Hispano and black women had lower incidence of endometrioid-clear cell tumors.

The incidence of non-epithelial cancers remains fairly constant between the races; especially germ cell tumors which has remained stable in incidence for three decades [44]. However, data from SEER suggest that the incidence of sex cord-stromal tumors is significantly lower among white women compared with black women (0.18 *vs.* 0.35 per 100,000 person years; relative risk, 0.53; 95% confidence interval (95% CI): 0.42–0.67) [46].

OC rates from Africa though reported to be low must be considered in the background of health circumstances in the region of lack of cancer registries, poor utilization of health facilities and rudimentary statistics.

Ovarian cancer is reported to be more common in developed countries than developing nations but over the last three decades, ovarian cancer incidence has remained stable in high-risk countries, while an increasing trend has been reported in low-risk countries.

5. Age as a risk factor

Increasing age is a risk factor for ovarian cancer which is generally considered a disease of the older women. Globally, the annual incidence regardless of age is 42 cases/100,000 women. Data from US SEER, ovarian cancer is rare before the age of 40 years and incidence rises steadily after the fifth decade to reach a peak at 80–84 years, when the age specific incidence is 61.3/100,000 women. More than half of cases of ovarian cancers are diagnosed in women over 65 year [47].

In the United States, the annual incidence is 61.3 per 100,000 for women aged 75 and 79 years.

In the UK, the overall incidence of a symptomatic ovarian cyst in a premenopausal female being malignant is approximately 1:1000 increasing to 3:1000 at the age of 50 years although 1000 women under the age of 50 years develop ovarian cancer annually in the UK [48–50]. Most diagnose are other histologic subtypes like borderline tumors and germ cell tumors. EOC are generally reported to be uncommon in young premenopausal women in the UK [50]. Women aged 65 years and above make 64% of mortality from OC [47, 50]. Young premenopausal women are more commonly affected by germ cell tumors and borderline tumors in most reports from European literature [35, 51].

Similarly, a meta-database analysis of 5055 ovarian cancer patients of 4 prospective phase III intergroup trials identified 294 (5.8%) patients under the age of 40 years from European studies. Young age appeared a strong independent protective on overall incidence of EOCs as well as prognostic factor for PFS and OS [52].

The issue of age and ovarian cancer diagnosis may however be different among non-Europeans races. Reports from India show much younger age affected than most European papers for EOC. Murtha et al. reported increased risk after 35 years with peak at ages of 55–64 years. Saini et al. have reported mean age of 55 years Basu et al. had 48.8 ± 11.2 years while Mondel had 48 years and Jindal et al. had a mean of 48 years. Malik from Pakistan found mean age for EOC to be 49.5 ± 13 years [53–57].

Mostafa et al. from Egypt reported a mean age of 47 years for epithelial ovarian cancers, with 1% of cases affecting women of 30 years and only 3% occurring in older women of 70 years [58].

From African subcontinent, findings contradict increasing age as a risk factor for EOC as reports show young premenopausal women to be mostly affected with serous cystadenocarcinoma, which is the most common histiotype. There is increasing report of rising incidence of ovarian cancer from Africa [38, 59–61].

Most reports suggest EOC to be the commonest but predominantly seen in young premenopausal, generally parous women [38, 60, 61].

A global report by the International Federation of Gynecology and Obstetrics (FIGO) has noted that the highest incidence of ovarian cancer was moving towards a younger age group, although the majority of patients with epithelial cancer were more than 50 years in age [38].

It is interesting that high grade serous cyst adenocarcinoma remains the commonest variety while literature from USA, Europe, Israel and Australia find it in older women above 65 years, in Asia, the Arab world and Africa, it is observed in young premenopausal women. Research for this important difference is worthwhile.

Early menarche is considered a weak predictor of ovarian cancer risk and women whose menarche was earlier than 12 years are at increased risk of epithelial tumors [62, 63]. Meta-analysis of 22 case–control studies and 5 cohort studies has reported a statistically significant inverse association between menarcheal age and ovarian cancer risk (RR = 0.85; 95% CI: 0.75–0.97) [62], but this association is most significant in invasive serous and borderline tumors. In this respect, 'incessant ovulation' theory as possible cause of tumor genesis provides plausible explanation [30, 34]. No association was found when menarche begins after age 16 years. Late menarche has not been shown to be protective [64].

Women who experience natural late menopause are at increased risk [13, 34, 65]. Odds ratios for late natural menopause were reported as low as 1.19 and as high as 1.25 (95% CI: 0.95–1.49) [65]. These findings may suggest that earlier menarcheal age and late natural menopause might increase risk of ovarian cancer by increasing a woman's lifetime number of ovulations. Results from the Nurses' Health Study (NHS) confirmed increased risk of endometrioid epithelial cancers with late natural menopause but not of serous or mucinous cancers (RR = 1.3, 95% CI: 1.04–1.22). Furthermore, the European Prospective Study into Cancer and Nutrition Cohort (EPIC) age at menopause >52 years was associated with increased risk compared with 45 years or less [66].

6. Infertility and use of ovulation induction drugs

Infertility either by itself or in association with some of its causes like endometriosis, is a risk factor and prolonged period of infertility is associated with higher risk [67].

A large cohort study, involving 54,362 women with infertility in the Danish fertility clinics (1963–1998) used parity specific cancer incidence and reported significantly increased from infertility (1.46, 95% CI: 1.24–1.71) [68].

Whittemore et al. analyzed 12 US case–control studies between 1957 and 1985, with 2197 cases of ovarian cancer and 4144 controls and confirmed higher risk in nulligravid subfertile women compared with controls [20].

However, study by Ness with 5207 cases of ovarian cancer and 7705 controls found only a weak association between infertility and epithelial ovarian cancer (OR 1.16, 95% CI: 1.02–1.31) [69].

Drug treatment of infertility may further increase risk as untreated infertile nulliparous women have 1.5–2-fold risk, while women who received treatment and failed to conceive have even higher risk [70].

Use of ovulation induction agents like clomiphene citrate, gonadotropins are associated with three times higher general population [69] particularly prolonged use of clomiphene (for more than 12 cycles). This is associated with rise in risk for invasive and borderline cases by about 11.1-fold compared with infertile women with no clomiphene use [67].

Use of gonadotropins is also associated with increased risk [31, 70]. There are, however, a number of studies that show no increased risk of OC with use of ovulation induction agents [71].

However, studies that report increased risk do of borderline tumors only not high grade serous.

7. Genetic factors

More than one-fifth of OC cases are hereditary from highly penetrant autosomal dominant genetic susceptibility [72]. Although accounting for only a limited number of cases, heredity is a strong risk factor for OC. The lifetime risk of a woman who has a first degree relative with OC is 5% compared with 1.4% in a woman without. The risk rises to 7% if two members of the family are affected [73]. These rate has been thought to be a probable underestimate as a British study has shown that where two close relatives (not necessarily first degree) are affected, the risk may be as high as 30–40% [73, 74]. The risk for confirmed carriers of BRCA at the age of 70 may be as high as 63% [73, 75]. Ovarian cancer in a first degree relative, has been shown to be a strong positive indicator of early onset epithelial cancer and positively associated with non-mucinous tumors [76].

The three main clinical types of genetic ovarian cancers include site-specific, hereditary breast and/or ovarian cancer (HBOC) and hereditary non-polyposis colorectal cancer (HNPCC) or Lynch II syndrome [77].

The first two syndromes are related to inheritance of BRCA1 and BRCA 2. Patients with HNPCC have inherited mismatch repair genes (MLH1, MLH2, MLH6, PMS1, PMS2 and possibly some other yet unidentified genes).

BRCA genes are common in the Ashkenazi Jewish population where 29–41% of ovarian cancer is believed to be secondary to inheriting one of three founder mutations in *BRCA*1 and *BRCA*2, against 10% in non-Ashkenazim [78].

BRCA 1 gene is an oncosuppressor gene located at chromosome 17q, it participates in chromatin remodeling and crucial steps in cell cycle [79].

OC associated with BRCA mutations are diagnosed at a younger age and are of high-grade serous type. In one study, the average age at diagnosis of OC in BRCA1 and BRCA2 mutation carriers was 52 and 62 years, respectively [77, 80]. BRCA mutations do not seem to play a significant role in the development of mucinous or borderline ovarian tumors. The BRCA associated OCs also tend to have better clinical outcome with longer overall survival and recurrence-free interval than sporadic cancers [77].

There is no standard clinical definition of hereditary breast and ovarian cancer syndrome but affected families may be identified from:

- Several cases of breast cancer diagnosed before the age of 50 years.
- One or more cases with ovarian cancer in the family.
- One or more relatives with both breast and ovarian cancer.
- The presence of a BRCA1 or BRCA 2.
- However, many women without a family history may still have a gene mutation associated with their BRCA1 or BRCA 2.

Lynch syndrome (LS) or hereditary non-polyposis colon cancer (HNPCC) refers to germline mutations in MMR genes (*MLH1*, *MSH2*, *MSH6*, *MLH3* and *PMS2*), which lead to the loss of expression of one of the MMR proteins. Clinically, LS is associated with higher risk of colorectal cancers that have specific predilection to location proximal to splenic flexure [72, 81]. Confirmed case of Lynch syndrome is associated with 6–10% life time risk of OC of early onset. MLH1 carriers are often diagnosed of ovarian cancer at average age of 52 years and MLH2 carriers at age of 45 years [82, 83].

HNPCC syndrome is also associated with cancers of the stomach, small bowel, hepatobiliary tract, pancreas, renal pelvis, ureter, breast, prostate and brain (particularly glioblastoma) [72, 84]. The OCs associated with LS are commonly endometrioid and clear cell varieties [82, 85] and tend to be diagnosed at a relatively early stage with high stage-specific survival rate compared with non LS type [86, 87].

The Li-Fraumeni syndrome is an autosomal dominant syndrome characterized by heterozygous germline mutation in TP53. It is the most frequently mutated gene in human cancer thus the syndrome is associated with development of multiple cancers at young age. About 50% will develop first tumor at age of 30 years [88] and up to 35% will develop multiple tumors in their lifetime [89]. Li-Fraumeni syndrome associated OC, though not the most common but tend to occur at around 39.5 years [90].

Peutz-Jeghers syndrome(PJS) is a rare autosomal dominant condition occurring in 1 in 25,000–30,000 livebirths [91] characterized by benign hamartomatous intestinal polyps with very low tendency to malignancy, cutaneous lesions increased risk of OC in addition to cancers of breast, colon, rectum, pancreas, stomach, testicles and lungs. Tumor suppressor gene STK11(LKB1), located on chromosome 19p13.3 is responsible for this syndrome. OC risk is as high as 18–21% [92]. The ovarian cancers associated with this syndrome are sex cord tumor with annular tubules (SCTATs) in addition to a range of other gynecological cancers [92, 93].

Mutations in double strand breaks repair system like *CHEK2, RAD51, BRIP1* and *PALB2* are also associated with increased risk of various types of ovarian cancer [89, 94]. To date, more than 16 genes are known to be involved in the mechanism of hereditary ovarian tumorigenesis and new ones are being discovered [77, 95].

8. Use of perineal talc

Talc, a metamorphic mineral composed of silicon, magnesium and oxygen, is a common component of genital powders. Applied by women for moisture absorption to prevent perineal chafing and rashes, talc has similarities to and co-occurs with asbestos in its natural form, which is a known carcinogen [96, 97]. Contamination of talc with asbestos was hypothesized to have a causal role in ovarian carcinogenesis [13, 98]. The finding of talc materials in ovarian cancer specimens supports this argument [99]. The International Agency for Research on Cancer(IARC) in 2006, classified genital talc use as possibly carcinogenic to humans based on evidence from epidemiologic studies (carcinogen group 2B) [100, 101].

Although the biological basis of talc carcinogenicity is not clear, direct physical contact with ovarian epithelium may cause chronic inflammation and retrograde transport of talc particles through the reproductive tract as suggested by some workers may occur [98]. An immune mechanism may also be the case.

Several case–control studies report association between perineal talc use and ovarian cancer and data from Women Health Initiative support this association also support this fact [98, 102–104]. Furthermore, a prospective study has confirmed association with serous cystadenocarcinoma and talc use. However asbestos-free talc has been in use in cosmetic products at least in most developed countries and later case–control studies show no association between use of talc and ovarian cancer [104]. Other case–control studies found increased risk by 92% that is a relative risk of 1.92 [98]. A study by Cook et al. reported 1.60 relative risk of ovarian cancer with use than non-use. This is an increase of 60%. Finally, a meta-analysis of about 20 published works reported 35% increased risk of cancer in women who used talc [102]. Scientific evidence has weighed heavily against the makers of talc products who recently lost over 4 billion dollars to a group of 22 women who developed ovarian cancer following talc use adding a court evidence to ovarian carcinogenesis by talc [105].

9. Diet and ovarian cancer

Diet has been directly or indirectly related to risk of ovarian cancer though very few studies specify the histologic subtype in relation to dietary types. Diet may be modifying the risk of ovarian cancer through effect on endogenous hormones, antioxidant activity or other anticarcinogenic mechanisms. There is however a unanimous finding of reduced incidence of ovarian cancer with higher intake of vegetables especially for epithelial ovarian cancer [106–111]. The average finding is a reduction of risk by about more than 50%. High dietary fiber, carotenoids total ligands and phytochemicals are associated with reduced risk [112].

Dairy products have received conflicting results. While over the years, studies showed no associations between dairy intake and ovarian cancer of any type [113, 114]. Faber et al. using the Danish population-based case–control studies reported increased risk especially with milk and lactose but decreased risk with cheese [115]. An interesting study by Merritt et al. using data from New England case–control study examined including histological subtypes and tumor aggression in relation to intake of dairy foods. They reported decreased risk of serous borderline and mucinous cancer with higher intake of calcium and vitamin D. High Vitamin D intake was also found to be inversely related to serous borderline and endometrioid cancers [116]. Merritt et al. found no evidence between lactose intake and risk of ovarian cancer [116].

High intake of total fat, animal fat, cholesterol and saturated fats may be associated with increased risk. Meta-analysis of 16 independent studies reported significant increase in risk of ovarian cancer with high intake of total saturated and trans fats with serous cancers being especially susceptible to dietary fats than other histologic subtypes [117, 118]. Huncharek and Kupelnick reported a RR of 1.70 or an increased risk of 70% in patients with high fat intake [117], however Bertone et al. found no association with intake of fats alone but associated increased with when combined with high intake of eggs [119]. High intake of eggs alone are reported to increase risk [111, 120]. This effect has been linked to high dietary cholesterol which may be increasing risk of ovarian cancer through increased circulating estrogens [111, 121].

Although the link between ovarian cancer and high intake of meat has been controversial with some studies finding no association [122], majority report positive association between high intake of red and processed meat with epithelial ovarian cancer, while poultry and fish have either no relative increase or observed reduction in risk [123–126].

High alcohol consumption has been studied in reasonable depth and only few studies show no association [127] while others show a reduction in risk with minimal and moderate intake of alcohol [128, 129]. The observed phenomenon may be due to the anti-oxidants in the wine and alcohol rather than the alcohol itself [130]. While tea consumption has not been associated with risk of ovarian cancer, coffee is associated with modest reduction of risk [131, 132].

High dietary intake of B carotene is reported to be protective against epithelial ovarian cancer; in a meta-analysis of over 3782 subjects, a modest 16% reduced risk was found [133]. Supplemental selenium (>20 μg daily) is associated with 30% risk reduction [134]. This fact, however, does not support use of selenium as a preventive strategy [135]. These antioxidants may be reducing risk by limiting oxidative stress to the ovarian epithelium.

The effect of vitamin D, particularly D3, has been of interest because of its ability to cause apoptosis of cancer cells in vitro and the demonstrated increased risk of ovarian cancer in vitamin D deficient Europeans [136], more research is necessary to define clinical implication of these findings as some researchers propose supplementation of vitamin D for preventive purposes [137].

10. Smoking

Association between cigarette smoking and ovarian cancer is not as clear as other cancers like lungs oropharynx and lungs that are very well documented [138]. However, metabolites of nicotine which are potent hydrocarbons and carcinogens like cotidine and benzopyrene have been isolated in follicular fluid and OC has been induced in rodents with cyclical hydrocarbons [139].

Cigarette smoking is associated with increased risk of mucinous ovarian cancers [140–143] but the effects on other histologic types is less clear. A Norwegian study, found increased risk of invasive borderline cancers in addition to mucinous [140]. Smokers however have a deficit of endometrioid tumors.

Survival of patients who smoke is also found to be worse than that of non-smokers [142, 144]. Studies have confirmed the increased risk of mucinous epithelial cancers in smokers to be directly proportional to the pack-years of smoking [145, 146]. A twofold increased risk of mucinous epithelial cancers is the generally observed phenomenon [141, 143, 146], but could be up to fourfold increase in women who have smoked for 40 years or more [146].

There is a suggestion however that with the deficit in clear cell and endometrioid cancer and despite the increase in borderline and mucinous cancer smoking may not be associated with overall increase in ovarian cancer mortality [144].

11. Endometriosis and risk of ovarian cancer

OC prevalence in women with endometriosis is higher than the general population 1.32–1.9 [147]. A recent systemic review agrees with this modest increase in risk of endometrioid, borderline and clear cell cancers with endometriosis [148]. Some reports suggest about two to threefold increase in risk [149]. This association between endometriosis and OC is not a proof of causality for the histiotypes.

It is more common in patients with longstanding or recurrent endometriosis and removal of endometrioma is not preventive towards development of OC [150]. The increased risk might be due to high estrogen concentration or due to gene mutations caused by oxidative stress due to iron in the endometriotic cyst [151].

12. Polycystic ovarian syndrome

PCOS is the commonest endocrine disease in women of reproductive age with incidence of about 20% [152]. Associated with infertility, obesity and abnormal gonadotropin secretion, PCOS is associated with 2.5-fold increased risk of epithelial ovarian cancer [153]. The risk of ovarian cancer in women with PCOS is greatest in lean women and those who never used oral contraceptive pills [153, 154].

A systemic review involving eight studies and a meta-analysis found increased incidence of borderline serous cancer in patients with PCOS [155]. Proteomic biomarkers for identification of patients with PCOS who are at increased risk of ovarian cancer may be useful for early diagnosis but the clinical use of these markers need further verification [156].

13. Pelvic inflammatory disease

Inflammation has been implicated in ovarian carcinogenesis but studies investigating the association between pelvic inflammatory disease (PID) and ovarian cancer risk are few and inconsistent with some studies reporting positive association [157, 158] and others excluding such association [159, 160]. A pooled reanalysis of 13 studies reported increased risk of borderline ovarian tumors in women who had multiple episodes of pelvic inflammation [157]. This association may be pronounced among Asian women [158]. Rasmussen et al. in a population-based cohort study recently reported increase in risk of serous ovarian cancer in patients with PID [157]. Therefore we can conclude that repeated episodes of PID is associated with statistically significant risk of borderline and serous cancers but not non-epithelial cancers which have been found not to be associated with PID [158].

14. Hormone replacement therapy (Hrt) and risk of ovarian cancer

Women who use menopausal hormone therapy are at an increased risk for ovarian cancer. A review and meta-analysis of data published between 1966 and 2006 concluded that current use of postmenopausal hormone therapy (HT) increased the risk of ovarian cancer by 30% compared with never use of HT [161]. Estrogen alone was thought to confer higher risk than combined estrogen and progesterone which is refuted by finding from data from million women study [162, 163]. Recent studies indicate that using a combination of estrogen and progestin for 5 or more years significantly increases the risk of serous and endometrioid OC in women with intact uterus, but for women who have had hysterectomy, 10 or more years of use is associated with increased risk [161, 164, 165]. In a recent pooled analysis of 52 epidemiological studies, the risk of serous cancer was 51.4% and that of endometrioid was 48.6% [164]. The increase has been interpreted to mean one extra OC in 1000 users and one extra mortality in 1700 user [166]. There is more risk with prolonged use irrespective of the type of HRT, regimes used or mode of administration.

15. Obesity

Obesity may be increasing risk of ovarian cancer significantly [166–168]. Obese women (BMI > 30 kg/m^2) who have not used menopausal hormone replacement therapy (MHR) had 25–80% increased risk compared with women with normal BMI (18.5–24.9) no relationship between BMI and OC in women with family history. Obesity is associated with an almost 80% higher risk of ovarian cancer in women 50–71 who had not taken hormones after menopause. For women who have not used HRT, evidence shows risk of ovarian cancer to increase by 10% with every 5 kg/m^2 increase in BMI (Collaborative Study). Higher BMI in young adulthood is reported to increase risk of premenopausal ovarian cancers [167].

Evidence from meta-analysis of 14 studies shows that slightly worse survival in obese women with ovarian cancer compared to non-obese women (pooled HR = 1.17, 95% CI: 1.03–1.32) [169].

Obesity may be increasing this risk for ovarian cancer through increasing inflammatory biomarkers and increase in hormonal factors especially androgens which is important in development of mucinous tumors [170].

Histologic subtypes associated with obesity include low-grade serous, mucinous tumors and endometrioid cancers. No association was found between high grade serous and obesity therefore reducing BMI is unlikely to reduce the incidence of high grade serous cancers [171]. Moreover, obese women with HGSC have poorer outcome than their non-obese counter parts [172].

Recent systemic review of 43 studies involving more than 3 million women concludes that the evidence is inconsistent that obesity is a definite risk factor for ovarian cancer [173]. This finding may be due to the dominance of HGSC which risk is not affected by obesity.

16. Protective factors that reduce risk of ovarian cancer.

16.1 Pregnancy

Pregnancy is thought to be protective against ovarian cancer [13, 47, 65]. Pregnancy whether uncompleted or term confers a protective benefit against epithelial ovarian cancer. Increasing parity is associated with a reduction in the risk of ovarian cancer [36, 63, 65, 174]. Pregnancy may be protective against all histological subtypes. A Swedish study has reported reduced risk for epithelial, stromal and germ cell tumors, but less consistent decrease in borderline cancers [63].

However, it appears that the protective effect of pregnancy (and breast feeding) so called reproductive factors, may be more significant in the West, parts of the US and among Jewish women as reports of ovarian cancer of all histologic subtypes in parous women in developing countries is so widespread and requires further research [38, 53, 55, 57, 59, 60]. The significance of this phenomenon is that the protective effect of pregnancy may be lost in the face of other more important risk factors that need to be defined.

All theories of ovarian carcinogenesis are not plausible explanation for the observed protective effect of pregnancy, therefore pregnancy-induced clearance of malignant cells has been proposed [63] which must to be case in all races to be an acceptable hypothesis.

16.2 Breastfeeding

Breast feeding exerts a strong protective effect with long-term breast feeding being more protective especially against epithelial cancers [175]. The mechanism may be by suppression of gonadotropins through unovulation, resulting in depressed production of plasma estradiol and unovulatory cycles [65, 176]. Breastfeeding also reduces the levels of gonadotropins, especially luteinizing hormone [176], which may be causal mechanism for ovarian carcinogenesis [177].

Meta-analysis of 12 US studies and 9 studies from developed countries showed an inverse association between breastfeeding and ovarian cancer risk [175]. Women who breast fed for up to 6 months showed duration-dependent benefit with women who breastfed for long having more protection. Breast feeding may be reducing risk of epithelial cancers by up to 30% compared with women who did not breast feed.

16.3 Oral contraceptives

The use of oral contraceptives decreases the risk of developing OC and the benefit may be enjoyed up to 25–30 years after stopping the pill [178, 179]. COCP use is associated with about a 40–50% lower risk compared with never use [178, 180]. Length of pill use appears to influence the degree of protection, with a relative risk of 0.4 for more than 5 years reported in pooled European and US studies [178, 181].

The protective benefit may be experienced even in high risk women though there is not enough evidence for use of the pill for chemoprophylaxis [180, 182, 183]. Women who use the pills for more than 5 years enjoy more protection of about 50% reduction [179]. This protection is enjoyed by women of all ages and parities.

Therefore while HRT is associated with increasing risk, the pills are associated with reduced risk a position both have similar active ingredients and estrogen has been blamed in ovarian carcinogenesis.

16.4 Hysterectomy/tubal ligation

Observational epidemiologic evidence strongly support tubal ligation and hysterectomy to be associated with a decrease in the risk of ovarian cancer, by approximately 26–30% [184]. Having fallopian tubes tied hysterectomy and unilateral oophorectomy may reduce risk by up to 67% [184, 185].

Patients with BRCA1 but not with BRCA2 are found to benefit from the protection conferred by tubal ligation to OC [186]. Tubal ligation and hysterectomy reduce risk of low grade more than high grade serous cancers. Risk of endometrioid cancer is almost halved. Tubal ligation is not observed to reduce the risk of mucinous tumors [187].

16.5 Physical activity and exercise

Physical activity may be beneficial in both risk reduction of inflammation, decreasing body fat and frequency of ovulation. Survivors of ovarian cancer may also experience general health benefit of physical activity [188]. The specific effect of physical exercise on ovarian cancer in general and the various histologic subtypes have shown inconsistent results. The most consistent result obtained by research is that of increasing risk by prolonged sedentary life style physical inactivity [188, 189].

Considering direct effect of physical activity however, some studies report no effect on the risk of ovarian cancer [190, 191] while other studies report risk reduction [190, 191]. The reduction of risk may be to epithelial cancers. Physical activity may not be affecting sex cord-stromal and germ cell cancers of the ovary.

17. Conclusion

The risk of ovarian cancer in women is modified by a number of biologic, hormonal, lifestyle and geographic factors the extent of which differs between the histologic varieties. There may be racial or regional variation in the extent to which these factor increase risk or protect against particularly the most common histologic subtype.

Author details

Marliyya S. Zayyan
Oncology Department of Obstetrics and Gynecology, Ahmadu Bello University, Zaria, Nigeria

*Address all correspondence to: marliyya.zayyan@gmail.com

References

[1] Bray F, Ferlay J, Soerjomataram I, Siegel RL, Torre LA, Jemal A. Global Cancer statistics 2018: GLOBOCAN estimates of incidence and mortality worldwide for 36 cancers in 185 countries. CA: A Cancer Journal for Clinicians. n.d. DOI: 10.3322/caac.21492

[2] Jacques F, Isabelle S, Rajesh D, Sultan E, Colin M, Marise R, et al. Cancer incidence and mortality worldwide: Sources, methods and major patterns in GLOBOCAN 2012. International Journal of Cancer. 2014;**136**:E359-E386. DOI: 10.1002/ijc.29210

[3] Malvezzi M, Carioli G, Rodriguez T, Negri E, La Vecchia C. Global trends and predictions in ovarian cancer mortality. 2016;**27**. DOI: 10.1093/annonc/mdw306

[4] Kumar B, Davies-Humphreys J. Tumour markers and ovarian cancer screening. The Obstetrician and Gynaecologist. 2011;**2**:41-44. DOI: 10.1576/toag.2000.2.4.41

[5] Alberico S, Facca MC, Millo R, Radillo L, Mandruzzato GP. Tumoral markers (CA 125--CEA) in the screening of ovarian cancer. European Journal of Gynaecological Oncology. 1988;**9**:485-489

[6] Bairey O, Blickstein D, Stark P, Prokocimer M, Nativ HM, Kirgner I, et al. Serum CA 125 as a prognostic factor in non-Hodgkin's lymphoma. Leukemia and Lymphoma. 2003;**44**:1733-1738. DOI: 10.1080/1042819031000104079

[7] Fritsche HA, Bast RC. CA 125 in ovarian cancer: Advances and controversy. Clinical Chemistry. 1998;**44**:1379-1380

[8] Pepin K, del Carmen M, Brown A, Dizon DS. CA 125 and epithelial ovarian cancer: Role in screening, diagnosis, and surveillance. Journal of Hematology and Oncology. 2014;**10**

[9] Eagle K, Ledermann JA. Tumor markers in ovarian malignancies. The Oncologist. 1997;**2**:324-329

[10] Berek JS, Bast RC. Ovarian cancer screening. The use of serial complementary tumor markers to improve sensitivity and specificity for early detection. Cancer. 1995;**76**:2092-2096

[11] Bast RC. Status of tumor markers in ovarian cancer screening. Journal of Clinical Oncology: Official Journal of the American Society of Clinical Oncology. 2003;**21**:200s-205s. DOI: 10.1200/JCO.2003.01.068

[12] La Vecchia C. Ovarian cancer: Epidemiology and risk factors. European Journal of Cancer Prevention. 2017;**26**:55-62. DOI: 10.1097/CEJ.0000000000000217

[13] Reid BM, Permuth JB, Sellers TA. Epidemiology of ovarian cancer: A review. Cancer Biology and Medicine. 2017;**14**:9-32

[14] Holschneider CH, Berek JS. Ovarian cancer: Epidemiology, biology, and prognostic factors. Seminars in Surgical Oncology. 2000;**19**:3-10. DOI: 10.1002/1098-2388(200007/08)19:1<3::AID-SSU2>3.0.CO;2-S

[15] Jacobs IJ, Menon U, Ryan A, Gentry-Maharaj A, Burnell M, Kalsi JK, et al. Ovarian cancer screening and mortality in the UK collaborative trial of ovarian cancer screening (UKCTOCS): A randomised controlled trial. Lancet (London, England). 2016;**387**:945-956. DOI: 10.1016/S0140-6736(15)01224-6

[16] Meinhold-Heerlein I, Fotopoulou C, Harter P, Kurzeder C, Mustea A, Wimberger P, et al. The new WHO

classification of ovarian, fallopian tube, and primary peritoneal cancer and its clinical implications. Archives of Gynecology and Obstetrics. 2016;**293**:695-700. DOI: 10.1007/s00404-016-4035-8

[17] Prat J, D'Angelo E, Espinosa I. Ovarian carcinomas: At least five different diseases with distinct histological features and molecular genetics. Human Pathology. 2018;**80**:11-27. DOI: 10.1016/j.humpath.2018.06.018

[18] A Soslow R. Histologic subtypes of ovarian carcinoma: An overview. International Journal of Gynecological Pathology. 2008;**27**:161-174. DOI: 10.1097/PGP.0b013e31815ea812

[19] Kurman R, Shih I-M. The origin and pathogenesis of epithelial ovarian cancer: A proposed unifying theory. The American Journal of Surgical Pathology. 2010;**34**:433-443. DOI: 10.1097/PAS.0b013e3181cf3d79

[20] Whittemore AS, Harris R, Itnyre J. Characteristics relating to ovarian cancer risk: Collaborative analysis of 12 US case-control studies. IV. The pathogenesis of epithelial ovarian cancer. Collaborative Ovarian Cancer Group. The The American Journal of Epidemiology 1992;136:1212-1220

[21] WHO classification of ovarian neoplasms n.d. Available from: http://www.pathologyoutlines.com/topic/ovarytumorwhoclassif.html [Accessed: 16 September 2018]

[22] Coburn SB, Bray F, Sherman ME, Trabert B. International patterns and trends in ovarian cancer incidence, overall and by histologic subtype. International Journal of Cancer. 2017;**140**:2451-2460. DOI: 10.1002/ijc.30676

[23] Ahn G, Folkins AK, McKenney JK, Longacre TA. Low-grade serous carcinoma of the ovary: Clinicopathologic analysis of 52 invasive cases and identification of a possible noninvasive intermediate lesion. The American Journal of Surgical Pathology. 2016;**40**:1165-1176. DOI: 10.1097/PAS.0000000000000693

[24] Vang R, Shih I-M, Kurman RJ. Ovarian low-grade and high-grade serous carcinoma: Pathogenesis, clinicopathologic and molecular biologic features, and diagnostic problems. Advances in Anatomic Pathology. 2009;**16**:267-282. DOI: 10.1097/PAP.0b013e3181b4fffa

[25] Lalwani N, Prasad SR, Vikram R, Shanbhogue AK, Huettner PC, Fasih N. Histologic, molecular, and cytogenetic features of ovarian cancers: Implications for diagnosis and treatment. Radiographics. 2011;**31**:625-646. DOI: 10.1148/rg.313105066

[26] Schultz KAP, Harris AK, Schneider DT, Young RH, Brown J, Gershenson DM, et al. Ovarian sex cord-stromal tumors. Journal of Oncology Practice/American Society of Clinical Oncology. 2016;**12**:940-946. DOI: 10.1200/JOP.2016.016261

[27] Boyd J. Specific keynote: Hereditary ovarian cancer: What we know. Gynecologic Oncology. 2003;**88**:S8-S10; discussion S11-13

[28] Low JJH, Ilancheran A, Ng JS. Malignant ovarian germ-cell tumours. Best Practice and Research. Clinical Obstetrics and Gynaecology. 2012;**26**:347-355. DOI: 10.1016/j.bpobgyn.2012.01.002

[29] Fathalla MF. Incessant ovulation—A factor in ovarian neoplasia? Lancet (London, England). 1971;**2**:163

[30] Fathalla MF. Incessant ovulation and ovarian cancer—A hypothesis re-visited. Facts Views Vis ObGyn. 2013;**5**:292-297

[31] Choi J-H, Wong AST, Huang H-F, PCK L. Gonadotropins and ovarian cancer. Endocrine Reviews. 2007;**28**:440-461. DOI: 10.1210/er.2006-0036

[32] Lee AW, Tyrer JP, Doherty JA, Stram DA, Kupryjanczyk J, Dansonka-Mieszkowska A, et al. Evaluating the ovarian cancer gonadotropin hypothesis: A candidate gene study. Gynecologic Oncology. 2015;**136**:542-548. DOI: 10.1016/j.ygyno.2014.12.017

[33] Ness RB, Cottreau C. Possible role of ovarian epithelial inflammation in ovarian cancer. Journal of the National Cancer Institute. 1999;**91**:1459-1467. DOI: 10.1093/jnci/91.17.1459

[34] Purdie DM, Bain CJ, Siskind V, Webb PM, Green AC. Ovulation and risk of epithelial ovarian cancer. International Journal of Cancer. 2003;**104**:228-232. DOI: 10.1002/ijc.10927

[35] Bray F, Loos AH, Tognazzo S, La Vecchia C. Ovarian cancer in Europe: Cross-sectional trends in incidence and mortality in 28 countries, 1953-2000. International Journal of Cancer. 2005;**113**:977-990. DOI: 10.1002/ijc.20649

[36] Albrektsen G, Heuch I, Kvåle G. Reproductive factors and incidence of epithelial ovarian cancer: A Norwegian prospective study. Cancer Causes and Control. 1996;7:421-427. DOI: 10.1007/BF00052668

[37] Keinan-Boker L, Silverman BG, Walsh PM, Gavin AT, Hayes C. Time trends in the incidence and mortality of ovarian cancer in Ireland, Northern Ireland, and Israel, 1994-2013. International Journal of Gynecological Cancer. 2017;**27**:1628-1636. DOI: 10.1097/IGC.0000000000001079

[38] Iyoke C, Ugwu G, Ezugwu E, Onah N, Ugwu O, Okafor O. Incidence, pattern and management of ovarian cancer at a tertiary medical center in Enugu, south East Nigeria. Annals of Medical and Health Sciences Research. 2013;**3**:417-421. DOI: 10.4103/2141-9248.117947

[39] Torre LA, Trabert B, DeSantis CE, Miller KD, Samimi G, Runowicz CD, et al. Ovarian cancer statistics, 2018. CA: A Cancer Journal for Clinicians. 2018;**68**:284-296. DOI: 10.3322/caac.21456

[40] Yamagami W, Nagase S, Takahashi F, Ino K, Hachisuga T, Aoki D, et al. Clinical statistics of gynecologic cancers in Japan. Journal of Gynecologic Oncology. 2017;**28**:e32. DOI: 10.3802/jgo.2017.28.e32

[41] Goodman MT, Howe HL, Tung KH, Hotes J, Miller BA, Coughlin SS, et al. Incidence of ovarian cancer by race and ethnicity in the United States, 1992-1997. Cancer. 2003;**97**:2676-2685. DOI: 10.1002/cncr.11349

[42] Weiderpass E, Sandin S, Inoue M, Shimazu T, Iwasaki M, Sasazuki S, et al. Risk factors for epithelial ovarian cancer in Japan—Results from the Japan public health center-based prospective study cohort. International Journal of Oncology. 2012;**40**:21-30. DOI: 10.3892/ijo.2011.1194

[43] Srivastava A, McKinnon W, Wood ME. Risk of breast and ovarian cancer in women with strong family histories. Oncology Williston Park N. 2001;**15**:889-902; discussion 902, 905-7, 911-3

[44] Weiss NS, Peterson AS. Racial variation in the incidence of ovarian cancer in the United States. American Journal of Epidemiology. 1978;**107**:91-95. DOI: 10.1093/oxfordjournals.aje.a112522

[45] Stewart SL, Harewood R, Matz M, Rim SH, Sabatino SA, Ward KC, et al.

Disparities in ovarian cancer survival in the United States (2001-2009): Findings from the CONCORD-2 study. Cancer. 2017;**123**(Suppl 24):5138-5159. DOI: 10.1002/cncr.31027

[46] SEER Cancer Statistics Review 1973-1997—Previous Version—SEER Cancer Statistics n.d. Available from: https://seer.cancer.gov/archive/csr/1973_1997/ [Accessed: 02 August 2018]

[47] Doufekas K, Olaitan A. Clinical epidemiology of epithelial ovarian cancer in the UK. International Journal of Women's Health. 2014;**6**:537-545. DOI: 10.2147/IJWH.S40894

[48] Morowitz M, Huff D, von Allmen D. Epithelial ovarian tumors in children: A retrospective analysis. Journal of Pediatric Surgery. 2003;**38**:331-335; discussion 331-335. DOI: 10.1053/jpsu.2003.50103

[49] Bhattacharyya NK, De A, Bera P, Mongal S, Chakraborty S, Bandopadhyay R. Ovarian tumors in pediatric age group—A clinicopathologic study of 10 years' cases in West Bengal, India. The Indian Journal of Medical and Paediatric Oncology. 2010;**31**:54

[50] Ovarian Cancer: Recognition and Initial Management | Guidance and Guidelines | NICE n.d. Available from: https://www.nice.org.uk/Guidance/cg122 [Accessed: 03 August 2018]

[51] Vecchia CL, Levi F, Lucchini F, Negri E, Franceschi S. Descriptive epidemiology of ovarian cancer in Europe. Gynecologic Oncology. 1992;**46**:208-215. DOI: 10.1016/0090-8258(92)90257-J

[52] Klar M, Hasenburg A, Hasanov M, Hilpert F, Meier W, Pfisterer J, et al. Prognostic factors in young ovarian cancer patients: An analysis of four prospective phase III intergroup trials of the AGO Study Group, GINECO and NSGO. The European Journal of Cancer. 1990, 2016;**66**:114-124. DOI: 10.1016/j.ejca.2016.07.014

[53] Murthy NS, Shalini S, Suman G, Pruthvish S, Mathew A. Changing trends in incidence of ovarian cancer—The Indian scenario. The Asian Pacific Journal of Cancer Prevention. 2009;**10**:1025-1030

[54] Saini SK. Clinical Cancer Investigation Journal n.d. Available from: http://www.ccij-online.org/article.asp?issn=2278-0513;year=2016;volume=5;issue=1;spage=20;epage=24;aulast=Saini [Accessed: 03 August 2018]

[55] Basu P, De P, Mandal S, Ray K, Biswas J. Study of "patterns of care" of ovarian cancer patients in a specialized cancer institute in Kolkata, eastern India. Indian Journal of Cancer. 2009;**46**:28-33

[56] Jindal D, Sahasrabhojanee M, Jindal M, D'Souza J. Epidemiology of epithelial ovarian cancer: A tertiary hospital based study in Goa, India. International Journal of Reproduction, Contraception, Obstetrics and Gynecology. 2017;**6**:2541. DOI: 10.18203/2320-1770.ijrcog20172348

[57] Malik IA. A prospective study of clinico-pathological features of epithelial ovarian cancer in Pakistan n.d.:8

[58] Mostafa MF, El-etreby N, Awad N. Retrospective analysis evaluating ovarian cancer cases presented at the clinical oncology department, Alexandria University. Alexandria Journal of Medicine. 2012;**48**:353-360. DOI: 10.1016/j.ajme.2012.07.001

[59] Zayyan MS, Ahmed SA, Oguntayo AO, Kolawole AO, Olasinde TA. Epidemiology of ovarian cancers in Zaria, northern Nigeria: A

10-year study. International Journal of Women's Health. 2017;**9**:855-860. DOI: 10.2147/IJWH.S130340

[60] Abuidris DO, Weng H-Y, Elhaj AM, Eltayeb EA, Elsanousi M, Ibnoof RS, et al. Incidence and survival rates of ovarian cancer in low-income women in Sudan. Molecular and Clinical Oncology. 2016;**5**:823-828. DOI: 10.3892/mco.2016.1068

[61] Akakpo PK, Derkyi-Kwarteng L, Gyasi RK, Quayson SE, Naporo S, Anim JT. A pathological and clinical study of 706 primary tumours of the ovary in the largest tertiary hospital in Ghana. BMC Womens Health. 2017;**17**:34. DOI: 10.1186/s12905-017-0389-8

[62] Gong T-T, Wu Q-J, Vogtmann E, Lin B, Wang Y-L. Age at menarche and risk of ovarian cancer: A meta-analysis of epidemiological studies. International Journal of Cancer. 2013;**132**:2894-2900. DOI: 10.1002/ijc.27952

[63] Adami HO, Hsieh CC, Lambe M, Trichopoulos D, Leon D, Persson I, et al. Parity, age at first childbirth, and risk of ovarian cancer. Lancet (London, England). 1994;**344**:1250-1254

[64] Yancik R. Ovarian cancer. Age contrasts in incidence, histology, disease stage at diagnosis, and mortality. Cancer. 1993;**71**:517-523

[65] Riman T, Nilsson S, Persson IR. Review of epidemiological evidence for reproductive and hormonal factors in relation to the risk of epithelial ovarian malignancies. Acta Obstetricia et Gynecologica Scandinavica. 2004;**83**:783-795. DOI: 10.1111/j.0001-6349.2004.00550.x

[66] Riboli E. The European Prospective Investigation into Cancer and Nutrition (EPIC): Plans and progress. The Journal of Nutrition. 2001;**131**:170S-175S. DOI: 10.1093/jn/131.1.170S

[67] Rossing MA, Daling JR, Weiss NS, Moore DE, Self SG. Ovarian tumors in a cohort of infertile women. The New England Journal of Medicine. 1994;**331**:771-776. DOI: 10.1056/NEJM199409223311204

[68] Jensen A, Sharif H, Frederiksen K, Kjær SK. Use of fertility drugs and risk of ovarian cancer: Danish population based cohort study. BMJ. 2009;**338**:580-583

[69] Ness RB, Cramer DW, Goodman MT, Kjaer SK, Mallin K, Mosgaard BJ, et al. Infertility, fertility drugs, and ovarian cancer: A pooled analysis of case-control studies. American Journal of Epidemiology. 2002;**155**:217-224

[70] Mosgaard BJ, Lidegaard Ø, Kjaer SK, Schou G, Andersen AN. Infertility, fertility drugs, and invasive ovarian cancer: A case-control study. Fertility and Sterility. 1997;**67**:1005-1012. DOI: 10.1016/S0015-0282(97)81431-8

[71] Tomao F, Lo Russo G, Spinelli GP, Stati V, Prete AA, Prinzi N, et al. Fertility drugs, reproductive strategies and ovarian cancer risk. Journal of Ovarian Research. 2014;**7**:51. DOI: 10.1186/1757-2215-7-51

[72] Lynch HT, Casey MJ, Snyder CL, Bewtra C, Lynch JF, Butts M, et al. Hereditary ovarian carcinoma: Heterogeneity, molecular genetics, pathology, and management. Molecular Oncology. 2009;**3**:97-137. DOI: 10.1016/j.molonc.2009.02.004

[73] Foulkes WD, Narod SA. Ovarian cancer risk and family history. The Lancet. 1997;**349**:878. DOI: 10.1016/S0140-6736(05)61782-5

[74] Kerlikowske K, Brown JS, Grady DG. Should women with familial ovarian cancer undergo prophylactic oophorectomy? Obstetrics and Gynecology. 1992;**80**:700-707

[75] Family History of Ovarian Cancer - an overview | ScienceDirect Topics n.d. Available from: https://www.sciencedirect.com/topics/medicine-and-dentistry/family-history-of-ovarian-cancer [Accessed: 03 November 2018]

[76] Soegaard M, Frederiksen K, Jensen A, Høgdall E, Høgdall C, Blaakaer J, et al. Risk of ovarian cancer in women with first-degree relatives with cancer. Acta Obstetricia et Gynecologica Scandinavica. 2009;**88**:449-456. DOI: 10.1080/00016340902807207

[77] Toss A, Tomasello C, Razzaboni E, Contu G, Grandi G, Cagnacci A, et al. Hereditary ovarian cancer: Not only BRCA 1 and 2 genes. BioMed Research International. 2015. DOI: 10.1155/2015/341723

[78] Robles-díaz L, Goldfrank DJ, Kauff ND, Robson M, Offit K. Hereditary ovarian cancer in Ashkenazi Jews. Familial Cancer. 2004;**3**:259-264. DOI: 10.1007/s10689-004-9552-0

[79] Villella JA, Parmar M, Donohue K, Fahey C, Piver MS, Rodabaugh K. Role of prophylactic hysterectomy in patients at high risk for hereditary cancers. Gynecologic Oncology. 2006;**102**:475-479. DOI: 10.1016/j.ygyno.2006.01.006

[80] Osman MA. Genetic cancer ovary. Clinical Ovarian and Other Gynecologic Cancer. 2014;7:1-7. DOI: 10.1016/j.cogc.2014.12.006

[81] Lynch HT, Krush AJ. Heredity and adenocarcinoma of the colon. Gastroenterology. 1967;**53**:517-527

[82] Watson P, Bützow R, Lynch HT, Mecklin JP, Järvinen HJ, Vasen HF, et al. The clinical features of ovarian cancer in hereditary nonpolyposis colorectal cancer. Gynecologic Oncology. 2001;**82**:223-228. DOI: 10.1006/gyno.2001.6279

[83] Vasen HF, Stormorken A, Menko FH, Nagengast FM, Kleibeuker JH, Griffioen G, et al. MSH2 mutation carriers are at higher risk of cancer than MLH1 mutation carriers: A study of hereditary nonpolyposis colorectal cancer families. Journal of Clinical Oncology: Official Journal of the American Society of Clinical Oncology. 2001;**19**:4074-4080. DOI: 10.1200/JCO.2001.19.20.4074

[84] Lynch HT, Boland CR, Gong G, Shaw TG, Lynch PM, Fodde R, et al. Phenotypic and genotypic heterogeneity in the Lynch syndrome: Diagnostic, surveillance and management implications. European Journal of Human Genetics. 2006;**14**:390-402. DOI: 10.1038/sj.ejhg.5201584

[85] Watson P, Vasen HFA, Mecklin J-P, Bernstein I, Aarnio M, Järvinen HJ, et al. The risk of extra-colonic, extra-endometrial cancer in the Lynch syndrome. The International Journal of Cancer. 2008;**123**:444-449. DOI: 10.1002/ijc.23508

[86] Liu J, Albarracin CT, Chang K-H, Thompson-Lanza JA, Zheng W, Gershenson DM, et al. Microsatellite instability and expression of hMLH1 and hMSH2 proteins in ovarian endometrioid cancer. Modern Pathology. 2004;**17**:75-80. DOI: 10.1038/sj.modpathol.3800017

[87] Chui MH, Gilks CB, Cooper K, Clarke BA. Identifying Lynch syndrome in patients with ovarian carcinoma: The significance of tumor subtype. Advances in Anatomic Pathology. 2013;**20**:378-386. DOI: 10.1097/PAP.0b013e3182a92cf8

[88] Beyond Li-Fraumeni syndrome: Clinical characteristics of families with p53 germline mutations. Journal of Clinical Oncology. n.d. 26(15_suppl). Available from: http://ascopubs.org/doi/abs/10.1200/jco.2008.26.15_suppl.11031 [Accessed: 12 November 2018]

[89] Hisada M, Garber JE, Fung CY, Fraumeni JF, Li FP. Multiple primary cancers in families with Li-Fraumeni syndrome. Journal of the National Cancer Institute. 1998;**90**:606-611

[90] Varley JM, Evans DG, Birch JM. Li-Fraumeni syndrome—A molecular and clinical review. British Journal of Cancer. 1997;**76**:1-14

[91] Oral and Maxillofacial Pathology. 3rd ed. n.d. Available from: https://www.elsevier.com/books/oral-and-maxillofacial-pathology/neville/978-1-4160-3435-3 [Accessed: 13 November 2018]

[92] Banno K, Kisu I, Yanokura M, Masuda K, Ueki A, Kobayashi Y, et al. Hereditary gynecological tumors associated with Peutz-Jeghers syndrome (review). Oncology Letters. 2013;**6**:1184-1188. DOI: 10.3892/ol.2013.1527

[93] Papp J, Kovacs ME, Solyom S, Kasler M, Børresen-Dale A-L, Olah E. High prevalence of germline STK11mutations in Hungarian Peutz-Jeghers syndrome patients. BMC Medical Genetics. 2010;**11**:169. DOI: 10.1186/1471-2350-11-169

[94] Prat J, Ribé A, Gallardo A. Hereditary ovarian cancer. Human Pathology. 2005;**36**:861-870. DOI: 10.1016/j.humpath.2005.06.006

[95] Fackenthal JD, Zhang J, Zhang B, Zheng Y, Hagos F, Burrill DR, et al. High prevalence of BRCA1 and BRCA2 mutations in unselected Nigerian breast cancer patients. International Journal of Cancer. 2012;**131**:1114-1123. DOI: 10.1002/ijc.27326

[96] Schmolz G. The carcinogenic effect of asbestos. Offentliche Gesundheitswesen. 1989;**51**:614-620

[97] Barrett JC, Lamb PW, Wiseman RW. Multiple mechanisms for the carcinogenic effects of asbestos and other mineral fibers. Environmental Health Perspectives. 1989;**81**:81-89

[98] Cramer DW, Vitonis AF, Terry KL, Welch WR, Titus LJ. The association between talc use and ovarian cancer: A retrospective case-control study in Two US States. Epidemiology (Cambridge, Mass.). 2016;**27**:334-346. DOI: 10.1097/EDE.0000000000000434

[99] Cramer DW, Welch WR, Berkowitz RS, Godleski JJ. Presence of talc in pelvic lymph nodes of a woman with ovarian cancer and long-term genital exposure to cosmetic talc. Obstetrics and Gynecology. 2007;**110**:498-501. DOI: 10.1097/01.AOG.0000262902.80861.a0

[100] IARC Monographs Volume 100C Asbestos (Chrysotile, Amosite, Crocidolite, Tremolite, Actinolite and Anthophyllite) – IARC n.d. Available from: https://monographs.iarc.fr/iarc-monographs-volume-100c-asbestos-chrysotile-amosite-crocidolite-tremolite-actinolite-and-anthophyllite/ [Accessed: 13 November 2018]

[101] Asbestos and Cancer Risk n.d. Available from: https://www.cancer.org/cancer/cancer-causes/asbestos.html [Accessed: 13 November 2018]

[102] Muscat JE, Huncharek MS. Perineal talc use and ovarian cancer: A critical review. The European Journal of Cancer Prevention. 2008;**17**:139-146. DOI: 10.1097/CEJ.0b013e32811080ef

[103] Gertig DM, Hunter DJ, Cramer DW, Colditz GA, Speizer FE, Willett WC, et al. Prospective study of talc use and ovarian cancer. The Journal of the National Cancer Institute. 2000;**92**:249-252. DOI: 10.1093/jnci/92.3.249

[104] Berge W, Mundt K, Luu H, Boffetta P. Genital use of talc and risk of ovarian cancer: A meta-analysis. European Journal of Cancer

Prevention. 2018;**27**:248. DOI: 10.1097/CEJ.0000000000000340

[105] Kennerly M, Esq. The Science Connecting Talcum Powder And Ovarian Cancer. Litig Trial Lawyer Blog 2016. Available from: https://www.litigationandtrial.com/2016/05/articles/attorney/consumer-protection/talcum-powder-ovarian-cancer/ [Accessed: 13 November 2018]

[106] Zhang M, Yang ZY, Binns CW, Lee AH. Diet and ovarian cancer risk: A case-control study in China. British Journal of Cancer. 2002;**86**:712-717. DOI: 10.1038/sj.bjc.6600085

[107] Plagens-Rotman K, Chmaj-Wierzchowska K, Pięta B, Bojar I. Modifiable lifestyle factors and ovarian cancer incidence in women. Annals of Agricultural and Environmental Medicine. 2018;**25**:36-40. DOI: 10.5604/12321966.1233565

[108] Schulz M, Lahmann PH, Boeing H, Hoffmann K, Allen N, Key TJA, et al. Fruit and vegetable consumption and risk of epithelial ovarian cancer: The European prospective investigation into cancer and nutrition. Cancer Epidemiology, Biomarkers and Prevention. 2005;**14**:2531-2535. DOI: 10.1158/1055-9965.EPI-05-0159

[109] Han B, Li X, Yu T. Cruciferous vegetables consumption and the risk of ovarian cancer: A meta-analysis of observational studies. Diagnostic Pathology. 2014;**9**:7. DOI: 10.1186/1746-1596-9-7

[110] Tang L, Lee AH, Su D, Binns CW. Fruit and vegetable consumption associated with reduced risk of epithelial ovarian cancer in southern Chinese women. Gynecologic Oncology. 2014;**132**:241-247. DOI: 10.1016/j.ygyno.2013.10.020

[111] Pan SY, Ugnat A-M, Mao Y, Wen SW, Johnson KC. A case-control study of diet and the risk of ovarian cancer. Cancer Epidemiology, Biomarkers and Prevention. 2004:8

[112] McCann SE, Freudenheim JL, Marshall JR, Graham S. Risk of human ovarian cancer is related to dietary intake of selected nutrients, phytochemicals and food groups. The Journal of Nutrition. 2003;**133**:1937-1942. DOI: 10.1093/jn/133.6.1937

[113] Genkinger JM, Hunter DJ, Spiegelman D, Anderson KE, Arslan A, Beeson WL, et al. Dairy products and ovarian cancer: A pooled analysis of 12 cohort studies. Cancer Epidemiology, Biomarkers and Prevention. 2006;**15**:364-372. DOI: 10.1158/1055-9965.EPI-05-0484

[114] Mommers M, Schouten LJ, Goldbohm RA, van den Brandt PA. Dairy consumption and ovarian cancer risk in the Netherlands cohort study on diet and cancer. British Journal of Cancer. 2006;**94**:165-170. DOI: 10.1038/sj.bjc.6602890

[115] Faber MT, Jensen A, Søgaard M, Høgdall E, Høgdall C, Blaakaer J, et al. Use of dairy products, lactose, and calcium and risk of ovarian cancer—Results from a Danish case-control study. Acta Oncologica (Stockholm, Sweden). 2012;**51**:454-464. DOI: 10.3109/0284186X.2011.636754

[116] Merritt MA, Cramer DW, Vitonis AF, Titus LJ, Terry KL. Dairy foods and nutrients in relation to risk of ovarian cancer and major histological subtypes. International Journal of Cancer. 2013;**132**:1114-1124. DOI: 10.1002/ijc.27701

[117] Huncharek M, Kupelnick B. Dietary fat intake and risk of epithelial ovarian cancer: A meta-analysis of 6,689 subjects from 8 observational studies. Nutrition and Cancer. 2001;**40**:87-91. DOI: 10.1207/S15327914NC402_2

[118] Qiu W, Lu H, Qi Y, Wang X. Dietary fat intake and ovarian cancer risk: A meta-analysis of epidemiological studies. Oncotarget. 2016;7:37390-37406. DOI: 10.18632/oncotarget.8940

[119] Bertone ER, Rosner BA, Hunter DJ, Stampfer MJ, Speizer FE, Colditz GA, et al. Dietary fat intake and ovarian cancer in a cohort of US women. American Journal of Epidemiology. 2002;**156**:22-31. DOI: 10.1093/aje/kwf008

[120] Keum N, Lee DH, Marchand N, Oh H, Liu H, Aune D, et al. Egg intake and cancers of the breast, ovary and prostate: A dose–response meta-analysis of prospective observational studies. The British Journal of Nutrition. 2015;**114**:1099-1107. DOI: 10.1017/S0007114515002135

[121] Risch HA, Jain M, Marrett LD, Howe GR. Dietary fat intake and risk of epithelial ovarian cancer. The Journal of the National Cancer Institute. 1994;**86**:1409-1415. DOI: 10.1093/jnci/86.18.1409

[122] Gilsing AM, Weijenberg MP, Goldbohm RA, van den Brandt PA, Schouten LJ. Consumption of dietary fat and meat and risk of ovarian cancer in the Netherlands cohort study. The American Journal of Clinical Nutrition. 2011;**93**:118-126. DOI: 10.3945/ajcn.2010.29888

[123] Meat consumption and cancer risk: A critical review of published meta-analyses. Critical Reviews in Oncology/Hematology. 2016;**97**:1-14. DOI: 10.1016/j.critrevonc.2015.11.008

[124] Kushi LH, Mink PJ, Folsom AR, Anderson KE, Zheng W, Lazovich D, et al. Prospective study of diet and ovarian cancer. American Journal of Epidemiology. 1999;**149**:21-31

[125] Wallin A, Orsini N, Wolk A. Red and processed meat consumption and risk of ovarian cancer: A dose-response meta-analysis of prospective studies. British Journal of Cancer. 2011;**104**:1196-1201. DOI: 10.1038/bjc.2011.49

[126] Kolahdooz F, van der Pols JC, Bain CJ, Marks GC, Hughes MC, Whiteman DC, et al. Meat, fish, and ovarian cancer risk: Results from 2 Australian case-control studies, a systematic review, and meta-analysis. The American Journal of Clinical Nutrition. 2010;**91**:1752-1763. DOI: 10.3945/ajcn.2009.28415

[127] Chang ET, Canchola AJ, Lee VS, Clarke CA, Purdie DM, Reynolds P, et al. Wine and other alcohol consumption and risk of ovarian cancer in the California Teachers Study cohort. Cancer Causes Control. 2007;**18**:91-103. DOI: 10.1007/s10552-006-0083-x

[128] Schouten LJ, Zeegers MPA, Goldbohm RA, van den Brandt PA. Alcohol and ovarian cancer risk: Results from the Netherlands cohort study. Cancer Causes and Control. 2004;**15**:201-209. DOI: 10.1023/B:CACO.0000019512.71560.2b

[129] Gwinn ML, Webster LA, Lee NC, Layde PM, Rubin GL. Alcohol consumption and ovarian cancer risk. American Journal of Epidemiology. 1986;**123**:759-766. DOI: 10.1093/oxfordjournals.aje.a114304

[130] Webb PM, Purdie DM, Bain CJ, Green AC. Alcohol, wine, and risk of epithelial ovarian cancer. Cancer Epidemiology, Biomarkers and Prevention. 2004;**13**:592-599

[131] Gosvig CF, Kjaer SK, Blaakær J, Høgdall E, Høgdall C, Jensen A. Coffee, tea, and caffeine consumption and risk of epithelial ovarian cancer and borderline ovarian tumors: Results from a Danish case-control study. Acta Oncologica. 2015;**54**:1144-1151. DOI: 10.3109/0284186X.2014.1001035

[132] Tworoger SS, Gertig DM, Gates MA, Hecht JL, Hankinson SE. Caffeine, alcohol, smoking, and the risk of incident epithelial ovarian cancer. Cancer. 2008;**112**:1169-1177. DOI: 10.1002/cncr.23275

[133] Huncharek M, Klassen H, Kupelnick B. Dietary beta-carotene intake and the risk of epithelial ovarian cancer: A meta-analysis of 3,782 subjects from five observational studies. Vivo Athens Greece. 2001;**15**:339-343

[134] Terry PD, Qin B, Camacho F, Moorman PG, Alberg AJ, Barnholtz-Sloan JS, et al. Supplemental selenium may decrease ovarian cancer risk in African-American women. The Journal of Nutrition. 2017;**147**:621-627. DOI: 10.3945/jn.116.243279

[135] Dennert G, Zwahlen M, Brinkman M, Vinceti M, Zeegers MPA, Horneber M. Selenium for preventing cancer. Cochrane Database of Systematic Reviews. 2011:CD005195. DOI: 10.1002/14651858.CD005195.pub2

[136] Ong J-S, Cuellar-Partida G, Lu Y, Fasching PA, Hein A, Burghaus S, et al. Association of vitamin D levels and risk of ovarian cancer: A Mendelian randomization study. International Journal of Epidemiology. 2016;**45**:1619-1630. DOI: 10.1093/ije/dyw207

[137] Guo H, Guo J, Xie W, Yuan L, Sheng X. The role of vitamin D in ovarian cancer: Epidemiology, molecular mechanism and prevention. Journal of Ovarian Research. 2018;**11**. DOI: 10.1186/s13048-018-0443-7

[138] Loeb LA. Tobacco causes human cancers—A concept founded on epidemiology and an insightful experiment now requires translation worldwide. Cancer Research. 2016;**76**:765-766. DOI: 10.1158/0008-5472.CAN-16-0149

[139] Marchbanks PA, Wilson H, Bastos E, Cramer DW, Schildkraut JM, Peterson HB. Cigarette smoking and epithelial ovarian cancer by histologic type. Obstetrics and Gynecology. 2000;**95**:255-260

[140] Licaj I, Jacobsen BK, Selmer RM, Maskarinec G, Weiderpass E, Gram IT. Smoking and risk of ovarian cancer by histological subtypes: An analysis among 300 000 Norwegian women. British Journal of Cancer. 2017;**116**:270-276. DOI: 10.1038/bjc.2016.418

[141] Zhang Y, Coogan PF, Palmer JR, Strom BL, Rosenberg L. Cigarette smoking and increased risk of mucinous epithelial ovarian cancer. American Journal of Epidemiology. 2004;**159**:133-139. DOI: 10.1093/aje/kwh015

[142] Faber MT, Kjær SK, Dehlendorff C, Chang-Claude J, Andersen KK, Høgdall E, et al. Cigarette smoking and risk of ovarian cancer: A pooled analysis of 21 case–control studies. Cancer Causes Control CCC. 2013;**24**. DOI: 10.1007/s10552-013-0174-4

[143] Gram IT, Lukanova A, Brill I, Braaten T, Lund E, Lundin E, et al. Cigarette smoking and risk of histological subtypes of epithelial ovarian cancer in the EPIC cohort study. International Journal of Cancer. 2012;**130**:2204-2210. DOI: 10.1002/ijc.26235

[144] Ovarian cancer and smoking: individual participant meta-analysis including 28 114 women with ovarian cancer from 51 epidemiological studies. The Lancet Oncology. 2012;**13**:946-956. DOI: 10.1016/S1470-2045(12)70322-4

[145] Modugno F, Ness RB, Cottreau CM. Cigarette smoking and the risk of mucinous and nonmucinous epithelial ovarian cancer. Epidemiology (Cambridge, Mass.). 2002;**13**:467-471

[146] Terry PD, Miller AB, Jones JG, Rohan TE. Cigarette smoking and the

risk of invasive epithelial ovarian cancer in a prospective cohort study. European Journal of Cancer (Oxford, England: 1990). 2003;**39**:1157-1164

[147] Sayasneh A, Tsivos D, Crawford R. Endometriosis and ovarian cancer: A systematic review. ISRN Obstetrics and Gynecology. 2011;**2011**. DOI: 10.5402/2011/140310

[148] Zafrakas M, Grimbizis G, Timologou A, Tarlatzis BC. Endometriosis and ovarian cancer risk: A systematic review of epidemiological studies. Frontiers in Surgery. 2014;**1**. DOI: 10.3389/fsurg.2014.00014

[149] Brinton LA, Gridley G, Persson I, Baron J, Bergqvist A. Cancer risk after a hospital discharge diagnosis of endometriosis. American Journal of Obstetrics and Gynecology. 1997;**176**:572-579

[150] Vercellini P, Somigliana E, Buggio L, Bolis G, Fedele L. Endometriosis and ovarian cancer. The Lancet Oncology. 2012;**13**:e188-e189. DOI: 10.1016/S1470-2045(12)70198-5

[151] Brilhante AVM, Augusto KL, Portela MC, Sucupira LCG, Oliveira LAF, Pouchaim AJMV, et al. Endometriosis and ovarian cancer: An integrative review (endometriosis and ovarian cancer). Asian Pacific Journal of Cancer Prevention. 2017;**18**:11-16. DOI: 10.22034/APJCP.2017.18.1.11

[152] The Rotterdam ESHRE/ASRM-Sponsored PCOS Consensus Workshop Group. Revised 2003 consensus on diagnostic criteria and long-term health risks related to polycystic ovary syndrome. Fertility and Sterility. 2004;**81**:19-25. DOI: 10.1016/j.fertnstert.2003.10.004

[153] Schildkraut J. Epithelial ovarian cancer risk among women with polycystic ovary syndrome. Obstetrics and Gynecology. 1996;**88**:554-559. DOI: 10.1016/0029-7844(96)00226-8

[154] Carmina E, Lobo RA. Polycystic ovary syndrome (PCOS): Arguably the most common endocrinopathy is associated with significant morbidity in women. The Journal of Clinical Endocrinology and Metabolism. 1999;**84**:1897-1899. DOI: 10.1210/jcem.84.6.5803

[155] Harris HR, Terry KL. Polycystic ovary syndrome and risk of endometrial, ovarian, and breast cancer: A systematic review. Fertility Research and Practice. 2016;**2**:14. DOI: 10.1186/s40738-016-0029-2

[156] Galazis N, Olaleye O, Haoula Z, Layfield R, Atiomo W. Proteomic biomarkers for ovarian cancer risk in women with polycystic ovary syndrome: A systematic review and biomarker database integration. Fertility and Sterility. 2012;**98**:1590-1601.e1. DOI: 10.1016/j.fertnstert.2012.08.002

[157] Rasmussen CB, Kjaer SK, Albieri V, Bandera EV, Doherty JA, Høgdall E, et al. Pelvic inflammatory disease and the risk of ovarian cancer and borderline ovarian tumors: A pooled analysis of 13 case-control studies. American Journal of Epidemiology. 2017;**185**:8-20. DOI: 10.1093/aje/kww161

[158] Zhou Z, Zeng F, Yuan J, Tang J, Colditz GA, Tworoger SS, et al. Pelvic inflammatory disease and the risk of ovarian cancer: A meta-analysis. Cancer Causes Control. 2017;**28**:415-428. DOI: 10.1007/s10552-017-0873-3

[159] Parazzini F, Vecchia CL, Negri E, Moroni S, Dal Pino D, Fedele L. Pelvic inflammatory disease and risk of ovarian cancer. Cancer Epidemiology, Biomarkers and Prevention. 1996;**5**:667-669

[160] Merritt MA, Green AC, Nagle CM, Webb PM, Australian Cancer study (ovarian Cancer), Australian ovarian Cancer study group. Talcum powder, chronic pelvic inflammation and NSAIDs in relation to risk of epithelial ovarian cancer. International Journal of Cancer. 2008;**122**:170-176. DOI: 10.1002/ijc.23017

[161] Greiser CM, Greiser EM, Dören M. Menopausal hormone therapy and risk of ovarian cancer: Systematic review and meta-analysis. Human Reproduction Update. 2007;**13**:453-463. DOI: 10.1093/humupd/dmm012

[162] Danforth KN, Tworoger SS, Hecht JL, Rosner BA, Colditz GA, Hankinson SE. A prospective study of postmenopausal hormone use and ovarian cancer risk. British Journal of Cancer. 2007;**96**:151-156. DOI: 10.1038/sj.bjc.6603527

[163] Beral V, Million Women Study Collaborators, Bull D, Green J, Reeves G. Ovarian cancer and hormone replacement therapy in the million women study. Lancet (London, England). 2007;**369**:1703-1710. DOI: 10.1016/S0140-6736(07)60534-0

[164] Lee AW, Ness RB, Roman LD, TerryKL, SchildkrautJM, Chang-ClaudeJ, et al. Association between menopausal estrogen-only therapy and ovarian carcinoma Risk. Obstetrics and Gynecology. 2016;**127**:828-836. DOI: 10.1097/AOG.0000000000001387

[165] Hormone Replacement Therapy May Increase Ovarian Cancer Risk. Medscape n.d. Available from: http://www.medscape.com/viewarticle/839758 [Accessed: 01 December 2018]

[166] Collaborative Group on Epidemiological Studies of Ovarian Cancer, Beral V, Gaitskell K, Hermon C, Moser K, Reeves G, et al. Menopausal hormone use and ovarian cancer risk: individual participant meta-analysis of 52 epidemiological studies. Lancet (London, England). 2015;**385**:1835-1842. DOI: 10.1016/S0140-6736(14)61687-1

[167] Olsen CM, Green AC, Whiteman DC, Sadeghi S, Kolahdooz F, Webb PM. Obesity and the risk of epithelial ovarian cancer: A systematic review and meta-analysis. European Journal of Cancer. 2007;**43**:690-709. DOI: 10.1016/j.ejca.2006.11.010

[168] Crosbie EJ, Zwahlen M, Kitchener HC, Egger M, Renehan AG. Body mass index, hormone replacement therapy, and endometrial cancer risk: A meta-analysis. Cancer Epidemiology, Biomarkers and Prevention. 2010;**19**:3119-3130. DOI: 10.1158/1055-9965.EPI-10-0832

[169] Olsen CM, Nagle CM, Whiteman DC, Ness R, Pearce CL, Pike MC, et al. Obesity and risk of ovarian cancer subtypes: Evidence from the Ovarian Cancer Association Consortium. Endocrine-Related Cancer. 2013;**20**:251-262. DOI: 10.1530/ERC-12-0395

[170] Tworoger SS, Huang T. Obesity and ovarian cancer. Recent Results in Cancer Research. 2016;**208**:155-176. DOI: 10.1007/978-3-319-42542-9_9

[171] Jochem C, Schlecht I, Leitzmann M. Epidemiologic relationship between obesity and ovarian cancer. In: Berger NA, Klopp AH, Lu KH, editors. Focus on Gynecologic Malignancies. Vol. 13. Cham: Springer International Publishing; 2018. pp. 21-30. DOI: 10.1007/978-3-319-63483-8_2

[172] Nagle CM, Dixon SC, Jensen A, Kjaer SK, Modugno F, deFazio A, et al. Obesity and survival among women with ovarian cancer: Results from the Ovarian Cancer Association Consortium. British Journal of Cancer.

2015;**113**:817-826. DOI: 10.1038/bjc.2015.245

[173] Foong KW, Bolton H. Obesity and ovarian cancer risk: A systematic review. Post Reproductive Health. 2017;**23**:183-198. DOI: 10.1177/2053369117709225

[174] Wentzensen N, Poole EM, Trabert B, White E, Arslan AA, Patel AV, et al. Ovarian cancer risk factors by histologic subtype: An analysis from the ovarian Cancer Cohort Consortium. Journal of Clinical Oncology: Official Journal of the American Society of Clinical Oncology. 2016;**34**:2888-2898. DOI: 10.1200/JCO.2016.66.8178

[175] Luan N-N, Wu Q-J, Gong T-T, Vogtmann E, Wang Y-L, Lin B. Breastfeeding and ovarian cancer risk: A meta-analysis of epidemiologic studies. The American Journal of Clinical Nutrition. 2013;**98**:1020-1031. DOI: 10.3945/ajcn.113.062794

[176] McNeilly AS. Lactational control of reproduction. Reproduction, Fertility, and Development. 2001;**13**:583-590

[177] Stadel BV. The etiology and prevention of ovarian cancer. American Journal of Obstetrics and Gynecology. 1975;**123**:772-774. DOI: 10.1016/0002-9378(75)90509-8

[178] Collaborative Group on Epidemiological Studies of Ovarian Cancer, Beral V, Doll R, Hermon C, Peto R, Reeves G. Ovarian cancer and oral contraceptives: Collaborative reanalysis of data from 45 epidemiological studies including 23,257 women with ovarian cancer and 87,303 controls. Lancet (London, England). 2008;**371**:303-314. DOI: 10.1016/S0140-6736(08)60167-1

[179] Why do Oral Contraceptives Prevent Ovarian Cancer? - Full Text View - ClinicalTrials.gov n.d. Available from: https://clinicaltrials.gov/ct2/show/NCT02155777 [Accessed: |19 November 2018]

[180] Tsilidis KK, Allen NE, Key TJ, Dossus L, Lukanova A, Bakken K, et al. Oral contraceptive use and reproductive factors and risk of ovarian cancer in the European prospective investigation into cancer and nutrition. 2011;**1442**. DOI: 10.1038/bjc.2011.371

[181] Bosetti C, Negri E, Trichopoulos D, Franceschi S, Beral V, Tzonou A, et al. Long-term effects of oral contraceptives on ovarian cancer risk. International Journal of Cancer. 2002;**102**:262-265. DOI: 10.1002/ijc.10696

[182] Moorman PG, Havrilesky LJ, Gierisch JM, Coeytaux RR, Lowery WJ, Peragallo Urrutia R, et al. Oral contraceptives and risk of ovarian cancer and breast cancer among high-risk women: A systematic review and meta-analysis. Journal of Clinical Oncology. 2013;**31**:4188-4198. DOI: 10.1200/JCO.2013.48.9021

[183] Ferris JS, Daly MB, Buys SS, Genkinger JM, Liao Y, Terry MB. Oral contraceptive and reproductive risk factors for ovarian cancer within sisters in the breast cancer family registry. British Journal of Cancer. 2014;**110**:1074-1080. DOI: 10.1038/bjc.2013.803

[184] Rice MS, Hankinson SE, Tworoger SS. Tubal ligation, hysterectomy, unilateral oophorectomy, and risk of ovarian cancer in the nurses' health studies. Fertility and Sterility. 2014;**102**:192-198.e3. DOI: 10.1016/j.fertnstert.2014.03.041

[185] Chan JK, Urban R, Capra AM, Jacoby V, Osann K, Whittemore A, et al. Ovarian cancer rates after hysterectomy with and without salpingo-oophorectomy. Obstetrics and Gynecology. 2014;**123**:65-72. DOI: 10.1097/AOG.0000000000000061

[186] Narod SA, Sun P, Ghadirian P, Lynch H, Isaacs C, Garber J, et al. Tubal ligation and risk of ovarian cancer in carriers of BRCA1 or BRCA2 mutations: A case-control study. The Lancet. 2001;**357**:1467-1470. DOI: 10.1016/S0140-6736(00)04642-0

[187] Gaitskell K, Green J, Pirie K, Reeves G. Tubal ligation and ovarian cancer risk in a large cohort: Substantial variation by histological type. International Journal of Cancer. 2016;**138**:1076-1084. DOI: 10.1002/ijc.29856

[188] Hannan LM, Leitzmann MF, Lacey JV, Colbert LH, Albanes D, Schatzkin A, et al. Physical activity and risk of ovarian cancer: A prospective cohort study in the United States. Cancer Epidemiology and Prevention Biomarkers. 2004;**13**:765-770

[189] Moorman PG, Jones LW, Akushevich L, Schildkraut JM. Recreational physical activity and ovarian cancer risk and survival. Annals of Epidemiology. 2011;**21**:178-187. DOI: 10.1016/j.annepidem.2010.10.014

[190] Tavani A, Gallus S, La Vecchia C, Dal Maso L, Negri E, Pelucchi C, et al. Physical activity and risk of ovarian cancer: An Italian case-control study. International Journal of Cancer. 2001;**91**:407-411

[191] Pan SY, Ugnat A-M, Mao Y. Physical activity and the risk of ovarian cancer: A case-control study in Canada. International Journal of Cancer. 2005;**117**:300-307. DOI: 10.1002/ijc.21157

Chapter 5

Appendiceal Neuroendocrine Tumors and Anorectal Melanoma

Marco Clementi, Renato Pietroletti, Andrea Ciarrocchi, Federica d'Ascanio, Guido Rindi and Francesco Carlei

Abstract

Tumor growth and spread are a complicated matter and are the result of many interconnected factors. The analysis of patterns emerging from highly numerous populations might help shed some light on such an intricate mechanism. In this respect, our studies are mostly based on the SEER database, a nation representative dataset collecting data regarding the US population, over a very long time span. This approach is revealed to be particularly useful for rare tumors, as prospective studies are not feasible. Here, we present the results and the clinical implications of our inquires: we show the impact on overall survival of several morphological and demographic characteristics of various malignancies including anorectal melanoma and neuroendocrine tumors of the appendix. The impact of surgical treatment is discussed as well. Finally, we endorse the need to find more reliable markers of tumor biology, such as genetic patterns, to tailor an effective multidisciplinary treatment.

Keywords: neuroendocrine tumors of the appendix, anorectal melanoma, multidisciplinary treatment, lymph node spread, carcinoid tumors

1. Introduction

Tumor progression is the result of several complex and interrelated mechanisms. Apart from stage of the disease, biologic features of the neoplastic cell play a relevant role. Size, location, grading, cell differentiation, genotype mutation, and expression of oncogene are well-known features of the primary tumor all responsible for tumor progression and disease aggressiveness. Progression of the disease may occur either as a result of local growth and invasion or by means of distant spread of the disease in targeted organs via lymphatic or venous outflow. The two phenomena are a consequence of specific biologic features of the neoplastic cell and thus may occur independently from each other.

Rare tumors are particularly difficult to investigate, since prospective analyses are not easy to plan due to the small number of patients observed and treated. Therefore, reliable prognostic information are lacking or are controversial. Neuroendocrine tumor in general and those located in the appendix in particular are subjected to several controversies. Size and histology of appendiceal carcinoids, for instance, seem to influence heavily lymphatic spread and thus prognosis. Surgical strategy is debated in consequence of such features with the aim of obtaining adequate lymph node harvesting to establish a correct stadiation and prognosis.

As far as recto-anal melanoma is concerned, prognosis is very poor due to frequent diagnostic delay and rarity of the disease leading to misdiagnosis and advanced stage at presentation. However, in spite of poor prognosis, extensive surgery is still advocated although the experiences reported in the literature are very limited and sparse, undoubtedly weak to support such aggressive approach.

Thus, since high-quality data regarding rare diseases such as appendiceal carcinoids or anorectal melanoma neither are presently available nor can be obtained prospectively in a short time, a reasonable approach to partially overcome such limitations is to analyze a pool of data in large tumor registry, collecting retrospective cases. In order to maximize the statistical power of the study, potential confounders by means of multivariate analysis must be taken into account. Mathematical models can be adopted to achieve such a goal; in particular Cox regression models or matching populations by the propensity score can be successfully adopted. Populations can be described by using descriptive statistical methods for categorical and continuous variables.

We planned a study on appendiceal carcinoids and anorectal melanoma accessing the Surveillance, Epidemiology, and End Results (SEER) database, a dataset collecting a large amount of data pertaining cancer in the US population over a time span of decades.

We were able to demonstrate the impact on overall survival of different morphological and demographic characteristics of anorectal melanoma and neuroendocrine tumors of the appendix [1–4], discussing their impact on surgical treatment and prognosis.

We accessed the SEER database to retrieve the data to analyze. Then, we selected the variables that we wanted to introduce in our models to assess their impact on survival. In any statistical test performed, $P < 0.05$ was considered significant. The covariates we focused on were demographic and morphologic. In most occasions, we retrieved data on age of the patients, gender, stage of disease, ethnicity, tumor size, and lymph node invasion.

2. Melanoma of the anorectum

Melanoma of the anorectum has a dismal prognosis since frequent early metastases make any treatment ineffective, despite a multimodal approach [5]. The rectum and anal canal represent the third most common primary site of origin [6]. The resemblance to benign common conditions such as hemorrhoids often delays the diagnosis, strongly impairing the possibility of treatment with intention to cure (**Figure 1**) (**Table 1**).

Site of origin is a determining prognostic factor for cutaneous melanoma [7]. With regard to mucosal melanomas, vulvar tumors proved a better outcome than those originating from the vagina [8]. Our interest was based on the fact that although most of the tumors arise in the anal canal, a not negligible percentage of the neoplasia is located more proximally in the rectum [9]. It seems reasonable that distal tumors could have a better prognosis, because they are clinically apparent sooner than more proximal masses. The latter, in fact, tend to become apparent only when symptoms of occlusion of the large intestine ensue. Moreover, anorectal melanomas arising in the anus/anal canal or rectum drain in different lymph node chains. To verify such hypothesis, we investigated the impact of site of origin on overall survival. Bello et al. [10] showed different patterns of local recurrence: anorectal melanoma recurred more often systemically, whereas tumors of the anal canal recurred first at inguinal lymph nodes. However, the overall survival did not vary between the groups. Our results confirmed that the site of origin along the rectum and anal canal does not influence survival ($P = 0.164$).

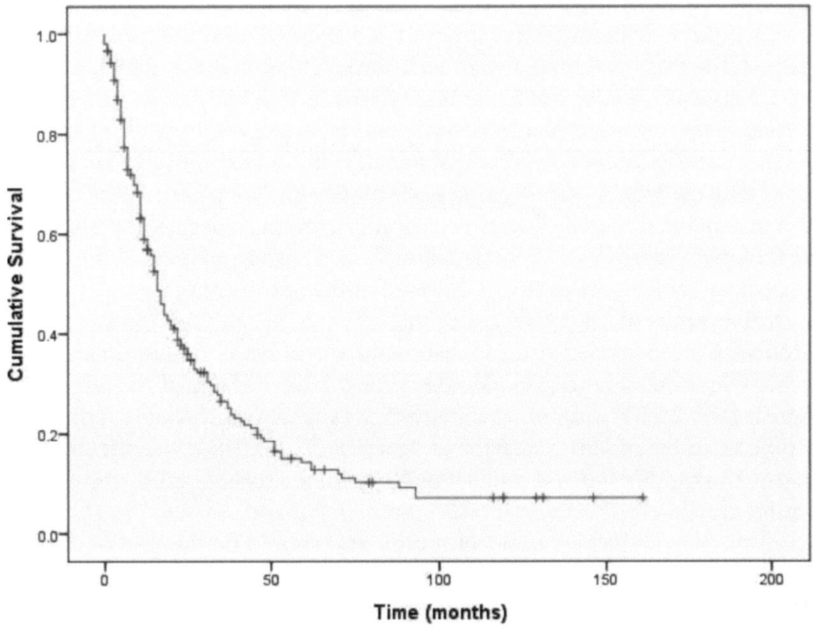

Figure 1.
Survival curve for patients affected by anorectal melanoma.

Category	P value	Hazard ratio	Confidence interval
Site of origin (rectum)	0.275	1.233	0.845–1.798
Gender (male)	0.707	0.932	0.646–1.344
Size	0.519	1.000	0.998–1.001
Race (other)	0.019	2.291	1.148–4.575
Race (White)	0.824	0.945	0.571–1.562
LN rate	0.027	1.873	1.076–3.261
Age	0.150	1.010	0.997–1.023
Surgical intervention (APR/AR)	0.194	0.783	0.541–1.133
Stage (regional)	0.880	1.035	0.659–1.628
Stage (distant)	0.347	1.241	0.792–1.945
Radiation (performed)	0.150	1.461	0.870–2.452
Lymphadenectomy (performed)	0.904	0.977	0.663–1.438

Table 1.
Cox regression model for anorectal melanoma.

Stage of disease did not prove to have an impact on survival (P = 0.880 for regional stage and P = 0.347 for distant stage). However, our results should be considered with caution, given that we had to use the SEER historical stage classification to obtain data consistent through time. In fact, the TNM has been changing over time, and we decided to avoid its use, in order to not reduce the overall number of cases available for final analysis. In other studies, stage showed a significant impact on survival [11, 12].

In addition, we inquired the prognostic value of locoregional metastatic lymph nodes and the impact of lymphadenectomy on overall survival. To better understand the role of lymph node metastasis on prognosis, we introduced the concept of lymph node ratio, defined as the ratio between metastatic lymph nodes and total lymph nodes harvested. This was necessary to avoid bias related to the extent of lymphadenectomy. In our series, performing lymphadenectomy did not improve survival (P = 0.904). This could be due to early tumor spread to distant sites, thus overcoming the potential benefits of local control. Sentinel lymph node biopsy has not proven to be useful in anorectal melanoma due to the low rate of positive findings, despite the presence of more distant metastases [13]. Therefore, lymph node spread of anorectal melanoma is far less predictable than, for example, the carcinoma of the breast.

Size of the tumor did not affect survival (P = 0.519), although it was previously associated with an increased risk of mesorectal and mesenteric lymph node metastases in anorectal melanoma [14]. Gender (P = 0.707) and age of the patient at time of diagnosis (P = 0.150) did not affect survival as well. Interestingly, ethnicity was found to be an independent predictor of survival (P = 0.019). Specifically, American Indian/Alaskan Native and Asian/Pacific Islander (other) ethnicity showed a worse outcome.

Radical surgery is the best option for cure and should be the goal of treatment [15, 16]. Optimal surgical strategies need to balance the need for radical excision including lymphadenectomy against increasing operative morbidity. Consistently with the recent literature, the type of surgical intervention was not a significant prognostic factor (P = 0.183). The fundamental dilemma regarding the treatment of anorectal melanoma is the choice between abdominoperineal/anterior resection and local wide excision. Previous studies suggested that aggressive treatment could provide better overall results by achieving local oncological control of the disease. More recently, another trend of treatment has been emerging. According to Matsuda et al. [17], no significant differences between the two options of treatment in terms of overall survival were apparent. Abdominoperineal resection has failed to show any advantage in terms of survival, adding a higher morbidity and poorer quality of life. Thus, local excision has now become the standard of treatment. In case of tumor recurrence, abdominoperineal or anterior resection can be performed as a salvage procedure [18, 19].

Radiation therapy did not influence prognosis (P = 0.864), although it has been demonstrated to provide better local control, especially in patients undergoing local excision [20]. The reason stands on the fact that multifocality of the disease and radial microscopic spread make effective radical excision difficult. Targeted or systemic immunotherapy as well as regional chemotherapy has been described to improve overall survival in patients with pelvic recurrences [21–23]. Molecular analysis of recurrence melanoma is an important factor in determining which type of therapy should be adopted [24]. However, better local control is ineffective when distant spread has occurred early in the natural history of the disease.

Interestingly, race resulted to be associated with prognosis. In particular, Spanish people showed a more than double hazard ratio of death as compared to African Americans. Although this result might be intriguing, we do not have sufficient data to discuss it, given the lack of genetic analyses regarding our series. Probably, both genetic and environmental factors may play a role.

3. Appendiceal neuroendocrine tumors

Current surgical strategy for primary neuroendocrine tumors of the appendix is mostly based on tumor size. Right hemicolectomy is warranted for neuroendocrine tumors larger than 2 cm in diameter, whereas appendectomy alone is performed for tumors smaller than 1 cm. Patients affected by neuroendocrine tumors with a diameter of 1–2 cm are candidates for hemicolectomy in case of invasion of the cecum or mesoappendix or infiltration of the lymph-vascular system [25]. This treatment algorithm was introduced on the basis of retrospective outcome data provided by Moertel and his colleagues. The disease is usually quite indolent, and overall survival is good [26] (**Table 2**).

At present, there is no proof of survival benefits of right hemicolectomy compared to appendectomy alone. In one of our studies, we wanted to verify whether 2 cm is a good cutoff value for identifying the best candidates for right hemicolectomy. The indication for such a procedure in patients with neuroendocrine tumors larger than 2 cm in diameter stands on the augmented risk of visceral lymph node involvement. In fact, tumor size is a predictor of nodal spread [27]. Assuming that there may be a progression from positive lymph nodes to distant metastases, hemicolectomy is recommended to achieve oncologic radicality. It has been argued that a more extended procedure may have a staging value, but not an actual impact on survival [28].

Our data showed that the type of surgical procedure did not reach statistical significance ($P = 0.513$), proving that an extended procedure does not confer a survival advantage. Such findings and the indolent course of the disease suggest that formal right hemicolectomy should be performed in young healthy patients, whereas those burdened with comorbidities can be treated with appendectomy without affecting oncologic outcomes. In other words, tumor size greater than 2 cm should not be considered an absolute indication for right hemicolectomy.

In another study, we focused on the natural history of metastatic lymph nodes and their clinical impact for primary pure and mixed neuroendocrine tumors of the appendix (**Figure 2**). The rationale for the surgical treatment is based on the risk of lymph node spread. However, the role of such an event on the natural history of the disease is not clear. First, the survival curve of our populations showed that pure carcinoids have a better prognosis than those with mixed variants ($P < 0.001$). After controlling for age, sex, tumor size, surgical intervention, and lymph nodes rate, a Cox proportional hazards model showed that histology was an independent predictor of overall survival ($P = 0.004$). This suggested that pure and mixed carcinoids differ with respect to their biological aggressiveness. For that reason, we analyzed patients having either pure or mixed carcinoids as two distinct series.

	Interaction* (P value)	Group	P value	Hazard ratio	Confidence interval
Gender (female)	0.066	Pure	0.154	0.538	0.229–1.263
		Mixed	0.347	1.201	0.820–1.758
Tumor size (≤2 cm)	0.017	Pure	0.896	0.937	0.355–2.474
		Mixed	<0.001	0.442	0.286–0.683
Surgical intervention (less than RHC)	0.017	Pure	0.029	0.241	0.067–0.867
		Mixed	0.019	1.675	1.088–2.578
Age	<0.001	Pure	<0.001	1.083	1.051–1.116
		Mixed	<0.001	1.041	1.026–1.056
LN rate	0.012	Pure	0.039	5.295	1.089–25.754
		Mixed	<0.001	17.471	10.47–33.382

Table 2.
Cox regression models for neuroendocrine tumors.

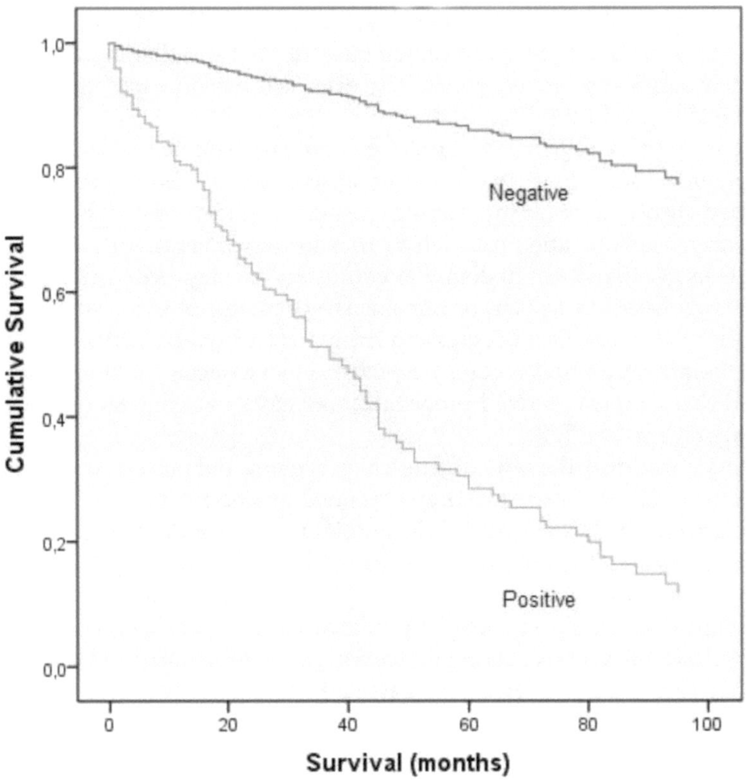

Figure 2.
Survival curve for patients affected by neuroendocrine tumors, according to lymph node status.

Age and surgical intervention (less than right hemicolectomy compared to hemicolectomy or more extended procedure) were found to be independent prognostic factors for both pure ($P < 0.001$ and $P < 0.001$) and mixed carcinoids ($P = 0.029$ and $P = 0.019$). In the latter group, tumor size ($P < 0.001$) was another independent predictor of survival. It is well established that the biological behavior of mixed neuroendocrine tumors can somewhat resemble that of adenocarcinoma, therefore showing a more aggressive behavior. Lymph node rate was found to have a strong independent negative impact on survival for both pure ($P = 0.039$) and mixed neuroendocrine tumors ($P < 0.001$). Metastatic spread to lymph nodes is thus of major importance to both groups. The presence of metastatic nodes largely affects overall survival and represents a reliable clinical hallmark of the aggressiveness of these tumors.

Right hemicolectomy or a more extended procedure exerted a significant protective effect with pure neuroendocrine tumors and a negative effect with mixed neuroendocrine tumors. This controversial result could be related to the higher frequency of distant metastases in the mixed group, although we were unable to test that idea because of the limitations of the SEER database.

Our studies however suffer from several limitations due to their retrospective nature and to well-known shortcomings of the SEER database. Some data were missing, thus limiting the numerosity of the populations. Moreover, the SEER database provides only a certain type of variable and no entries regarding aspects related to molecular biology. However, these are the best data available, when it is not feasible to design randomized prospective studies.

4. Conclusion

Tumor growth and spread are complex processes. Rare diseases are the most difficult to analyze, due to controversial issues and lack of data. Moreover, morphologic data retrieved from large databases do not always provide accurate results regarding the biologic aggressiveness and survival. Therefore, molecular biology markers and genetic profiling should be the basis of future investigations.

Author details

Marco Clementi[1]*, Renato Pietroletti[2], Andrea Ciarrocchi[2], Federica d'Ascanio[2], Guido Rindi[3] and Francesco Carlei[1]

1 Department of Biotechnological and Applied Clinical Sciences, University of L'Aquila, San Salvatore Hospital, L'Aquila, Italy

2 Surgical Coloproctology University of L'Aquila, Hospital Val Vibrata-Sant'Omero (TE), Italy

3 Unit of Pathology Fondazione Universitaria A Gemelli, Catholic University of Rome, Italy

*Address all correspondence to: marco.clementi@univaq.it

References

[1] Ciarrocchi A, Pietroletti R, Carlei F, Amicucci G. Extensive surgery and lymphadenectomy do not improve survival in primary melanoma of the anorectum: Results from analysis of a large database (SEER). Colorectal Diseases. Feb 2016;**19**(2):158-164

[2] Ciarrocchi A, Pietroletti R, Carlei F, Necozione S, Amicucci G. Propensity adjusted appraisal of the surgical strategy for appendiceal carcinoids. Techniques in Coloproctology. Jan 2014; **19**(1):35-41

[3] Ciarrocchi A, Pietroletti R, Carlei F, Amicucci G. Clinical significance of metastatic lymph nodes in the gut of patients with pure and mixed primary appendiceal carcinoids. Diseases of the Colon and Rectum. Jun 2016;**59**(6): 508-512

[4] Ciarrocchi A, Pietroletti R, Carlei F, Amicucci G. Outcome of anal and rectal melanoma: Has site of origin a prognostic value? Analysis of 287 patients. European Surgery. Oct 2015; **47**(5):262-265

[5] Thibault C, Sagar P, Nivatvongs S, Ilstrup DM, Wolff BG. Anorectal melanoma: An incurable disease? Diseases of the Colon and Rectum. 1997; **40**:661-668

[6] Chang AE, Karnell LH, Menck HR. The National Cancer Data Base report on cutaneous and noncutaneous melanoma: A summary of 84,836 cases from the past decade. The American College of Surgeons Commission on cancer and the American Cancer Society. Cancer. 1998; **83**:1664-1678

[7] Lachiewicz AM, Berwick M, Wiggins CL, Thomas NE. Survival differences between patients with scalp or neck melanoma and those with melanoma of other sites in the surveillance, epidemiology, and end results (SEER) program. Archives of Dermatology. 2008;**144**:515-521

[8] Smyth EC, Flavin M, Barbi A, Bogdatch K, Wolchok JD, Chapman PB, et al. Memorial Sloan-Kettering Cancer Center (MSKCC) single institutional vulvovaginal mucosal melanoma (VVMM) experience from 1995 to 2010. The European Journal of Cancer. 2011; **47**:661

[9] Cagir B, Whiteford MH, Topham A, Rakinic J, Fry RD. Changing epidemiology of anorectal melanoma. Diseases of the Colon and Rectum. 1999; **42**:1203-1208

[10] Bello DM, Smyth E, Perez D, Khan S, Temple LK, Ariyan CE, et al. Anal versus rectal melanoma: Does site of origin predict outcome? Diseases of the Colon and Rectum. 2013;**56**:150-157

[11] Pessaux P, Pocard M, Elias D, Duvillard P, Avril MF, Zimmerman P, et al. Surgical management of primary anorectal melanoma. The British Journal of Surgery. 2004;**244**:1183-1187

[12] Yeh JJ, Shia J, Hwu WJ, Busam KJ, Paty PB, Guillem JG, et al. The role of abdominoperineal resection as surgical therapy for anorectal melanoma. The Annals of Surgery. 2006;**244**:1012-1017

[13] Kelly P, Zagars GK, Cormier JN, Ross MI, Guadagnolo BA. Sphincter-sparing local excision and hypofractionated radiation therapy for anorectal melanoma: A 20-year experience. Cancer. 2011;**117**:4747-4755

[14] Wang M, Zhang Z, Zhu J, Sheng W, Lian P, Liu F, et al. Tumour diameter is a predictor of mesorectal and mesenteric lymph node metastases in anorectal melanoma. Colorectal Disease. 2013;**15**:1086-1092

[15] Nilsson PJ, Ragnarsson-Olding BK. Importance of clear resection margins in anorectal malignant melanoma. The British Journal of Surgery. 2010;**97**: 98-103

[16] Choi BM, Kim HR, Yun HR, Choi SH, Cho YB, Kim HC, et al. Treatment outcomes of anorectal melanoma. Journal of the Korean Society of Coloproctology. 2011;**27**: 27-30

[17] Matsuda A, Miyashita M, Matsumoto S, Takahashi G, Matsutani T, Yamada T, et al. Abdominoperineal resection provides better local control but equivalent overall survival to local excision of anorectal malignant melanoma: A systematic review. Annals of Surgery. 2015;**261**:670-677

[18] Bullard KM, Tuttle TM, Rothenberger DA, Madoff RD, Baxter NN, Finne CO, et al. Surgical therapy for anorectal melanoma. Journal of the American College of Surgeons. 2003;**196**:206-211

[19] Belli F, Gallino GF, Vullo SL, Mariani L, Poiasina E, Leo E. Melanoma of the anorectal region: The experience of the National Cancer Institute of Milano. European Journal of Surgical Oncology. 2009;**35**:757-762

[20] Meguerditchian AN, Meterissian SH, Dunn KB. Anorectal melanoma: Diagnosis and treatment. Diseases of the Colon and Rectum. 2011; **54**:638-644

[21] Guadagni S, Palumbo G, Fiorentini G, Clementi M, Marsili L, Giordano AV, et al. Surgical versus percutaneous isolated pelvic perfusion (IPP) for advanced melanoma: Comparison in terms of melphalan pharmacokinetic pelvic bio-availability. BMC Research Notes. 2017;**10**:411

[22] Guadagni S, Fiorentini G, Clementi M, Palumbo G, Masedu F, Deraco M, et al. MGMT methylation correlates with melphalan pelvic perfusion survival in stage III melanoma patients: A pilot study. Melanoma Research. 2017;**27**(5):439-447

[23] Guadagni S, Fiorentini G, Clementi M, Palumbo G, Chiominto A, Cappelli S, et al. Melphalan hypoxic perfusion with hemophiltration for melanoma locoregional metastases in the pelvis. Journal of Surgical Research. 2017;**215**:114-124

[24] Guadagni S, Fiorentini G, Clementi M, Palumbo G, Palumbo P, Chiominto A, et al. Does locoregional chemotherapy still matter in the treatment of advanced pelvic melanoma? International Journal of Molecular Sciences. 2017;**18**(11):2382

[25] Pape UF, Perren A, Niederle B, Gross D, Gress T, Costa F, et al. ENETS consensus guidelines for the management of patients with neuroendocrine neoplasms from the jejuno-ileum and appendix including goblet cell carcinomas. Neuroendocrinology. 2012;**95**:135-156

[26] Moertel CG, Weiland LH, Nagorney DM, Dockerty MB. Carcinoid tumor of the appendix: Treatment and prognosis. The New England Journal of Medicine. 1987;**317**:1699-1701

[27] Groth SS, Virnig BA, Al-Refaie WB, Jarosek SL, Jensen EH, Tuttle TM. Appendiceal carcinoid tumors: Predictors of lymph node metastasis and the impact of right hemicolectomy on survival. Journal of Surgical Oncology. 2011;**103**:39-45

[28] Bamboat ZM, Berger DL. Is right hemicolectomy for 2.0-cm appendiceal carcinoids justified? Archives of Surgery. 2006;**142**:349-352

Chapter 6

Neuroimmunoendocrine Interactions in Tumorigenesis and Breast Cancer

Rocío Alejandra Ruiz-Manzano,
Tania de Lourdes Ochoa-Mercado, Mariana Segovia-Mendoza,
Karen Elizabeth Nava-Castro, Margarita Isabel Palacios-Arreola
and Jorge Morales-Montor

Abstract

Organism homeostasis is regulated through the tri-directional relationships between immune, endocrine, and nervous systems. These relationships are established by a complex network of chemokines, cytokines, hormones (peptide and non-peptide), neurotransmitters, and neurohormones that act onto its target cells, through common receptors. Despite initial attribution of the exclusive action of each molecule group (neurotransmitters, hormones, and cytokines), to the function of one specific system (nervous, endocrine, and immune, respectively), ligand and receptor pleiotropy and redundancy showed the multidirectional communication between systems. Cancer and metabolic and autoimmune diseases get established when homeostasis is disrupted. These interactions act in different disease levels, in cancer, since initial immunosurveillance phase, until immunosubversion and metastasis, in all cases is crucial for tumor development, cancer outcome, and patient prognosis.

Keywords: neuroimmunoendocrine network, breast cancer, neuroimmunoregulation, endocrinoimmune regulation, tumor, cytokines, steroids, neurotransmitters

1. Introduction

Cancer is one of the most common health issues worldwide. According to the World Health Organization (WHO), in 2018 18,078,957 new cases and 9,555,027 related deaths were reported. Breast cancer is the second leading cancer, after lung cancer, but is the first in women incidence and prevalence [1]. An estimation made in 2009 calculated that one out of eight American women could develop breast cancer in their life course [2].

There are several risk factors associated with breast cancer. The first and most important is gender; as mentioned before, women get breast cancer more often than males. Other risk factors are early menarche, first terminal pregnancy after 30 years old, late menopause, nulliparity, no breastfeeding, overweight or obesity, family or personal history of breast cancer, alcohol abuse, consumption of hormone oral

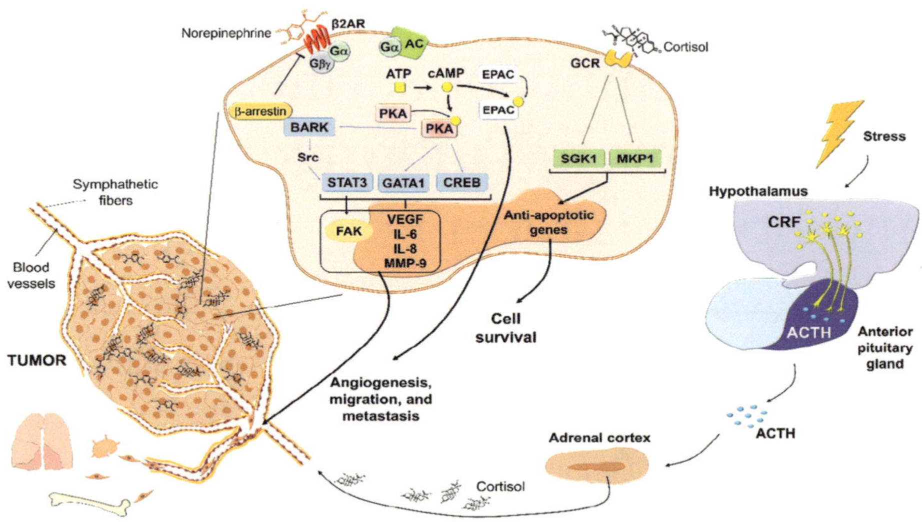

Figure 1.
Nervous regulation during breast tumor growth and metastasis. Sympathetic fibers and blood vessels infiltrate tumor and are responsible for tumor communication with the nervous system. Sympathetic fibers release norepinephrine in tumor, which binds to β_2-adrenergic receptor in the tumor cell membrane and activates adenylate cyclase through G-protein-coupled receptor subunit α. AC promotes ATP-cAMP conversion, and cAMP activates protein kinase A and exchange protein activated by adenylyl cyclase. PKA phosphorylates β-adrenergic receptor kinase, CREB, and GATA1 transcription factors. BARK recruits β-arrestin, inhibits β-adrenergic signal, and activates Src kinase, which in turn activates STAT3 and downstream focal adhesion kinase. FAK enhances migration. CREB, GATA1, and STAT3 promote VEGF, IL-6, IL-8, and MMP-9 expression, enhancing angiogenesis, migration, and invasion. In the other pathway activated through cAMP, EPAC also promotes cell migration. Stress stimulates hypothalamic-pituitary-adrenocortical axis, and the hypothalamus secretes corticotropin-releasing factor (CRF) that stimulates the adrenocorticotropic hormone (ACTH) secretion into blood vessels and systemic circulation. ACTH in adrenal gland cortex stimulates cortisol release. In tumor, cortisol binds to glucocorticoid receptor (GCR) in breast cancer cells and promotes the expression of MAPK phosphatase-1 (MKP1) and serine/threonine protein kinase 1 (SGK1) and other genes related to cell survival and apoptosis protection.

contraceptives or menopausal hormone therapy, and environmental pollution with compounds such as bisphenols and phthalates, among others [3–5].

To classify breast cancer, the actualized TNM anatomical staging system categorizes primary tumor (T), regional lymph node invasion (N), and distant metastases (M), to determine the actual stage group of breast cancer. This classification is very useful, not only for diagnosis and prognosis but also for treatment. In addition to the anatomical staging system, factor-based prognostic stage groups that include tumor grade (histological), hormone receptor status, and a multigene panel status (when is available) were added in the 2017 TNM meeting [2, 3, 6].

Hormone receptor status takes into account the presence of estrogen receptor (ER), progesterone receptor (PR), and human epidermal growth factor receptor 2 (HER-2) in tumor mammary cells. There are some characteristics that determine the status of the tumor, such as anatomical localization, tumor grade, hormone receptor status, and, with it, the prognostic and treatment of breast cancer [6].

A normal breast is composed of mammary glands (lobules and ducts), fibrous connective and adipose tissues, blood and lymph vessels, lymph nodes, nerves, and ligaments [7]. Duct branches form each mammary gland epithelium whose caliber is decreased until it forms ductules that flow into lobes [7, 8]. The epithelium is formed by luminal epithelial cells and basal epithelial cells, also known as myoepithelial cells, adjacent to the basement membrane [9]. Proliferation and apoptosis of mammary epithelia are regulated by the extracellular matrix (ECM) signals [10]. Either lobules or ducts can become dysplastic and eventually neoplastic, a phenomenon also regulated by ECM, and adjacent cell interactions, including stromal, vascular, fibroblasts, and immune cells, may favor the transformation and uncontrolled proliferation of cells in the breast tissue.

In breast cancer progression, there are three phases: benign disease and noninvasive and invasive cancer (**Figure 1**). By definition, benign disease and noninvasive cancer share the same condition, where transformed cells do not trespass the basal membrane but are differentiated by histological grade. An example of this is the lobular carcinoma in situ, classified as a benign tumor, with associated risk in developing carcinoma [6]. On the other hand, in the invasive cancer, cells migrate through basal membrane to stromal breast and/or adjacent tissues and organs [11].

Several interactions determine different outcomes in tumor development, including the interactions among nervous, immune, and endocrine systems with the tumor. Next, we described the overall function of these systems in breast cancer and finally the interactions between them.

2. System interactions in breast cancer

2.1 The role of the nervous system on tumor growth and metastasis

Nervous regulation during cancer is mainly mediated through the sympathetic nervous system (SNS) and the hypothalamic-pituitary-adrenocortical (HPA) axis [12].

2.1.1 Sympathetic nervous system

The sympathetic nervous system regulates the organism's vital involuntary functions and is in charge of the "fight-or-flight" response in danger and stressful situations and modulates the connection between the central nervous system and immune system [13].

SNS nerve fibers emerge from the thoracolumbar spinal cord, innervate different tissues, and produce norepinephrine [12, 14]. Nowadays, it is known that sympathetic nerve fibers innervate the bone marrow, thymus (primary lymphoid organs), spleen and lymph nodes (secondary lymphoid organs), and mucosa- (MALT), bronchus- (BALT), and gut- (GALT) associated lymphoid tissues [15–17]. Epinephrine arrives to the target tissue through blood circulation after being produced in the adrenal gland. Both norepinephrine and epinephrine bind with different affinities to adrenergic receptors α (α_1/α_2) and β ($\beta_1/\beta_2/\beta_3$) in target cells in different tissues and organs, such as the heart, brain, adipose tissue, mammary gland, ovaries, prostate, lymphoid tissue, bones, and different types of cancer cells [13, 14].

These adrenergic receptors are expressed differentially. In smooth muscles α_1AR and α_2AR can be found, although the latter also is expressed in platelets and neurons [14]. Regarding β receptors, of which noradrenaline is the main ligand, β_1AR can be found in the adipose tissue and cardiac muscle. And β_2-adrenergic receptors (β_2ARs) are expressed in tumor and immune cells, in the heart, lung tissue, and smooth muscle. At least, β_3AR can be found in the adipose tissue. Either β_1AR, β_2AR, or β_3AR activates cAMP and in turn stimulates protein kinase A (PKA) [14].

2.1.2 Adrenergic signaling in tumors

β_2AR expression has been detected in breast cancer cell lines, with different densities among them [18], and also in human breast tumor biopsies [19, 20]. Therefore, β_2AR expression should be considered if a β_2AR agonist treatment is going to be performed [21].

It is known that β_2AR signaling regulates proliferation and tumor cell invasion; this is evidenced with β_2AR blockers and the associated beneficial effect in breast cancer recurrence and bone, lung, and brain metastasis [13, 22]. Interestingly, primary TN tumor cells expressed lesser β_2AR mRNA and protein than TN brain metastatic cells from primary breast tumor; these metastatic cells exhibited increased proliferation and migration. In vivo and in vitro, invasive and metastatic potential of these cells was diminished when treated with propranolol [22].

There have been different mechanisms described that regulate invasion and metastasis through β_2AR signaling in tumor cells. Norepinephrine, epinephrine, or agonists bind β_2AR and activate adenylate cyclase (AC) through G-protein-coupled receptor subunit α ($G\alpha_s$). AC activation promotes ATP-cAMP conversion (**Figure 1**) and Ca^{2+} intracellular increase [23]. In highly metastatic breast tumor cells (MDA-MB-231HM), another G-protein subunit, Gβγ, also promotes intracellular Ca^{2+} augmentation through β_2AR signaling. Either through Gβγ or $G\alpha_s$, cAMP activates effector PKA and exchange protein activated by adenylyl cyclase (EPAC) and inhibits pERK1/pERK2; therefore, cell proliferation is mediated independently by ERK phosphorylation [23]. PKA phosphorylates CREB/ATF, GATA1 transcription factors, and β-adrenergic receptor kinase (BARK). BARK recruits β-arrestin which activates Src kinase, and this activates STAT3 [24]. Focal adhesion kinase (FAK) activated by STAT3 enhances migration and apoptosis resistance. CREB/ATF, GATA1, and STAT3 promote VEGF, IL-6, IL-8, and MMP-9 expression and enhance angiogenesis, migration, and invasion (**Figure 1**) [24]. Meanwhile, in breast tumor cells (MCF-7 and MDA-MB-231) treated with an EPAC inhibitor (ESI-09), migration inhibition was found associated with mislocalization of the A-kinase anchoring protein 9 (AKAP9); therefore, EPAC also promotes cell migration [25].

Another way in which β_2AR signaling stimulates tumor growth is through promoting DNA damage and p53-associated apoptosis suppression [26].

2.1.3 Tumor innervation

During tumor initial innervation, nearby healthy tissue provides sympathetic fibers that infiltrate the periphery of the growing tumor [27], in response to neurotropic factors secreted by tumor cells, such as neurotrophic growth factor (NGF) [28] and brain-derived neurotrophic factor (BDNF) [29]. These factors increase nerve fiber growth and thereby tumor innervation [28]. Tumor innervation is associated with vasculature; therefore, together with nerve fibers, blood vessels go through the tumor mass [30] (**Figure 1**). Sympathetic innervation in tumor is the main catecholamine source [30, 31]; this is evidenced because its local concentration is higher than plasma [31]. In this sense, innervation is a feature of tumor microenvironment associated with tumor aggressiveness [28].

Therefore, β-receptor antagonists could have an important role in the development of new therapies that diminish metastasis risk and promote a slow tumor progression.

2.1.4 HPA axis

The HPA axis also plays an important role in stress response in mammals. In the hypothalamus, the paraventricular nucleus neurons secrete corticotropin-releasing factor into hypophyseal portal blood. CRF stimulates the release of adrenocorticotropic hormone by the anterior pituitary gland, to the blood vessels and systemic circulation. When ACTH reaches adrenal glands, the cortex stimulates the corticosterone production (in rodents) or cortisol (humans) (**Figure 1**) [32].

Cortisol and corticosterone (glucocorticoids) exert their effects through glucocorticoid receptor. Different immune and breast cancer cells express this receptor, and glucocorticoids exert different effects in these cells.

GCR in breast cancer cells, especially in triple-negative lines (MDA-MB-231), promotes the expression of genes related to cell survival and apoptosis protection, for example, MAPK phosphatase-1 and serine/threonine protein kinase 1 (**Figure 1**) [33, 34]. In addition, the activation of the GCR induces the expression of genes related to cell survival, adhesion, and EMT in a premalignant breast [35]. Correspondingly, in xenograft MDA-MB-231 breast tumors in mice pre-treated with systemic dexamethasone, the paclitaxel treatment effect was inhibited [36]. Therefore, glucocorticoids protect breast cancer cells from apoptosis and enhance their survival capabilities, favoring tumor growth.

2.1.5 Stress and tumor growth

Stress is largely linked to cancer development. Stressor exposition and SNS activation promote noradrenaline release into the tumor that regulates tumor progression [30]. In animals under social isolation (a stress experimental model), there is an increased tumor size and reduced survival [37]. Also in other stress models, increased tumor progression and metastasis have been observed [38, 39].

During metastatic establishment, β_2AR overexpression enhances cell proliferation and invasion, to ensure metastatic establishment, and, maybe, that is why in primary tumor resection, the surgery induces stress and releases norepinephrine and epinephrine that enhance tumor metastasis. Thus, the use of treatments that antagonize the effect of these neurotransmitters may reduce metastasis [22].

Thus, nervous control of tumor growth is regulated by the sympathetic and HPA systems. The sympathetic regulation is via tumor innervation with sympathetic fibers and the adrenergic signaling in tumor, through local and peripheral catecholamine (epinephrine and norepinephrine) production and the β_2AR expression in tumor and immune cells. Meanwhile, HPA system regulates glucocorticoid production, which enhances tumor cell survival and downmodulates inflammatory response, thus enhancing tumor growth and metastasis (**Figure 1**).

3. Immune response in mammary tumors

Tumorigenesis usually courses a slow development during years, and the immune response depends on the different stages of the disease and the tumor microenvironment [40].

Every day, immune cells detect and destroy transformed cells, in a phenomenon called immunosurveillance. But, when transformed cells evade elimination mechanisms (immunoescape), survive and proliferate. At this point, tumor can remain in a state of dormancy, partially by the action of immune cells, but when the balance between stromal, immune, and tumor cells with their secretory products leads to local immunosuppression, the immunosubversion is established, and the tumor grows (**Figure 2**) [41, 42].

3.1 Immune innate cells in mammary tumors

3.1.1 Dendritic cells

Dendritic cells are antigen-presenting cells (APCs) that recognize, uptake, process, and present antigens to different cells including T cells. In the immunosurveillance

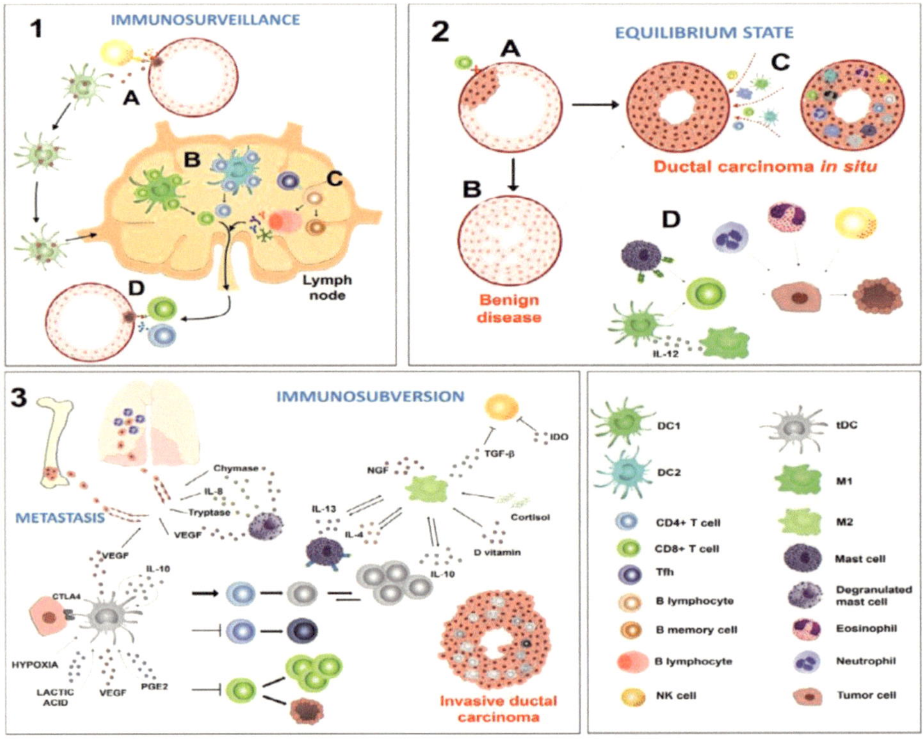

Figure 2.

Immune response in breast tumor development. (1) In immunosurveillance, breast tissue-resident conventional dendritic cells (cDC) capture antigens released by transformed cell after recognition and destruction by cytotoxic cells (NK cells). cDC migrate to peripheric lymph node and as DC type 1 (DC1) or DC type 2 (DC2) present antigens to CD8⁺ T cells or CD4⁺ T cells, respectively. In lymph nodes T follicular cells activate B lymphocytes into plasma (antibody producer) or B memory cells. After the activation and subsequent proliferation, CD8⁺ T cytotoxic and CD4⁺ T helper cells migrate. Cytotoxic cells induce apoptosis to transformed cells, and T helper cells produce cytokines and chemokines to enhance cytotoxic effect. (2) In the equilibrium state, transformed cells evade immune recognition and proliferate to hyperplasia (benign disease) and eventually to ductal carcinoma in situ (DCIS). In these phases immune cells are recluted, and cytotoxic cells (CD8⁺, neutrophils, and eosinophils) may eliminate transformed cells in an equilibrium phase. Indirectly, other cells enhance cytotoxic response, for example, M1 macrophages produce IL-12 that enhances dendritic cell antigen presentation to CD8⁺ cells. Also mast cells MHC-I⁺ stimulate CD8⁺ T-cell proliferation. (3) In immunosubversion and metastasis, when invasive ductal carcinoma is established, tumor dendritic cells (tDC) are induced through IL-10, vascular endothelial factor (VEGF), prostaglandin E2 (PGE2), hypoxia, and lactic acid and by direct contact with tumor CTLA4⁺. tDC produce IL-10, which in turn induces their own expansion as well as T regulatory cell (Tregs) proliferation and the inhibition of effector CD4⁺ and CD8⁺ T cells, Th1 differentiation, and CD8⁺ T cells function. Also, IL-10, D vitamin, and cortisol activate M2. M2 macrophages produce IL-4, IL-10, IL-13 (that feedback M2 generation), NGF, and TGF-β that with IDO inhibit cytotoxic NK function. Mast cells secrete VEGF, tryptase, chymase, and IL-8 that enhance metastasis to different organs (lung and bone). Neutrophils may enhance metastasis because they form premetastatic niches that promote tumor cell migration and metastasis establishment.

phase, dendritic cells resident in the breast tissue sense and capture different antigens released by transformed cells and then migrate to draining lymph nodes, where, as a mature cell, antigens to naïve T cells are present [43–45]. After the activation and subsequent proliferation, the $CD8^+$ T and $CD4^+$ T cells migrate to the site where transformed neoplastic cells reside. The cytotoxic response is carried out mainly by $CD8^+$ T cells and NK cells, which detect and induce apoptosis to transformed cells; meanwhile, $CD4^+$ T helper cells produce cytokines and chemokines that modulate the immune response and recruit other immune cells (**Figure 2**).

Two lineages of dendritic cells are responsible for T-cell priming. The first are DC1s that express chemokine receptor CXR1 and present antigens through MHC-I preferentially to CD8$^+$ T cells. The second are the DC2s that express CD172a and MHC-II (high), to activate CD4$^+$ T cells [43]. DC1s can be lymphoid-resident DC1s (CD8α in mice) or migratory DC1s (CD103$^+$ in mice), being the latter mentioned as the main subset of DC that can induce a strong cytotoxic response against tumor through the activation of CD8$^+$ T cells [46]. Meanwhile, DC2s (CD11$^+$ in mouse) seem to fail in tumor antigen presentation to CD4$^+$ T cells in lymph nodes, but it is unclear why. A possibility is an inadequate process of antigen or the nature of tumor antigen. These DC2s cells can be tolerogenic, because they cannot generate an adequate activation and stimulation [43].

Three features lead to the induction of suppressive or tumor phenotype DC. The first is the presence of tumor cell neoantigens that leads eventually to immuno-escape and the failure of immunosurveillance. The second is the degree of DC maturation, in which immature DC acquire a tolerogenic phenotype and generate regulatory T cells. And the third is related to the immune suppression in the tumor microenvironment mediated by other cells and soluble factors. The balance of stimulatory and suppressive signals determines tumor progression and is related to cell tumor phenotype and the interaction among cells [43].

There are many tumor microenvironment factors that suppress DC activation in vitro, for example, IL-10, vascular endothelial factor, prostaglandin E2, hypoxia, and lactic acid [47]. Another important interaction is when breast tumor and DC are in contact. Chen et al. showed a decreased expression of CD40, CD80, CD86 (costimulatory molecules), HLA-DR, and CD83 and a reduced production of IFN-γ, TNF-α, IL-1β, IL-2, IL-6, and IL-12, in lipopolysaccharide (LPS)-stimulated human DC, when co-cultured with CTLA4$^+$ breast cancer cells. These suppressive DC inhibit CD4$^+$ and CD8$^+$ T-cell proliferation, Th1 differentiation, and cytotoxic lymphocyte (CTL) function (**Figure 2**) [48].

When a transformed cell escapes of the immune recognition and destruction, and starts proliferating, it recruits different immune cells and promotes a pro-tumoral and suppressor microenvironment. Among these tumor-recruited cells are DCs, which migrate to local lymph nodes and present tumor antigens to lymphocytes. Meanwhile some recruited DC go to lymph nodes, and another subset of DC remains in tumor and developed suppressor functions through the direct inhibition of the local activation of CD4$^+$ and CD8$^+$ T cells or through suppressive cytokine production (IL-10) (**Figure 2**) [43, 49]. These DC may have an important role in lymphocyte priming in tumor, associated with the presence of tertiary lymphoid structures (TLS) in breast tumors, specially placed in stroma and with naïve T cells in tumors that are activated in situ [50, 51].

3.1.2 Neutrophils

Neutrophils are polymorphonuclear (PMN) cells and the most abundant leukocyte in human. These cells are responsible for host defense to bacterial, fungal, and viral infections and support wound healing [52]. Neutrophils can phagocyte, form neutrophil extracellular traps (NETs) to eliminate invasive microorganisms, and synthesize and store in cytoplasmic granules neutrophil elastase, cathepsin G, proteinase 3, neutrophil collagenase (MMP-8), gelatinase B (MMP-9), reactive oxygen species (ROS), and antimicrobial peptides [53–55]. Through chemotactic stimuli, neutrophils arrive to the inflammation site and phagocyte the invading microorganism. Thereafter, cytoplasmic granules in the neutrophil get fused with the phagolysosome where the microorganism is destroyed [52]. Under adverse circumstances, neutrophil can release proteinases through microbursts, to the extracellular space, or produce NETs to fix the microorganisms, stop their migration, and concentrate on toxic factors [56].

Some authors mentioned a neutrophil polarization similar to classical activated macrophages (M1) and alternative activated macrophages (M2), named N1 and N2; also, neutrophils present different degrees of activation, and according to it, there are four types of PMN: naïve circulating, mildly activated, activated (acute inflammation), and highly activated (sepsis, unsuccessful phagocytosis). Among mildly activated neutrophils are tumor-associated neutrophils (TANs) that in mice express $CD11b^{+}$ and $Ly\text{-}6G^{hi}$ markers [52, 57].

Cellular cytotoxic role in cancer is traditionally associated with cytotoxic T cells, NK cells, and macrophages, and little attention is focused on neutrophils, but nowadays, reports are linking neutrophils to different stages of cancer [56]. Naïve neutrophils are recruited to the tumor, mainly by macrophages, and display the same repertory to kill a microorganism for the destruction of a tumor cell, and eventually a pro-host or pro-tumoral effect in situ is developed (**Figure 2**) [52].

The presence or absence and quantity of neutrophils within the tumor, associated with tumor type, determine the prognostic of the disease [57]. In an orthotopic murine model of breast cancer with 4T1 (metastatic cells) and 4T07 (nonmetastatic cells), more neutrophils within 4T1 tumors in comparison to 4T07 tumors were detected. Also in 4T1 tumors, higher mRNA expression of CXCL1, a neutrophil-recruiting chemokine, was detected [58]. For example, a pre-metastatic niche has been reported in remote organs, where neutrophils come together and shape a microenvironment that favored the migration of tumor cells (**Figure 2**) [59]. One of the mechanisms that shape a pre-metastatic niche could be mediated by NETs, as has been demonstrated in an experiment where neutrophils were co-cultured with 4T1 cells in a transwell chamber assay and produced more NETs than neutrophils co-cultured with 4T07 cells. In the same report, authors proved the presence of NET structures located next to 4T1 cells, which was assumed to contribute to support metastasis [58].

3.1.3 Eosinophils

Eosinophils are granulocyte cells that can be found in the spleen, lymph nodes, thymus, and gastrointestinal tract [60] and are able to phagocyte and act as antigen-presenting cell in lymph nodes, through the expression of major compatibility complex and costimulatory molecules (CD40, CD80, CD86) [61]. Furthermore, eosinophils produce cytokines, chemokines, growth factors, lipid mediators, and cytotoxic granules (**Table 1**).

Eosinophils are usually related to parasitic infections, especially helminthiases, in which eosinophilia is a characteristic feature. But recently their role in cancer has become relevant. Depending on its cytokine profile production, a new classification of eosinophils has been proposed; the eosinophils that secrete Th1 cytokines (IL-8, TNF-α, and IFN-γ) are called E1, and the ones that produce Th2 cytokines (IL-4, IL-5, and IL-13) are E2. Despite this classification, in breast cancer it is unknown if the eosinophils secrete any of those cytokines, although blood eosinophilia is related to a good or poor prognostic of the disease, depending on the cancer type [79]. Related to eosinophil infiltration into the breast cancer tumor, the presence of eosinophils is one indicator of increased survival, maybe because these cells participate in host-tumor interactions and because of their cytotoxic activity [83].

3.1.4 Mast cells

Mast cells originate in bone marrow, then circulate and migrate to tissues, and in nearby blood vessels mature into effector cells, in which along with DC and macrophages, are the first cells to recognize and interact with pathogens or allergens [84, 85]. Inside mast cells there are granules with preformed substances that included histamine

		General functions	Cancer-related features
Cytokines	IL-8	Supports endothelial cell proliferation and survival [62]	Breast cancer tissue expresses higher concentrations of IL-8 than normal tissue[63]
	TNF-α	Pro-inflammatory cytokine	Chronic expression sustains breast tumor growth [64]
	IL-4	Promotes a Th2 profile, B-cell differentiation, and IgE isotype switch	
	IL-5	Stimulates proliferation, differentiation, recruitment, and activation of eosinophils [65]	
	IL-13	Regulates IgE synthesis and mucus production [66]	A higher tumor stage correlates with higher serum levels and lymph node metastasis [67]
Chemokines	CCL3, CCL5, CCL11, CCL24; CXCL8, CCL7	Chemoattractant for eosinophils	Recruitment of eosinophils to tumor
	CCL3, CCL5, CCL11, CCL17, CCL22, CCL23; CXCL1, CXCL5, CXCL8, CXCL9, CXCL10, CXCL11	Chemokines secreted by eosinophils to recruit other immune cells	Recruitment of immune cells to tumor
Growth factors	TGF-α		In mammary mouse tissue, overexpression of TGF-α induces hyperplasia and proliferation [68]
	TGF-β	Regulates cellular differentiation, proliferation, apoptosis, and migration [69]	In early stages suppresses tumor progression but in late stages favors tumor growth [69]
	VEGF	Promotes angiogenesis	Promotes tumor angiogenesis
Lipid mediators	Leukotrienes	Pro-inflammatory	Elevated levels in colon, pancreatic, and prostate cancer [70]
	Prostaglandin E2	Shifts Th2 response and downregulates $CD8^+$ T-cell activity and tumor cell antigen presentation [71]	Promotes tumor growth in breast cancer Is associated with poor prognosis [72]
	Thromboxanes		Overexpression is associated with poor prognosis in urothelial cancer [73]
	Lipoxins (lipoxin A4)		Suppressing the polarization of B regulatory cells [74]

		General functions	Cancer-related features
Cytotoxic granules	Eosinophil cationic protein	Tissue remodeling, suppression of T-cell proliferation, mast cell degranulation, and secretion of airway mucus [75]	Proliferation inhibition in colorectal carcinoma and oral squamous cell carcinoma cell lines, via osmotic lysis [76, 77]
	Major basic protein	Tissue damage	Cytotoxic effect in human cancer cell lines [78]
	Eosinophil-derived neurotoxin	Cytotoxic activity and chemoattractant of DC, monocytes, neutrophils, mast cells, and T cells [79]	Cytotoxic activity in colorectal carcinoma cell line [80]
	Eosinophil peroxidase	Related to inflammatory tissue injury [81]	Absent in normal breast tissue but present in breast cancer tumor stroma [82]

CCL5 or RANTES, regulated on activation normal T expressed and secreted; CCL3 or MIP-1α, macrophage inflammatory protein; CCL7 or MCP-3, monocyte-specific chemokine protein; TGF-α, transforming growth factor α; TGF-β, transforming growth factor β; VEGF, vascular endothelial cell growth factor; GM-CSF, granulocyte macrophage colony-stimulating factor

Table 1.
Functions and related cancer features of cytokines and chemokines.

(vasodilator), heparin (anticoagulant), serotonin, dopamine, tryptase, and chymase. The mast cell activation stimulates the production of leukotrienes and cytokines (e.g., TNF-α) and the cell degranulation [86].

Mast cells may perform both immunosuppressive and inflammatory functions depending on the interaction with the effector or regulatory immune cells [85]. For example, the expression of MHC-II in mast cells can be induced by the exposure of LPS and IFN-γ, and the interaction of MHC-II-expressing mast cells with effector T cells induces the expansion of Treg cells; meanwhile, mast cells expressing MHC-I can enhance the proliferation of $CD8^+$ T cells [87, 88]. Besides direct contact with T cell, an alternative activation mechanism could be the mast cell production of IFN. This cytokine enhances the proliferation of T cells, depending on the number of mast cells within the microenvironment, for example, at low numbers proliferation is enhanced, but in higher numbers proliferation is inhibited, in a mechanism mediated by the H1 histamine receptor [89, 90].

On the other hand, for naïve B-cell survival and activation and for plasma cell proliferation and differentiation, mast cells interact with B cell through superficial CD40L. Also for the B-cell synthesis of IgE, the secretion of IL-4 and IL-13, among others, by mast cells is necessary [85].

Despite mast cells releasing angiogenic factors, as VEGF, chymase, tryptase, heparin, fibroblast growth factor-2 (FGF-2), IL-8, TGF-β, and nerve growth factor, the inhibition of mast cell degranulation did not change the mammary tumor vascularization, but that does not mean that degranulation may enhance angiogenesis [91]. In this regard, a study informed that tryptase did not stimulate the proliferation of MDA-MB-231 breast cancer cells but indeed enhances its migration and invasion [92]. In malignant breast carcinomas, there are more tryptase-containing mast cells detected through immunohistochemistry assay than that in benign lesions [93]. Given the prominent angiogenic character of mast cells, to date, their presence has not been strongly associated with the enhancement of the tumor vascularization, and it is not clear if comorbidities favoring increased quantities of mast cells may improve tumor vascularization and metastasis.

3.1.5 Macrophages

Macrophages are mononuclear phagocytic cells that according to environment signals turn into different phenotypes. One of these phenotypes is the classically activated macrophages or M1, induced by Toll-like receptors (TLR) and IFN-γ. These cells are characterized by the expression of IL-12, the major histocompatibility complex class II (MHC-II) and TNF-α, and ROS and nitric oxide (NO) production and are associated with microorganisms and cell destruction [94]. The second phenotype is the "alternatively or selectively" activated macrophages, which are characterized by the secretion of IL-4, IL-10, IL-13, and TGF-β and the expression of arginase-1 and VEGF and are related to wound healing and humoral response [94, 95].

Macrophages, monocytes, and DC can be found in tumor microenvironment, being the macrophages the most abundant phagocytic population. Tumor-associated macrophages (TAMs) are characterized by the cell surface expression of CD68 and have been related to invasion and migration of cancer cells, being a prognostic factor in cancer [95, 96]. Some reports have shown that the density of TAMs in breast cancer samples is related to hormone receptor status, lymph node metastasis, stage, and prognosis. Higher concentrations of TAMs are associated with a poor prognosis, and the worse prognostic group is the one with a high proportion of CD163 and CD206 (M2 markers) [95].

TAMs are related to immunosuppressive features, for example, low antigen-presenting capability, low tissue remodeling activity, and low toxicity functions that promote tumor growth and metastasis [97]. These immunosuppressive TAMs function as M2 macrophages and are activated by IL-4, IL-10, IL-13, glucocorticoids, and vitamin D_3 [98].

3.1.6 NK cells

The innate immune system recognizes and kills infected and transformed cells; NK cells are responsible for this task, through granzyme b-perforin system, TNF-related apoptosis-inducing ligand (TRAIL), and the expression of CD95 ligand [99]. NK cells produce IFN-γ, granulocyte/macrophage colony-stimulating factor (GM-CSF), and TNF [100] and are one of the main cells in antitumoral response.

Depending on the signals that NK cells receive, activation or inhibition receptors or coreceptors are expressed [101, 102].

NK cell cytotoxicity is activated by different ligands upregulated during cellular stress, also with the recognition of antibodies in the antibody-dependent cellular toxicity (ADCC) through the expression of CD16 (Fc immunoglobulin fragment low-affinity receptor) and with the detection of cells that underexpressed HLA-class I molecules [101, 103]. In immunosurveillance, tumor cells are detected and destroyed by NK cells, through these mechanisms (**Figure 2**). In immunosubversion, tumor cells evade NK cell recognition, and tumor microenvironment leads to NK cell impairment, through the inhibition of surface-activating receptor expression, such as NKp46 and NKG2D or NKp30 and NKG2D mediated by indoleamine 2,3-dioxygenase (IDO) and TGF-β1, respectively (**Figure 2**) [101, 104, 105].

In breast cancer patients, tumor NK cells possess a more prominent inhibitory phenotype than peripheral NK cells. Also depending on disease progression, for example, in late stages, NK cells lose their cytotoxic activity and express inhibitory receptors (NKG2A); meanwhile, in early stages NK cells express activating receptors (NKp30, NKG2D, DNAM-1, and CD16). One of the stroma-derived suppressor factors that induced NK cell function impairment is TGF-β1 [101].

3.2 Immune adaptive cells in mammary tumors

3.2.1 T lymphocytes

T lymphocytes are one of the most important cell populations in cancer. The activation of T cells is performed, firstly, through TCR stimulation with its specific antigen, presented in the context of MHC, by a dendritic cell or another professional antigen-presenting cell; secondly, with the binding of "costimulatory" molecules in the dendritic cell; and, thirdly, by the cytokine milieu and soluble factors [106, 107]. In addition, antigen presentation is performed by immature DCs, resulting in a non-responsive or anergic T cells [108]. In breast cancer tertiary lymphoid structures and germinal centers were detected next to tumor in extensively infiltrated tumors. This TLS possesses a similar structure to lymph node, including a T-cell zone with $CD3^+/CD4^+$ T cells and a germinal center with B cells and T follicular helper (Tfh) cells [109].

3.2.2 T helper cells

Different factors such as the expression of transcription factors, chemokine receptors, signal transduction activators, and the chemokine and cytokine secretion regulate the effector phenotype and function of these cells [107]. Regarding human breast cancer, different effector phenotypes have been reported, for example, through flow cytometry of invasive breast tumors, Tfh, Th1, Th2, Th17, and Tregs were found [109].

3.2.3 T follicular helper (Tfh) cell

The effector phenotype Tfh cell stays in the lymph node and induces activation and differentiation of affine B cells into plasma or memory cells [110]. But, in advanced stages of invasive breast cancer, $CD4^+$ Tfh cells were detected in the T-cell zone and germinal centers of TLS. This localization is may be due to their function in tumor, because Tfh cells were localized near to B cells [111].

3.2.4 T helper 1 (Th1)

$CD4^+$ T helper 1 (Th1) cell differentiation and IFN-γ production are modulated by IL-12 produced by APCs (monocytes/macrophages, DCs, and even NK cells) and IFN-γ (**Figure 2**) [112–114]. Th1 cells express the transcription factor T-bet; secrete IFN-γ, TNF-α, and IL-2; and function as regulators of monocyte activation and T lymphocyte differentiation induction [115, 116]. Th1 cells are associated with early tumor phases, because of their IFN-γ production that activates $CD8^+$ cytotoxic T cells (**Figure 2**) [117]. Therefore, there is an association between improving survival and the infiltration of Th1 and $CD8^+$ T cells in breast tumors [118].

3.2.5 T helper 2 (Th2)

A T helper subset related to immunosubversion and tumor progression is the $CD4^+$ T helper 2 (Th2) cells, characterized by the expression of transcription factor GATA3 and the secretion of IL-4, IL-5, IL-10, and IL-13 [121]. Th2 cells are related to nematode response, tissue repair, and antibody production. In breast cancer, Th2 cells have been found in human mammary tumors [109], and IL-13 is reported to be present also in human breast tumors, promoting tumor development (**Figure 2**) [119].

3.2.6 T helper 17 (Th17)

$CD4^+$ Th17 (T helper 17) cells are related to autoimmunity, tissue inflammation, and host defense against bacteria, fungi, viruses, and protozoa and play an important role in mucosal immunity [120]. Th17 cells produce IL-17 and IL-22 and express transcription factor RORγt [121]. Regarding Th17 cells in tumor, it is not recognized if they could be induced in tumor or be recruited from other places, but their presence has been detected in breast tumors [109]. Th17 cell tumor infiltration mediates an inflammatory microenvironment [122].

3.2.7 Regulatory T cells (Tregs)

Tregs are a subset of T helper cells that express Foxp3 transcription factor and have an important role in controlling inflammation and autoimmunity in mouse and man [123]. These cells normally are residents in the secondary lymphoid organs, lung, peripheral blood, gastrointestinal tract, liver, and skin and can be recruited to other tissues, under inflammatory conditions [124]. Tregs are $CD4^+$, $CD127^{low}$, $CD25^{hi}$, and also $CTLA^+$ and exert immune suppression through different mechanisms, for example, the production of tolerogenic cytokines (IL-10, IL-35, and TGF-β), the induction of arginine depletion that leads to T-cell dysfunction, the expression of suppressive molecules (CTLA-4, CD80/CD86), and the direct cytolysis through granzyme b-perforin system and through local consumption of IL-2 (with the constitutive expression of high-affinity receptor CD25) [125, 126].

IL-10 is a suppressive cytokine secreted by macrophages, NK cells, NKT cells, B cells, DCs, and $CD4^+$ T cell (specially Treg cells), that suppress inflammatory responses, prevent autoimmune diseases, and enhance tumor growth (**Figure 2**) [127–129].

3.2.8 T cytotoxic lymphocytes (CTLs)

$CD8^+$ cytotoxic T lymphocytes play an important role in adaptive antitumor response; therefore, when tumor immunosubversion is stablished, the cytotoxicity of $CD8^+$T cells gets compromised (**Figure 2**). During immunosurveillance, in secondary lymphoid organs (lymph nodes and spleen), APCs present tumor-associated antigens and tumor neoantigens to CTLs, which in the presence of costimulatory and cytokine signals, such as IL-12 (produced by DCs) and IFN-γ (produced by Th1 cells), undergo activation, maturation, and clonal expansion [117, 130]. After, CTLs migrate through the body, search for specific antigen, and kill the tumor antigen-specific cell through IFN-γ release and perforin and granzyme system (**Figure 2**) [117, 131, 132]. Also, through the activation of its receptor, IL-12 promotes the differentiation of effector CD8 cells and inhibits at the same time the development of memory CD8 cells [133, 134]. When effector CTL cells failed in killing target cell and are exposed to persistent antigen stimulation (in chronic infectious diseases or in tumors), CTL express inhibitory cell surface receptors, PD-1, LAG3, TIM3, TIGIT, and CTLA-4, and became exhausted $CD8^+$ T cells. During tumor immunosubversion $CD8^+$ T cell exhausted profile is generated; therefore, cytolysis or IFN-γ secretion mediated through CTLs is inhibited (**Figure 2**) [135].

Another important cytokine related to $CD8^+$ T cells is IL-2, which is described not only as a growth factor, secreted by $CD4^+$- and $CD8^+$-activated T cells, but also as a differentiation inducer for $CD8^+$ effector cells [115]. $CD8^+$ T cells cultured with IL-2 presented an upregulation in perforin (Prf1) transcription and a suppressed expression of Bcl6 and IL-7Rα (memory $CD8^+$ markers). Meanwhile, in $CD8^+$ T cells with deficiency of IL-2 receptor (IL-2Rα or CD25), cell differentiation impairment was shown in vivo, demonstrated with granzyme B and perforin diminished expression and a poor ex vivo cytotoxicity [136].

In regard to $CD8^+$ T cell antitumor activity, an experiment in tumor from four T1 mammary gland tumor cells in syngeneic mice showed that in mice injected with IL-12, tumor growth was suppressed through an increased $CD8^+$ cell infiltration and production of IFN-γ and the induction of apoptosis of tumor cells [137]. This effect correlates with good prognosis in $CD8^+$ T cell infiltration in breast tumors in women [138]. With the time, CTLs lose their cytotoxic phenotype and acquired an exhausted phenotype that needs further characterization in breast tumors but is likely to be associated with late stages (triple-negative breast cancer).

4. Endocrine factors related to the development of breast cancer

Mammary gland epithelium is highly dynamic, characterized by proliferation, differentiation, and apoptosis cycles, regulated in part by hormones. Breast cancer is associated with an abnormal proliferation of epithelial cells, related to genetic mutations and epigenetic modifications in suppressor and DNA repair genes and oncogenes [139].

4.1 Estrogens and progesterone

During life, the mammary gland development is divided by different stages and modulated by hormones such as estrogens (17β estradiol) and progesterone. These stages are related to sexual development and includes embryonic and prepuberal phase, puberty, pregnancy, lactation, and involution. Epidermal growth factor (EGF) and estrogens that arrive through the breast stroma during puberty induce ductal elongation and branching. Meanwhile, the lobes formed by secretory epithelial cells organized in alveoli develop during gestation and probably in lactation, through the placental lactogens, progesterone, and prolactin signaling [140]. In lactation, milk secretion is promoted by the contraction of rounding epithelium smooth muscle cells mediated by oxytocin [8].

Estrogen effects are regulated through alpha and beta estrogen receptors (ERα and ERβ), both expressed in mammary normal tissue [141]. ERα signaling is responsible for ductal elongation in puberty and the stromal invasion in normal breast tissue [142].

The sharing ERα-ERβ distribution suggests that ERβ may be related to a negative ERα regulation, through antiestrogen or non-habitual effects [143]. The ERα or ERβ receptor dimerization is induced by ligand-receptor union and leads to the formation of homodimers (ERα/α, Erβ/β) or heterodimers (ERα/β). Recently, it was described that the dimer conformation is associated with their function. ERα/α is linked with proliferation induced by estrogen, and ERβ/β homodimer is linked with antiproliferative and pro-apoptotic functions; meanwhile, ERα/β effects are not elucidated as well (**Figure 3**) [144].

Proliferation in breast tumor cells is ligand-dependent in early stages and ligand-independent in late stages. In the estrogen-dependent pathway, cell proliferation is activated through cytoplasmic or membrane estrogen receptors. Intracellular signaling begins with estrogen-receptor union, their consequent translocation to nuclei, where the estrogen-receptor complex binds to specific

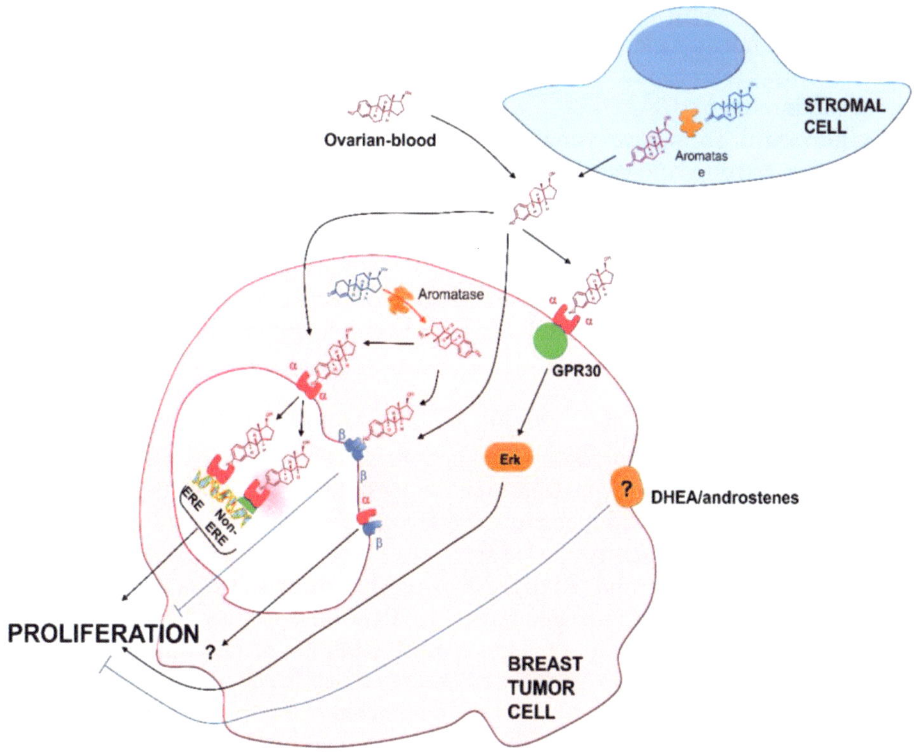

Figure 3.
Endocrine interactions in breast cancer. In the estrogen-dependent pathway, cell proliferation is activated through cytoplasmic or membrane estrogen receptors. Intracellular signaling begins with estrogen-receptor union, their consequent translocation to nuclei, where the estrogen-receptor complex binds to specific estrogen-response elements (ERE) in estrogen-responsive genes, in a non-ERE way, functioning as gene transcription co-regulator. Furthermore, estrogen-membrane ER signals through GPR30 and Erk to elicit proliferation. Estrogen sources to breast tumor cell are intracrine, endocrine (blood supply), and paracrine (stromal adjacent cells). Dehydroepiandrosterone (DHEA) and other androstenes inhibit tumor cell proliferation.

estrogen-response elements in estrogen-responsive genes or to other transcription factors, such as AP1 or Sp1, in a non-ERE way, functioning as gene transcription co-regulator [145, 146]. Furthermore, estrogen-membrane ER signals through GPR30 and Erk to elicit proliferation (**Figure 3**) [145]. Meanwhile, the estrogen-independent pathway is mediated through ligand binding and activation of growth factor receptors (GFRs), such as epithelial growth factor receptor (EGFR), insulin-like growth factor receptor (IGF), and HER-2, among others. This activation promotes ER phosphorylation and activation through PI3K/AKT and Ras/Raf/MAPK pathways [145, 147].

On the other hand, progesterone exerts its action through two receptors (PRA and PRB), both signaling and activating gene transcription [148]. ERα and PR are co-expressed in the mammary gland in 15–30% of epithelial cells [149]. Meanwhile, estradiol and progesterone drive epithelial mammary gland proliferation directly through the hormone-receptor union and have been proposing a second control mechanism in which epithelial cells sense hormone concentrations through their estrogen and progesterone receptors and, in consequence, secrete or not growth factors to promote nearby cell proliferation [148].

In breast cancer staging, ER and/or PR expression loss is associated with more aggressive tumors, with self-sufficiency of growth signals independently of estrogen or progesterone receptors. Additionally, positive ERα tumor is related to a better prognostic, as well as ERβ tumor expression [150].

Besides the receptor's presence in tumor cells, another important issue to consider is the hormone levels within the tumor. Intratumoral estradiol concentration in normal breast tissue was lower than in ductal carcinoma in situ and invasive ductal carcinoma [151].

In this regard, aromatase is an important enzyme responsible for the production of estrogens, estrone, and estradiol, through the aromatization and conversion of androstenedione and testosterone [152]. Invasive ductal carcinoma expresses a higher amount of aromatase mRNA than DCIS and normal breast tissue, and both epithelial and stromal cells expressed aromatase mRNA [151]. Therefore, tumor cells have different sources of estrogen, called endocrine (ovary), intracrine, and paracrine, which enhance cell proliferation of tumor target cells.

4.2 Androgens

Meanwhile estrogens stimulate mammary gland development, and androgens inhibit it. For example, estrogen treatment in prostate cancer patients promotes mammary gland growth and ingestion of androgens by athletes or transsexuals and produces mammary gland atrophy [153].

Androgens as testosterone (T) and dihydrotestosterone (DHT) exert their effects through the union to their androgen receptor (AR). This receptor has been colocalized with ER and PR in mammary gland epithelia, but not in adjacent stromal cells; therefore, androgen-mediated proliferation is regulated in the mammary epithelium [154]. The androgen receptor (AR) has been reported to be present in 80% of primary breast tumors, and its presence is associated with a favorable response to endocrine treatment and a better prognostic, especially if ER is also present [155].

In this sense, the union of BRCA1 gene product with AR activates AR functions; therefore, the mutation of this BRCA1 may interfere with AR antiproliferative functions and allow cell proliferation [156].

4.3 Adrenal steroids

Dehydroepiandrosterone, an estrogen and testosterone precursor [157], is an adrenal steroid which is metabolized into active metabolites, such as Δ5-androstene-3β, 17β-diol (17β-androstenediol), Δ5-androstene-3β17α-diol (17α-androstenediol), and Δ5-androstene-3β,7β,17β-triol (17β-androstenetriol) [158]. DHEA is able to activate ERα, ERβ, AR, and glucocorticoid receptor (GR); meanwhile, its metabolites showed a weaker activation [159]. All of androstene hormones (DHEA, 17β-androstenediol, 17α-androstenediol, and 17β-androstenetriol) have been shown to have an antiproliferative effect in cellular lines, including breast cancer (**Figure 3**) [160]. Only DHEA presented a protective effect in vivo, but the other androstenes have not been tested in vitro [160]; therefore, there is a promising search field around androstenes and the development of breast cancer.

5. Tumor development and neuroimmunoendocrine interactions

The relation between nervous and immune systems is importantly transduced through β_2AR and GCR localized in immune cells, such as B lymphocytes, T lymphocytes, NK cells, and macrophages, which regulate cytokine production, molecule expression, development, survival, proliferation, circulation, and cell recruitment [161]. Meanwhile, interactions among endocrine and immune or nervous systems are regulated through the hormone receptor expression (ER, PR, and AR) and the effects driving in immune and/or nervous cells (**Figure 4**).

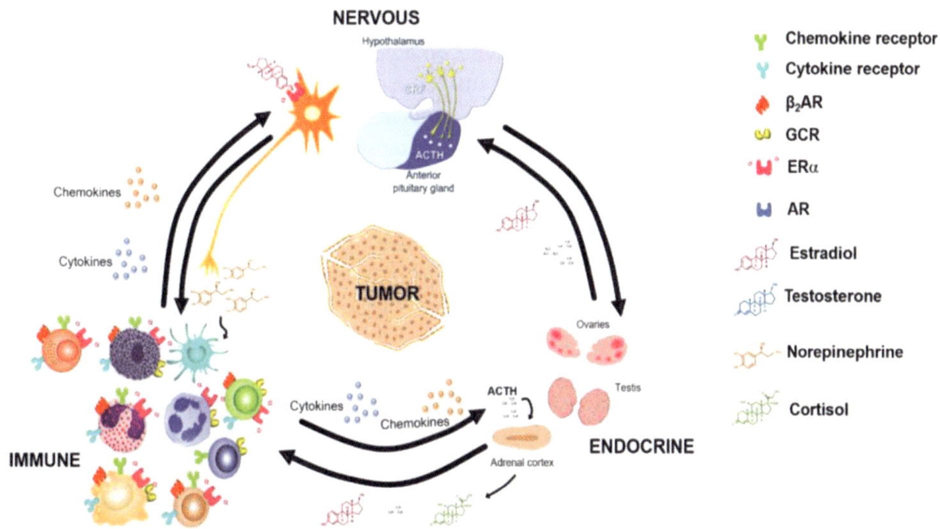

Figure 4.
Neuroimmunoendocrine interactions in breast cancer. Bidirectional interactions among nervous, immune, and endocrine systems are stablished by soluble factors and receptors in cells of the three systems.

In mice treated with selective β_2AR agonists, such as clenbuterol or salbutamol, to stimulate these receptors, the lymph node egress of $CD4^+$, $CD8^+$ T lymphocytes, and antigen-primed T cells and B cells is retarded and is associated with lymphopenia. This lymphocyte retention is mediated through CXC chemokine receptor 4 (CXCR4) in T cells and B cells and is thought to explain the reduction of T-cell-mediated inflammation and lymphopenia [161]. CXCR4 is also expressed in monocytes and dendritic cells. CXCR4 ligand is the stromal cell-derived factor 12 (CXCL12), and both are linked to breast cancer metastasis. CXCR4-CXCL12 union promotes cell migration and adhesion and angiogenesis [162].

In lymph nodes with breast cancer metastasis, an increased level of CXCR4 transcript was detected compared to nonmetastatic lymph nodes. Also, a higher mRNA expression was found in breast cancer tumor stages III–IV than in stages I–II. Interestingly, in tumor tissues with HER-2 expression, CXCR4 transcription levels are also more elevated than in HER-2-negative tumors; therefore, there is a positive correlation between CXCR4 and HER-2 expression in breast tumors [163]. This phenomenon is explained because HER-2 enhances and impedes CXCR4 degradation [164]. CXCR4-CXCL12 axis is evolved in organ-directed metastasis, mainly associated with a higher CXCL12 expression in lymph nodes and lung, liver, and bone tissues where breast cancer metastasis is very common. CXCL12 acts as a chemoattractant for breast cancer cells that express CXCR4, promoting the arrival of these cells [165, 166].

Another group of immune cells, in which β_2AR produces an inhibitory effect, is the DCs. The stimulation of β_2AR with salbutamol inhibited the NF-κB transcription [167]. This transcription factor is required for DC antigen presentation; for the expression of CD80, CD86, and CD40 (costimulatory molecules); and for IL-12 secretion [168]. Also, salmeterol (β_2AR agonist) diminishes the IL-1, IL-6, and TNF-α production, in LPS-activated DCs [169].

On the other hand, in human monocytes primed during 16 hours with IFN-γ and stimulated with LPS, the addition of salbutamol diminished the IL-12 and TNF-α secretion, but not the IL-1α, IL-1β, or IL-10 production. Also, in neonatal $CD4^+$ lymphocytes, the Th1 cell differentiation in vitro was inhibited; instead, these $CD4^+$ T cells, stimulated with β_2AR agonists, produce IL-4 (Th2 cytokine), but not

IFN-γ (Th1 cytokine) [168]. Meanwhile in rats, adrenaline or metaproterenol (β_2AR agonist) in physiologic doses inhibited NK cell activation [170].

Either by directly action on tumor or immune cells, sympathetic signals regulate tumor progression. In this regard, as mentioned before, immune cell recruitment is a crucial step in immunosurveillance and immunosubversion. Sympathetic innervation in distant organs such as bone marrow promotes noradrenaline secretion that activates bone marrow-resident cells and promotes immune cell development and trafficking [171] and the posterior cell recruitment to tumor microenvironment mediated through tumor chemokine release and chemokine receptor expression in immune cells [166]. In this sense, tumor primary macrophage recruitment [39] and tumor cells increasing cytokine pro-inflammatory expression [21] are β_2AR mediated and influencing tumor progression [37, 39].

Despite the differences in β_2AR breast tumor cell expression that as an example in MB-231 cell line is higher than in MB-231BR cell line, the treatment with a β_2AR agonist (terbutaline or norepinephrine) modulates VEGF secretion through cAMP-PKA pathway, which is diminished in MB-231 cell line and augmented in MB-231BR cell line (metastatic to mouse brain). Meanwhile, IL-6 production in both cell lines was increased, in a cAMP-dependent and PKA-independent pathway [21]. These differences in VEGF secretion are maybe associated with the brain metastatic potential of MB-231BR cell line, because VEGF enhances blood vessel neoformation for tumor growth.

As mentioned before, immunosuppressive TAM works as M2 macrophages and, in this sense, has been found that epinephrine induces M2 macrophage polarization, in RAW 264.7 cells. This polarization is regulated through β_2AR. Also, in breast tumors co-expression of CD163$^+$ (M2 macrophages human marker) and β_2AR cell has been demonstrated; thus, macrophages in tumor microenvironment are influenced by adrenergic signals [37]. The relationship between M1 or M2 macrophages and hormone receptor status in breast cancer is due to the development of the disease. Hollmen et al. reported that when a cell line positive for the estrogen receptor (ER) is co-cultured with human monocytes, they acquire an M1 phenotype; meanwhile, the co-culture of them with ER- breast cancer cell line induced an M2 phenotype. The above indicates that ER governs the changes of the macrophages phenotype [172]. ER$^+$ breast cancer is related with an "early" development and a better prognostic, maybe associated with a M1 acute phase inflammatory response that effectively controls tumor progression. Meanwhile, TNBC usually presents a worse prognosis, and the presence of M2 exerts an immunosuppressive intratumoral effect that allows breast tumor growth and metastasis. Therefore, the macrophage phenotype is due to microenvironmental conditions and is associated consequently with tumor staging and prognosis.

Overexpression of HER-2 is correlated with β_2AR expression levels in breast tumor samples. In this sense, in MCF-7 cells overexpressing HER-2 (MCF-7/HER-2), β_2AR expression was also elevated, in an autocrine way through MCF-7/HER-2 epinephrine secretion. Interestingly, β_2AR activation with epinephrine, with norepinephrine, or with β_2AR agonists (isoproterenol and salmeterol) induces HER-2 expression in MCF-7 breast cancer cells. These findings are important because in HER-2$^+$ breast cancer cells, the activation of this surface tyrosine kinase may improve epinephrine secretion, through ERK signaling. Epinephrine may upregulate either β_2AR expression or HER-2 [173].

Concerning to breast cancer, in more aggressive tumors (TNBC), an increased amount of Foxp3$^+$ lymphocytes can be found in than less aggressive tumors (ER$^+$ or HER$^+$ tumors); this higher Treg tumor infiltration is also related to an increased risk of recurrence and a poor prognosis [174].

Ali et al. reported that in ER^- and HER^+ breast tumors, $CD8^+$ cell infiltration in tumor was associated with a reduction (28%) of mortality risk, but if these cells were in the tumor stroma, the risk reduction was lower (21%). A similar risk reduction (27%) was found in ER^+/HER^+ breast tumors [138]. The $CD8^+$ T-cell presence in tumor is associated then with the induction of tumor cell apoptosis that improve the prognosis and in some point is still acting as an effector-killing cell rather than a memory cell.

6. Conclusion

In breast cancer development, tumor cell proliferation is extensively studied, and almost all the treatments are encouraged to diminish it. Tumor cell interactions with other immune, nervous, tumor, and stromal cells, through the production of soluble factors and the expression of receptors, are the drivers of this proliferation. These relations may be driven inside the tumor or across the organism in distant places that respond to tumor signals. Therefore, elucidating not only molecular mechanisms but interactions among cells may enhance the development of new and more effective therapies against breast cancer.

Acknowledgements

The authors are grateful for the financial support received from the following agencies: Grant IN-209719 from Programa de Apoyo a Proyectos de Innovación Tecnológica (PAPIIT), Dirección General de Asuntos del Personal Académico (DGAPA), and Universidad Nacional Autónoma de México (UNAM) and Grant 2125 from Fronteras en la Ciencia, Consejo Nacional de Ciencia y Tecnología (CONACYT), both to J. Morales-Montor. Grant IA-202919 from Programa de Apoyo a Proyectos de Innovación Tecnológica (PAPIIT), Dirección General de Asuntos del Personal Académico (DGAPA), and Universidad Nacional Autónoma de México (UNAM) to KE. Nava-Castro. Rocío Alejandra Ruiz-Manzano is a PhD student at Programa de Doctorado en Ciencias Biomédicas, Universidad Nacional Autónoma de México, and received a fellowship from CONACyT. Mariana Segovia-Mendoza and Margarita Isabel Palacios-Arreola are postdoctoral fellows from DGAPA, UNAM.

Conflict of interest

The authors declare that there is no conflict of interest.

Author details

Rocío Alejandra Ruiz-Manzano[1], Tania de Lourdes Ochoa-Mercado[1], Mariana Segovia-Mendoza[1], Karen Elizabeth Nava-Castro[2], Margarita Isabel Palacios-Arreola[2] and Jorge Morales-Montor[1]*

1 Immunology Department, Biomedical Research Institute, National Autonomous University of Mexico, Mexico City, Mexico

2 Ambiental Genotoxicity and Mutagenesis Laboratory, Environmental Sciences Department, Atmospheric Sciences Center, National Autonomous University of Mexico, Mexico City, Mexico

*Address all correspondence to: jmontor66@biomedicas.unam.mx; jmontor66@hotmail.com

References

[1] Globocan W. Breast Cancer Fact Sheet Lyon [updated]. France: WHO; 2018 Available from: http://gco.iarc.fr/today/fact-sheets-cancers

[2] Jemal A, Siegel R, Ward E, Hao Y, Xu J, Thun MJ. Cancer statistics, 2009. CA: A Cancer Journal for Clinicians. 2009;**59**(4):225-249

[3] Barnard ME, Boeke CE, Tamimi RM. Established breast cancer risk factors and risk of intrinsic tumor subtypes. BBA Reviews on Cancer. 2015;**1856**(1):73-85

[4] Nava-Castro KE, Morales-Montor J, Ortega-Hernando A, Camacho-Arroyo I. Diethylstilbestrol exposure in neonatal mice induces changes in the adulthood in the immune response to taenia crassiceps without modifications of parasite loads. BioMed Research International. 2014;**2014**:498681

[5] Palacios-Arreola MI, Nava-Castro KE, Rio-Araiza VHD, Perez-Sanchez NY, Morales-Montor J. A single neonatal administration of bisphenol a induces higher tumour weight associated to changes in tumour microenvironment in the adulthood. Scientific Reports. 2017;**7**(1):10573

[6] Giuliano AE, Connolly JL, Edge SB, Mittendorf EA, Rugo HS, Solin LJ, et al. Breast cancer-major changes in the American joint committee on cancer eighth edition cancer staging manual. CA: A Cancer Journal for Clinicians. 2017;**67**(4):291-303

[7] Macias H, Hinck L. Mammary gland development. WIREs Developmental Biology. 2012;**1**(4):533-557

[8] Hennighausen L, Robinson GW. Signaling pathways in mammary gland development. Developmental Cell. 2001;**1**(4):467-475

[9] Gusterson BA, Warburton MJ, Mitchell D, Ellison M, Munro Neville A, Rudland PS. Distribution of myoepithelial cells and basement membrane proteins in the normal breast and in benign and malignant breast diseases. Cancer Research. 1982;**42**(11):4763-4770

[10] Barcellos-Hoff MH, Aggeler J, Ram TG, Bissell MJ. Functional differentiation and alveolar morphogenesis of primary mammary cultures on reconstituted basement membrane. Development. 1989;**105**(2):223-235

[11] Hanahan D, Coussens LM. Accessories to the crime: Functions of cells recruited to the tumor microenvironment. Cancer Cell. 2012;**21**(3):309-322

[12] Hanoun M, Maryanovich M, Arnal-Estapé A, Frenette PS. Neural regulation of hematopoiesis, inflammation, and cancer. Neuron. 2015;**86**(2):360-373

[13] Elefteriou F. Chronic stress, sympathetic activation and skeletal metastasis of breast cancer cells. BoneKEy Reports. 2015;**4**:693

[14] Cole SW, Nagaraja AS, Lutgendorf SK, Green PA, Sood AK. Sympathetic nervous system regulation of the tumour microenvironment. Nature Reviews. Cancer. 2015;**15**:563

[15] Bellinger DL, Lorton D. Autonomic regulation of cellular immune function. Autonomic Neuroscience: Basic & Clinical. 2014;**182**:15-41

[16] Bellinger DL, Millar BA, Perez S, Carter J, Wood C, Thyagarajan S, et al. Sympathetic modulation of immunity: Relevance to disease. Cellular Immunology. 2008;**252**(1-2):27-56

[17] Nance DM, Sanders VM. Autonomic innervation and regulation of the immune system (1987-2007). Brain, Behavior, and Immunity. 2007;**21**(6):736-745

[18] Madden KS. Sympathetic neural-immune interactions regulate hematopoiesis, thermoregulation and inflammation in mammals. Developmental and Comparative Immunology. 2017;**66**:92-97

[19] Du YY, Zhou LH, Wang YH, Yan TT, Jiang YW, Shao ZM, et al. Association of alpha2a and beta2 adrenoceptor expression with clinical outcome in breast cancer. Current Medical Research and Opinion. 2014;**30**(7):1337-1344

[20] Powe DG, Voss MJ, Habashy HO, Zanker KS, Green AR, Ellis IO, et al. Alpha- and beta-adrenergic receptor (AR) protein expression is associated with poor clinical outcome in breast cancer: An immunohistochemical study. Breast Cancer Research and Treatment. 2011;**130**(2):457-463

[21] Madden KS, Szpunar MJ, Brown EB. Beta-adrenergic receptors (beta-AR) regulate VEGF and IL-6 production by divergent pathways in high beta-AR-expressing breast cancer cell lines. Breast Cancer Research and Treatment. 2011;**130**(3):747-758

[22] Choy C, Raytis JL, Smith DD, Duenas M, Neman J, Jandial R, et al. Inhibition of beta2-adrenergic receptor reduces triple-negative breast cancer brain metastases: The potential benefit of perioperative beta-blockade. Oncology Reports. 2016;**35**(6):3135-3142

[23] Pon CK, Lane JR, Sloan EK, Halls ML. The beta2-adrenoceptor activates a positive cAMP-calcium feedforward loop to drive breast cancer cell invasion. The FASEB Journal. 2016;**30**(3):1144-1154

[24] Cole SW, Sood AK. Molecular pathways: Beta-adrenergic signaling in cancer. Clinical Cancer Research. 2012;**18**(5):1201-1206

[25] Kumar N, Gupta S, Dabral S, Singh S, Sehrawat S. Role of exchange protein directly activated by cAMP (EPAC1) in breast cancer cell migration and apoptosis. Molecular and Cellular Biochemistry. 2017;**430**(1-2):115-125

[26] Hara MR, Kovacs JJ, Whalen EJ, Rajagopal S, Strachan RT, Grant W, et al. A stress response pathway regulates DNA damage through beta (2)-adrenoreceptors and beta-arrestin-1. Nature. 2011;**477**(7364):349-U129

[27] Ayala GE, Dai H, Powell M, Li R, Ding Y, Wheeler TM, et al. Cancer-related axonogenesis and neurogenesis in prostate cancer. Clinical Cancer Research. 2008;**14**(23):7593-7603

[28] Pundavela J, Roselli S, Faulkner S, Attia J, Scott RJ, Thorne RF, et al. Nerve fibers infiltrate the tumor microenvironment and are associated with nerve growth factor production and lymph node invasion in breast cancer. Molecular Oncology. 2015;**9**(8):1626-1635

[29] Kowalski PJ, Paulino AFG. Perineural invasion in adenoid cystic carcinoma: Its causation/promotion by brain-derived neurotrophic factor. Human Pathology. 2002;**33**(9):933-936

[30] Szpunar MJ, Belcher EK, Dawes RP, Madden KS. Sympathetic innervation, norepinephrine content, and norepinephrine turnover in orthotopic and spontaneous models of breast cancer. Brain, Behavior, and Immunity. 2016;**53**:223-233

[31] Lutgendorf SK, DeGeest K, Dahmoush L, Farley D, Penedo F, Bender D, et al. Social isolation is associated with elevated tumor

norepinephrine in ovarian carcinoma patients. Brain, Behavior, and Immunity. 2011;**25**(2):250-255

[32] Stephens MA, Wand G. Stress and the HPA axis: Role of glucocorticoids in alcohol dependence. Alcohol Research: Current Reviews. 2012;**34**(4):468-483

[33] Melhem A, Yamada SD, Fleming GF, Delgado B, Brickley DR, Wu W, et al. Administration of glucocorticoids to ovarian cancer patients is associated with expression of the anti-apoptotic genes SGK1 and MKP1/DUSP1 in ovarian tissues. Clinical Cancer Research. 2009;**15**(9):3196-3204

[34] Mikosz CA, Brickley DR, Sharkey MS, Moran TW, Conzen SD. Glucocorticoid receptor-mediated protection from apoptosis is associated with induction of the serine/threonine survival kinase gene, sgk-1. The Journal of Biological Chemistry. 2001;**276**(20):16649-16654

[35] Pan D, Kocherginsky M, Conzen SD. Activation of the glucocorticoid receptor is associated with poor prognosis in estrogen receptor-negative breast cancer. Cancer Research. 2011;**71**(20):6360-6370

[36] Pang D, Kocherginsky M, Krausz T, Kim SY, Conzen SD. Dexamethasone decreases xenograft response to paclitaxel through inhibition of tumor cell apoptosis. Cancer Biology & Therapy. 2006;**5**(8):933-940

[37] Qin JF, Jin FJ, Li N, Guan HT, Lan L, Ni H, et al. Adrenergic receptor beta2 activation by stress promotes breast cancer progression through macrophages M2 polarization in tumor microenvironment. BMB Reports. 2015;**48**(5):295-300

[38] Armaiz-Pena GN, Cole SW, Lutgendorf SK, Sood AK. Neuroendocrine influences on cancer progression. Brain, Behavior, and Immunity. 2013;**30**(Suppl):S19-S25

[39] Sloan EK, Priceman SJ, Cox BF, Yu S, Pimentel MA, Tangkanangnukul V, et al. The sympathetic nervous system induces a metastatic switch in primary breast cancer. Cancer Research. 2010;**70**(18):7042-7052

[40] Zou W, Restifo NP. T(H)17 cells in tumour immunity and immunotherapy. Nature Reviews. Immunology. 2010;**10**(4):248-256

[41] Emens LA, Silverstein SC, Khleif S, Marincola FM, Galon J. Toward integrative cancer immunotherapy: Targeting the tumor microenvironment. Journal of Translational Medicine. 2012;**10**(1):70

[42] Zitvogel L, Tesniere A, Kroemer G. Cancer despite immunosurveillance: Immunoselection and immunosubversion. Nature Reviews. Immunology. 2006;**6**(10):715-727

[43] Gardner A, Ruffell B. Dendritic cells and cancer immunity. Trends in Immunology. 2016;**37**(12):855-865

[44] Steinman RM. Decisions about dendritic cells: Past, present, and future. Annual Review of Immunology. 2012;**30**:1-22

[45] Steinman RM, Inaba K, Turley S, Pierre P, Mellman I. Antigen capture, processing, and presentation by dendritic cells: Recent cell biological studies. Human Immunology. 1999;**60**(7):562-567

[46] Segura E, Amigorena S. Cross-presentation in mouse and human dendritic cells. Advances in Immunology. 2015;**127**:1-31

[47] Gottfried E, Kreutz M, Mackensen A. Tumor-induced modulation of dendritic cell function. Cytokine & Growth Factor Reviews. 2008;**19**(1):65-77

[48] Chen X, Shao Q, Hao S, Zhao Z, Wang Y, Guo X, et al. CTLA-4 positive breast cancer cells suppress dendritic cells maturation and function. Oncotarget. 2017;**8**(8):13703-13715

[49] Ruffell B, Chang-Strachan D, Chan V, Rosenbusch A, Ho CMT, Pryer N, et al. Macrophage IL-10 blocks CD8(+) T cell-dependent responses to chemotherapy by suppressing IL-12 expression in Intratumoral dendritic cells. Cancer Cell. 2014;**26**(5):623-637

[50] Buisseret L, Desmedt C, Garaud S, Fornili M, Wang X, Van den Eyden G, et al. Reliability of tumor-infiltrating lymphocyte and tertiary lymphoid structure assessment in human breast cancer. Modern Pathology: An Official Journal of the United States and Canadian Academy of Pathology, Inc. 2017;**30**(9):1204-1212

[51] Thompson ED, Enriquez HL, Fu YX, Engelhard VH. Tumor masses support naive T cell infiltration, activation, and differentiation into effectors. The Journal of Experimental Medicine. 2010;**207**(8):1791-1804

[52] Houghton AM. The paradox of tumor-associated neutrophils fueling tumor growth with cytotoxic substances. Cell Cycle. 2010;**9**(9):1732-1737

[53] Brinkmann V, Reichard U, Goosmann C, Fauler B, Uhlemann Y, Weiss DS, et al. Neutrophil extracellular traps kill bacteria. Science. 2004;**303**(5663):1532-1535

[54] Kolaczkowska E, Kubes P. Neutrophil recruitment and function in health and inflammation. Nature Reviews. Immunology. 2013;**13**(3):159-175

[55] Pham CTN. Neutrophil serine proteases: Specific regulators of inflammation. Nature Reviews. Immunology. 2006;**6**(7):541-550

[56] Garley M, Jablonska E, Dabrowska D. NETs in cancer. Tumor Biology. 2016;**37**(11):14355-14361

[57] Treffers LW, Hiemstra IH, Kuijpers TW, van den Berg TK, Matlung HL. Neutrophils in cancer. Immunological Reviews. 2016;**273**(1):312-328

[58] Park J, Wysocki RW, Amoozgar Z, Maiorino L, Fein MR, Jorns J, et al. Cancer cells induce metastasis-supporting neutrophil extracellular DNA traps. Science Translational Medicine. 2016;**8**(361):1-21

[59] Wels J, Kaplan RN, Rafii S, Lyden D. Migratory neighbors and distant invaders: Tumor-associated niche cells. Genes & Development. 2008;**22**(5):559-574

[60] Kato M, Kephart GM, Talley NJ, Wagner JM, Sarr MG, Bonno M, et al. Eosinophil infiltration and degranulation in normal human tissue. The Anatomical Record. 1998;**252**(3):418-425

[61] Akuthota P, Wang HB, Weller PF. Eosinophils as antigen-presenting cells in allergic upper airway disease. Current Opinion in Allergy and Clinical Immunology. 2010;**10**(1):14-19

[62] Hamed EA, Zakhary MM, Maximous DW. Apoptosis, angiogenesis, inflammation, and oxidative stress: Basic interactions in patients with early and metastatic breast cancer. Journal of Cancer Research and Clinical Oncology. 2012;**138**(6):999-1009

[63] Snoussia K, Mahfoudha W, Bouaouinaac N, Ahmedd SB, Helalb AN, Chouchane L. Genetic variation in IL-8 associated with increased risk and poor prognosis of breast carcinoma. Human Immunology. 2006;**67**(1-2):13-21

[64] Kamel M, Shouman S, El-Merzebany M, Kilic G, Veenstra T, Saeed M et al. Effect of tumour necrosis factor-alpha on estrogen metabolic pathways in breast cancer cells. Journal of Cancer. 2012;**3**:310-321

[65] Sanderson CJ. Interleukin-5, eosinophils, and disease. Blood. 1992;**79**(12):3101-3109

[66] Grencis RK, Bancroft AJ. Interleukin-13—A key mediator in resistance to gastrointestinal-dwelling nematode parasites. Clinical Reviews in Allergy and Immunology. 2004;**26**(1):51-60

[67] Srabovic N, Mujagic Z, Mujanovic-Mustedanagic J, Muminovic Z, Softic A, Begic L. Interleukin 13 expression in the primary breast cancer tumour tissue. Biochemia Medica. 2011;**21**(2):131-138

[68] Humphreys RC, Hennighausen L. Transforming growth factor alpha and mouse models of human breast cancer. Oncogene. 2000;**19**(8):1085-1091

[69] Esquivel-Velazquez M, Ostoa-Saloma P, Palacios-Arreola MI, Nava-Castro KE, Castro JI, Morales-Montor J. The role of cytokines in breast cancer development and progression. Journal of Interferon and Cytokine Research. 2015;**35**(1):1-16

[70] Hennig R, Ding XZ, Tong WG, Schneider MB, Standop J, Friess H et al. 5-Lipoxygenase and leukotriene B(4) receptor are expressed in human pancreatic cancers but not in pancreatic ducts in normal tissue. The American Journal of Pathology. 2002;**161**(2):421-428

[71] Wang D, Dubois RN. Eicosanoids and cancer. Nature Reviews Cancer. 2010;**10**(3):181-193

[72] Wang D, Dubois RN. Cyclooxygenase-2: A potential target in breast cancer. Seminars in Oncology. 2004;**31**(1 Suppl 3):64-73

[73] Sobolesky PM, Halushka PV, Garrett-Mayer E, Smith MT, Moussa O. Regulation of the tumor suppressor FOXO3 by the thromboxane-A2 receptors in urothelial cancer. PLoS One. 2014;**9**(9):e107530

[74] Wang Z, Cheng Q, Tang K, Sun Y, Zhang K, Zhang Y, et al. Lipid mediator lipoxin A4 inhibits tumor growth by targeting IL-10-producing regulatory B (Breg) cells. Cancer Letters. 2015;**364**(2):118-124

[75] Rothenberg ME, Hogan SP. The eosinophil. The Annual Review of Immunology. 2006;**24**:147-174

[76] Gatault S, Legrand F, Delbeke M, Loiseau S, Capron M. Involvement of eosinophils in the anti-tumor response. Cancer Immunology, Immunotherapy. 2012;**61**(9):1527-1534

[77] De Lima PO, Dos Santos FV, Oliveira DT, De Figueredo RC, Pereira MC. Effect of eosinophil cationic protein on human oral squamous carcinoma cell viability. Molecular and Clinical Oncology. 2015;**3**(2):353-356

[78] Kubo H, Loegering DA, Adolphson CR, Gleich GJ. Cytotoxic properties of eosinophil granule major basic protein for tumor cells. International Archives of Allergy and Immunology. 1999;**118**(2-4):426-428

[79] Sakkal S, Miller S, Apostolopoulos V, Nurgali K. Eosinophils in cancer: Favourable or unfavourable? Current Medicinal Chemistry. 2016;**23**(7):650-666

[80] Davis BP, Rothenberg ME. Eosinophils and cancer. Cancer Immunology Research. 2014;**2**(1):1-8

[81] Wu W, Samoszuk MK, Comhair SA, Thomassen MJ, Farver CF, Dweik RA, et al. Eosinophils generate brominating oxidants in allergen-induced asthma. The Journal of Clinical Investigation. 2000;**105**(10):1455-1463

[82] Samoszuk M, Sholly S, Epstein AL. Eosinophil peroxidase is detectable with a monoclonal antibody in collagen bands of nodular sclerosis Hodgkin's disease. Laboratory Investigation. 1987;**56**(4):394-400

[83] Gouon-Evans V, Lin EY, Pollard JW. Requirement of macrophages and eosinophils and their cytokines/chemokines for mammary gland development. Breast Cancer Research. 2002;**4**(4):155-164

[84] Galli SJ, Borregaard N, Wynn TA. Phenotypic and functional plasticity of cells of innate immunity: Macrophages, mast cells and neutrophils. Nature Immunology. 2011;**12**(11):1035-1044

[85] Mekori YA, Hershko AY, Frossi B, Mion F, Pucillo CE. Integrating innate and adaptive immune cells: Mast cells as crossroads between regulatory and effector B and T cells. European Journal of Pharmacology. 2016;**778**:84-89

[86] Della Rovere F, Granata A, Monaco M, Basile G. Phagocytosis of cancer cells by mast cells in breast Cancer. Anticancer Research. 2009;**29**(8):3157-3161

[87] Kambayashi T, Allenspach EJ, Chang JT, Zou T, Shoag JE, Reiner SL, et al. Inducible MHC class II expression by mast cells supports effector and regulatory T cell activation. Journal of Immunology. 2009;**182**(8):4686-4695

[88] Stelekati E, Bahri R, D'Orlando O, Orinska Z, Mittrucker HW, Langenhaun R, et al. Mast cell-mediated antigen presentation regulates CD8(+) T cell effector functions. Immunity. 2009;**31**(4):665-676

[89] Khan MM, Strober S, Melmon KL. Regulatory effects of mast-cells on lymphoid-cells—The role of histamine Type-1 receptors in the interaction between mast-cells, helper T-cells and natural suppressor cells. Cellular Immunology. 1986;**103**(1):41-53

[90] Nakae S, Suto H, Kakurai M, Sedgwick JD, Tsai M, Galli SJ. Mast cells enhance T cell activation: Importance of mast cell-derived TNF. Proceedings of the National Academy of Sciences of The United States of America. 2005;**102**(18):6467-6472

[91] Faustino-Rocha AI, Gama A, Oliveira PA, Katrien VE, Saunders JH, Pires MJ, et al. Modulation of mammary tumor vascularization by mast cells: Ultrasonographic and histopathological approaches. Life Sciences. 2017;**176**:35-41

[92] Xiang M, Gu Y, Zhao F, Lu H, Chen S, Yin L. Mast cell tryptase promotes breast cancer migration and invasion. Oncology Reports. 2010;**23**(3):615-619

[93] Kankkunen JP, HArvima IT, Naukkarinen A. Quantitative analysis of tryptase and chymase containing mast cells in benign and malignant breast lesions. International Journal of Cancer. 1997;**72**(3):385-388

[94] Qian BZ, Pollard JW. Macrophage diversity enhances tumor progression and metastasis. Cell. 2010;**141**(1):39-51

[95] Zhao X, Qu J, Sun Y, Wang J, Liu X, Wang F, et al. Prognostic significance of tumor-associated macrophages in breast cancer: A meta-analysis of the literature. Oncotarget. 2017;**8**(18):30576-30586

[96] Wu P, Wu D, Zhao L, Huang L, Chen G, Shen G, et al. Inverse role of distinct subsets and distribution of macrophage in lung cancer prognosis: A meta-analysis. Oncotarget. 2016;**7**(26):40451-40460

[97] Noy R, Pollard JW. Tumor-associated macrophages: From mechanisms to therapy. Immunity. 2014;**41**(1):49-61

[98] Mantovani A, Biswas SK, Galdiero MR, Sica A, Locati M. Macrophage plasticity and polarization in tissue repair and remodelling. The Journal of Pathology. 2013;**229**(2):176-185

[99] Lodoen MB, Lanier LL. Natural killer cells as an initial defense against pathogens. Current Opinion in Immunology. 2006;**18**(4):391-398

[100] Arase H, Arase N, Saito T. Interferon gamma production by natural killer (NK) cells and NK1.1(+) T cells upon NKR-P1 cross-linking. The Journal of Experimental Medicine. 1996;**183**(5):2391-2396

[101] Mamessier E, Sylvain A, Thibult ML, Houvenaeghel G, Jacquemier J, Castellano R, et al. Human breast cancer cells enhance self tolerance by promoting evasion from NK cell antitumor immunity. The Journal of Clinical Investigation. 2011;**121**(9):3609-3622

[102] Moretta L, Moretta A. Unravelling natural killer cell function: Triggering and inhibitory human NK receptors. The EMBO Journal. 2004;**23**(2):255-259

[103] Madjd Z, Spendlove I, Pinder SE, Ellis IO, Durrant LG. Total loss of MHC class I is an independent indicator of good prognosis in breast cancer. International Journal of Cancer. 2005;**117**(2):248-255

[104] Castriconi R, Cantoni C, Della Chiesa M, Vitale M, Marcenaro E, Conte R, et al. Transforming growth factor beta 1 inhibits expression of NKp30 and NKG2D receptors: Consequences for the NK-mediated killing of dendritic cells. Proceedings of the National Academy of Sciences of the United States of America. 2003;**100**(7):4120-4125

[105] Della Chiesa M, Carlomagno S, Frumento G, Balsamo M, Cantoni C, Conte R, et al. The tryptophan catabolite L-kynurenine inhibits the surface expression of NKp46- and NKG2D-activating receptors and regulates NK-cell function. Blood. 2006;**108**(13):4118-4125

[106] Curtsinger JM, Mescher MF. Inflammatory cytokines as a third signal for T cell activation. Current Opinion in Immunology. 2010;**22**(3):333-340

[107] Kohlhapp FJ, Zloza A. $CD4^+$ T cells. In: Marshall JL, editor. Cancer Therapeutic Targets. New York, NY: Springer, New York; 2017. pp. 117-129

[108] Mescher MF, Agarwal P, Casey KA, Hammerbeck CD, Xiao Z, Curtsinger JM. Molecular basis for checkpoints in the CD8 T cell response: Tolerance versus activation. Seminars in Immunology. 2007;**19**(3):153-161

[109] Gu-Trantien C, Willard-Gallo K. Tumor-infiltrating follicular helper T cells: The new kids on the block. Oncoimmunology. 2013;**2**(10):e26066

[110] Tangye SG, Ma CS, Brink R, Deenick EK. The good, the bad and the ugly—TFH cells in human health and disease. Nature Reviews Immunology. 2013;**13**(6):412-426

[111] Gu-Trantien C, Loi S, Garaud S, Equeter C, Libin M, de Wind A et al. $CD4^+$ follicular helper T cell infiltration predicts breast cancer survival. The Journal of Clinical Investigation. 2013;**123**(7):2873-2892

[112] Gollob JA, Ritz J. CD2-CD58 interaction and the control of T-cell interleukin-12 responsiveness. Adhesion molecules link innate and acquired immunity. Annals of the New York Academy of Sciences. 1996;**795**:71-81

[113] Manetti R, Parronchi P, Giudizi MG, Piccinni MP, Maggi E, Trinchieri G, et al. Natural killer cell stimulatory factor (interleukin 12

[IL-12]) induces T helper type 1 (Th1)-specific immune responses and inhibits the development of IL-4-producing Th cells. The Journal of Experimental Medicine. 1993;**177**(4):1199-1204

[114] Trinchieri G. Interleukin-12: A cytokine produced by antigen-presenting cells with immunoregulatory functions in the generation of T-helper cells type 1 and cytotoxic lymphocytes. Blood. 1994;**84**(12):4008-4027

[115] Malek TR, Castro I. Interleukin-2 receptor signaling: At the interface between tolerance and immunity. Immunity. 2010;**33**(2):153-165

[116] Mosmann TR, Coffman RL. TH1 and TH2 cells: Different patterns of lymphokine secretion lead to different functional properties. Annual Review of Immunology. 1989;**7**:145-173

[117] Pruneri G, Vingiani A, Denkert C. Tumor infiltrating lymphocytes in early breast cancer. Breast (Edinburgh, Scotland). 2018;**37**:207-214

[118] Mahmoud S, Lee A, Ellis I, Green A. CD8(+) T lymphocytes infiltrating breast cancer: A promising new prognostic marker? Oncoimmunology. 2012;**1**(3):364-365

[119] Aspord C, Pedroza-Gonzalez A, Gallegos M, Tindle S, Burton EC, Su D, et al. Breast cancer instructs dendritic cells to prime interleukin 13-secreting $CD4^-$ T cells that facilitate tumor development. The Journal of Experimental Medicine. 2007;**204**(5):1037-1047

[120] Guglani L, Khader SA. Th17 cytokines in mucosal immunity and inflammation. Current Opinion in HIV and AIDS. 2010;**5**(2):120-127

[121] Zhu J, Paul WE. Peripheral $CD4^+$ T-cell differentiation regulated by networks of cytokines and transcription factors. Immunological Reviews. 2010;**238**(1):247-262

[122] Ye J, Livergood RS, Peng G. The role and regulation of human Th17 cells in tumor immunity. The American Journal of Pathology. 2013;**182**(1):10-20

[123] Josefowicz SZ, Lu L-F, Rudensky AY. Regulatory T cells: Mechanisms of differentiation and function. Annual Review of Immunology. 2012;**30**:531-564

[124] Sather BD, Treuting P, Perdue N, Miazgowicz M, Fontenot JD, Rudensky AY, et al. Altering the distribution of Foxp3(+) regulatory T cells results in tissue-specific inflammatory disease. The Journal of Experimental Medicine. 2007;**204**(6):1335-1347

[125] Khor B, Regulatory T. Cells: Central concepts from ontogeny to therapy. Transfusion Medicine Reviews. 2017;**31**(1):36-44

[126] Vignali DAA, Collison LW, Workman CJ. How regulatory T cells work. Nature Reviews. Immunology. 2008;**8**(7):523-532

[127] Hamidullah CB, Konwar R. Role of interleukin-10 in breast cancer. Breast Cancer Research and Treatment. 2012;**133**(1):11-21

[128] Saraiva M, O'Garra A. The regulation of IL-10 production by immune cells. Nature Reviews. Immunology. 2010;**10**(3):170-181

[129] Trandem K, Zhao J, Fleming E, Perlman S. Highly activated cytotoxic CD8 T cells express protective IL-10 at the peak of coronavirus-induced encephalitis. Journal of Immunology. 2011;**186**(6):3642-3652

[130] Curtsinger JM, Lins DC, Mescher MF. Signal 3 determines tolerance versus full activation of naive

CD8 T cells: Dissociating proliferation and development of effector function. The Journal of Experimental Medicine. 2003;**197**(9):1141-1151

[131] Varn FS, Mullins DW, Arias-Pulido H, Fiering S, Cheng C. Adaptive immunity programmes in breast cancer. Immunology. 2017;**150**(1):25-34

[132] Zhang N, Bevan MJ. CD8(+) T cells: Foot soldiers of the immune system. Immunity. 2011;**35**(2):161-168

[133] Maimela NR, Liu S, Zhang Y. Fates of CD8+ T cells in tumor microenvironment. Computational and Structural Biotechnology Journal. 2019;**17**:1-13

[134] Tugues S, Burkhard SH, Ohs I, Vrohlings M, Nussbaum K, Vom Berg J, et al. New insights into IL-12-mediated tumor suppression. Cell Death and Differentiation. 2015;**22**(2):237-246

[135] Schietinger A, Greenberg PD. Tolerance and exhaustion: Defining mechanisms of T cell dysfunction. Trends in Immunology. 2014;**35**(2):51-60

[136] Pipkin ME, Sacks JA, Cruz-Guilloty F, Lichtenheld MG, Bevan MJ, Rao A. Interleukin-2 and inflammation induce distinct transcriptional programs that promote the differentiation of effector cytolytic T cells. Immunity. 2010;**32**(1):79-90

[137] Yang SX, Wei WS, Ouyan QW, Jiang QH, Zou YF, Qu W, et al. Interleukin-12 activated CD8(+) T cells induces apoptosis in breast cancer cells and reduces tumor growth. Biomedicine & pharmacotherapy = Biomedecine & Pharmacotherapie. 2016;**84**:1466-1471

[138] Ali HR, Provenzano E, Dawson SJ, Blows FM, Liu B, Shah M, et al. Association between CD8+ T-cell infiltration and breast cancer survival in 12,439 patients. Annals of Oncology: Official Journal of the European Society for Medical Oncology. 2014;**25**(8):1536-1543

[139] Nava-Castro KE, Palacios-Arreola MI, Ostoa-Saloma P, Muñiz-Hernández S, Cerbón MA, Gomez-Icazbalceta G, et al. The immunoendocrine network in breast cancer. Advances in Neuroimmune Biology. 2014;**5**(2):109-131

[140] Brisken C, Park S, Vass T, Lydon JP, O'Malley BW, Weinberg RA. A paracrine role for the epithelial progesterone receptor in mammary gland development. Proceedings of the National Academy of Sciences of the United States of America. 1998;**95**(9):5076-5081

[141] Pelletier G, El-Alfy M. Immunocytochemical localization of estrogen receptors alpha and beta in the human reproductive organs. The Journal of Clinical Endocrinology and Metabolism. 2000;**85**(12):4835-4840

[142] Mallepell S, Krust A, Chambon P, Brisken C. Paracrine signaling through the epithelial estrogen receptor alpha is required for proliferation and morphogenesis in the mammary gland. Proceedings of the National Academy of Sciences of the United States of America. 2006;**103**(7):2196-2201

[143] Hall JM, McDonnell DP. The estrogen receptor beta-isoform (ERbeta) of the human estrogen receptor modulates ERalpha transcriptional activity and is a key regulator of the cellular response to estrogens and antiestrogens. Endocrinology. 1999;**140**(12):5566-5578

[144] Coriano CG, Liu F, Sievers CK, Liang M, Wang Y, Lim Y, et al. A computational-based approach to identify estrogen receptor alpha/beta heterodimer selective ligands. Molecular Pharmacology. 2018;**93**(3):197-207

[145] Khan D, Ansar AS. The immune system is a natural target for estrogen action: Opposing effects of estrogen in two prototypical autoimmune diseases. Frontiers in Immunology. 2015;**6**:635

[146] Osborne CK, Schiff R, Fuqua SA, Shou J. Estrogen receptor: Current understanding of its activation and modulation. Clinical Cancer Research. 2001;**7**(12 Suppl):4338s-4342s; discussion 411s-412s

[147] Nemere I, Pietras RJ, Blackmore PF. Membrane receptors for steroid hormones: Signal transduction and physiological significance. Journal of Cellular Biochemistry. 2003;**88**(3):438-445

[148] Scarpin KM, Graham JD, Mote PA, Clarke CL. Progesterone action in human tissues: Regulation by progesterone receptor (PR) isoform expression, nuclear positioning and coregulator expression. Nuclear Receptor Signaling. 2009;**7**:e009-e

[149] Clarke RB, Spence K, Anderson E, Howell A, Okano H, Potten CS. A putative human breast stem cell population is enriched for steroid receptor-positive cells. Developmental Biology. 2005;**277**(2):443-456

[150] Fox EM, Davis RJ, Shupnik MA. ERbeta in breast cancer—Onlooker, passive player, or active protector? Steroids. 2008;**73**(11):1039-1051

[151] Shibuya R, Suzuki T, Miki Y, Yoshida K, Moriya T, Ono K, et al. Intratumoral concentration of sex steroids and expression of sex steroid-producing enzymes in ductal carcinoma in situ of human breast. Endocrine-Related Cancer. 2008;**15**(1):113-124

[152] Sasano H, Harada N. Intratumoral aromatase in human breast, endometrial, and ovarian malignancies. Endocrine Reviews. 1998;**19**(5):593-607

[153] Dimitrakakis C, Bondy C. Androgens and the breast. Breast Cancer Research: BCR. 2009;**11**(5):212

[154] Yeh S, Hu YC, Wang PH, Xie C, Xu Q, Tsai MY, et al. Abnormal mammary gland development and growth retardation in female mice and MCF7 breast cancer cells lacking androgen receptor. The Journal of Experimental Medicine. 2003;**198**(12):1899-1908

[155] Vera-Badillo FE, Templeton AJ, de Gouveia P, Diaz-Padilla I, Bedard PL, Al-Mubarak M, et al. Androgen receptor expression and outcomes in early breast cancer: A systematic review and meta-analysis. Journal of the National Cancer Institute. 2014;**106**(1):djt319

[156] Spurdle AB, Antoniou AC, Duffy DL, Pandeya N, Kelemen L, Chen X, et al. The androgen receptor CAG repeat polymorphism and modification of breast cancer risk in BRCA1 and BRCA2 mutation carriers. Breast Cancer Research. 2005;**7**(2):R176-R183

[157] Labrie F, Belanger A, Luu-The V, Labrie C, Simard J, Cusan L, et al. DHEA and the intracrine formation of androgens and estrogens in peripheral target tissues: Its role during aging. Steroids. 1998;**63**(5-6):322-328

[158] Oberbeck R, Kobbe P. Dehydroepiandrosterone (DHEA): A steroid with multiple effects. Is there any possible option in the treatment of critical illness? Current Medicinal Chemistry. 2010;**17**(11):1039-1047

[159] Shaak TL, Wijesinghe DS, Chalfant CE, Diegelmann RF, Ward KR, Loria RM. Structural stereochemistry of androstene hormones determines interactions with human androgen, estrogen, and glucocorticoid receptors. International Journal of Medicinal Chemistry. 2013;**2013**:203606

[160] Lopez-Marure R, Contreras PG, Dillon JS. Effects of

dehydroepiandrosterone on proliferation, migration, and death of breast cancer cells. European Journal of Pharmacology. 2011;**660**(2-3):268-274

[161] Nakai A, Hayano Y, Furuta F, Noda M, Suzuki K. Control of lymphocyte egress from lymph nodes through beta2-adrenergic receptors. The Journal of Experimental Medicine. 2014;**211**(13):2583-2598

[162] Luker KE, Luker GD. Functions of CXCL12 and CXCR4 in breast cancer. Cancer Letters. 2006;**238**(1):30-41

[163] Dayer R, Babashah S, Jamshidi S, Sadeghizadeh M. Upregulation of CXC chemokine receptor 4-CXC chemokine ligand 12 axis ininvasive breast carcinoma: A potent biomarker predicting lymph node metastasis. Journal of Cancer Research and Therapeutics. 2018;**14**(2):345-350

[164] Li YM, Pan Y, Wei Y, Cheng X, Zhou BP, Tan M, et al. Upregulation of CXCR4 is essential for HER2-mediated tumor metastasis. Cancer Cell. 2004;6(5):459-469

[165] Mukherjee D, Zhao J. The role of chemokine receptor CXCR4 in breast cancer metastasis. American Journal of Cancer Research. 2013;**3**(1):46-57

[166] Palacios-Arreola MI, Nava-Castro KE, Castro JI, Garcia-Zepeda E, Carrero JC, Morales-Montor J. The role of chemokines in breast cancer pathology and its possible use as therapeutic targets. Journal of Immunology Research. 2014;**2014**:849720

[167] Herve J, Dubreil L, Tardif V, Terme M, Pogu S, Anegon I, et al. beta2-Adrenoreceptor agonist inhibits antigen cross-presentation by dendritic cells. Journal of Immunology. 2013;**190**(7):3163-3171

[168] Panina-Bordignon P, Mazzeo D, Lucia PD, D'Ambrosio D, Lang R, Fabbri L, et al. Beta2-agonists prevent Th1 development by selective inhibition of interleukin 12. The Journal of Clinical Investigation. 1997;**100**(6):1513-1519

[169] Abdi K, Singh NJ, Matzinger P. Lipopolysaccharide-activated dendritic cells: "exhausted" or alert and waiting? Journal of immunology (Baltimore, MD: 1950). 2012;**188**(12):5981-5989

[170] Ben-Eliyahu S, Shakhar G, Shakhar K, Melamed R. Timing within the oestrous cycle modulates adrenergic suppression of NK activity and resistance to metastasis: Possible clinical implications. British Journal of Cancer. 2000;**83**(12):1747-1754

[171] Scanzano A, Cosentino M. Adrenergic regulation of innate immunity: A review. Frontiers in Pharmacology. 2015;**6**:171

[172] Hollmen M, Karaman S, Schwager S, Lisibach A, Christiansen A, Maksimow M, et al. G-CSF regulates macrophage phenotype and associates with poor overall survival in human triple-negative breast cancer. Scandinavian Journal of Immunology. 2016;**83**(5):373-374

[173] Shi M, Liu D, Duan H, Qian L, Wang L, Niu L, et al. The beta2-adrenergic receptor and Her2 comprise a positive feedback loop in human breast cancer cells. Breast Cancer Research and Treatment. 2011;**125**(2):351-362

[174] Plitas G, Konopacki C, Wu K, Bos PD, Morrow M, Putintseva EV, et al. Regulatory T cells exhibit distinct features in human breast cancer. Immunity. 2016;**45**(5):1122-1134

Section 3

Prediction of Response to Therapy and Drug Resistance

Chapter 7

Recent Approaches Encompassing the Phenotypic Cell Heterogeneity for Anticancer Drug Efficacy Evaluation

Aurimas Stulpinas, Aušra Imbrasaitė, Natalija Krestnikova and Audronė Valerija Kalvelytė

Abstract

Despite the advancements in biomarker-based personalized cancer therapy, the inadequacy of molecular and genetic profiling in identifying effective drug combinations was defined in most cases. Drug resistance remains a major limitation of the current predictive oncology. Emerging reports indicate that the success of anticancer therapy is usually limited by intratumoral heterogeneity which is not captured by the existing cancer cell biomarker-based approaches. Cell heterogeneity, not only genetic but also phenotypic, is considered to be the root cause of resistance to anticancer treatment, cancer progression, and the presence of cancer stem cells. Therefore, functional testing of live cells representing various cell types within the tumor exposed to potential therapies is needed for identification of effective drug combinations. Here we look at the different existing model systems, including ex vivo models of the patient's tumor cells, 2D/3D in vitro cultures/cocultures, patient-derived cellular organoids, single-cell models, ex vivo tumor platforms containing tumor microenvironment and extracellular matrix, etc., scoping at drug efficacy evaluation and solving the problem of cancer resistance.

Keywords: ex vivo model, cancer heterogeneity, tumor microenvironment, cancer stem cells, anticancer therapy, drug resistance, plasticity

1. Introduction

Fighting cancer is a major challenge for scientists and clinicians. As a result of human population aging, today cancer is the most common cause of death in the world. One of the most promising measures to reduce cancer deaths is believed to be prevention. However, only smaller part of cancers can be prevented by avoiding environmental risk factors. The recent results presented in Science suggest that only one-third of the cancer risk is attributable to environmental factors or inherited predispositions, and that unavoidable random errors or mutations (bad-luck mutations), occurring during DNA replication in normal stem cells, are a major contributing factor in cancer development [1]. Authors suggest that this stochastic factor is the major contributor to cancer overall. The results are consistent with epidemiological estimates of the fraction of cancers that can be prevented by changes in the environment.

Therefore, random, replicative errors every time a cell divides can contribute to cancers all along tumorigenesis, and at the same time, environmental factors can play a role during all phases. Authors suggest two prevention strategies in cancer: primary and secondary [2].

The importance of spontaneous endogenously generated DNA damage in oncogenesis is supported by the other recent studies [3, 4]. This understanding is vital for designing strategies to reduce deaths from cancer, suggesting the essential role of intervention. From that point of view, choosing the most effective medication and the treatment strategy as well as the ability to predict the treatment outcome is of particular importance.

Nowadays, biomarker-driven personalized cancer therapy has emerged as a powerful concept and significantly improved the results of cancer therapy. However, although discoveries in tumor genomics have led to the identification of a number of new cellular targets and the development of novel targeted drugs, currently available FDA-approved targeted therapies fall over time due to the development of drug resistance after impressive initial response. Intrinsic and acquired resistances remain the major limitation of the current predictive oncology.

Data presented in Nature indicate that precision oncology strategy to target the specific mutations in a tumor (to link genetic testing of patients with the drugs that would work best for them) has not been shown to work well, and perhaps it never will [5–7]. Therefore, in addition to more targeted agents, there is a great need for new approaches and for more predictive model systems to substantially improve in vitro drug testing.

Emerging reports indicate that the success of anticancer therapy is usually limited by intratumoral heterogeneity which is not captured by the existing cancer cell biomarker-based approaches. Cell heterogeneity in the tumor is considered to be the root cause of resistance (both intrinsic and acquired) to anticancer treatment including conventional chemotherapy, radiation therapy, and molecularly targeted therapy. Traditionally, it is thought that it arises from distinct mutations in "driver" oncogenes; however, intratumoral heterogeneity depends not only on genetic modifications but also on nongenetic processes involving either stochastic events or epigenetic modifications [8].

The development of tumor cell heterogeneity is believed to be related to cancer stem cells (CSCs). Reversible transitions between CSCs and non-CSCs within the tumor contribute to intratumoral heterogeneity. The heterogeneity of cellular states in cancer has been linked to drug resistance, cancer progression, and the presence of cancer stem cells [9, 10]. Therefore, subpopulations of cancer cells can be morphologically and/or functionally distinct, and this phenotypic diversity of cancer cells may account for differences in drug resistance. These data propose a different strategy in treating cancer by exploiting the observed phenotypic heterogeneity in cellular types.

Although current therapies rarely take intratumoral heterogeneity into account when predicting clinical response, the future oncology will likely require designing new innovative approaches involving ex vivo platforms that consider intratumoral heterogeneity in the context of therapy resistance mechanisms [11]. Detailed analysis of the response of phenotypically different cancer cells to the applied drugs is required in each individual patient's case. This analysis could be performed by using ex vivo patient-derived cancer cell lines and functional testing of different tumor cells exposed to potential therapies. Patient-derived models are needed to identify effective drug combinations for cancer treatment. New research, combining large-scale molecular studies data from patients, laboratory cancer cell lines, and drug sensitivity tests, showed that patient-derived cell lines did carry the same genetic alterations that drove cancer in patients, and thus are suitable to predict how tumor will respond to a drug [12]. This means that cell lines can be used to create tools for physicians to select the best available drugs for each patient individually. *A reliable patient-specific model system, which includes patient's ex vivo heterogeneous cancer cells as an experimental model, for the identification of effective drug combinations in individual cells in each individual cancer case should appear.*

In any case, before running complex and expensive trials of individualized cancer treatment (including clinical trials, genetic, epigenetic, cellular, and immunological research), studies involving the development of appropriate experimental cell culture models must be carried out. Only then the models can be used for the evaluation of cellular response of different tumor subpopulations to the chemotherapy/targeted therapy treatment in every individual case, as well as for the identification of the best cell-type-specific treatment along with a proposed molecular mechanism and characteristic markers of the case.

Currently, various models are used for tumor resistance studies. Most popular methods are these: in vitro acquired resistance models using commercial cancer cell lines, while the other is searching for presumptive biomarkers. However, the first strategy does not reflect the actual situation of the individual patient, whereas the second strategy, without live cancer cells, lacks functional component. Experimental models of mouse tumors, including genetically modified mice and human tumor xenografts, due to large requirement of space, duration, and relatively high price, are not very promising for use in the clinic. Also, these methods do not consider tumor cell heterogeneity. It is believed that cell-based functional studies and methods, once optimized, could bypass the need for whole animal cancer avatars [13].

Single-cell models (e.g., circulating tumor cells), being very promising for genomic, transcriptomic, and multiplex proteomic analyses, however, also have a disadvantage: functional studies in models of single cancer cells do not estimate the importance of extracellular interactions within a solid tumor, especially in response to the treatment [14]. Over the last few years, Science and other journals have published works on the use of patient-derived cell lines in the selection of targeted medicines in specific cases of resistant tumors, but cell subpopulations were not included in the studies [15, 16]. The most advanced model systems that contextually conserve the personalized tumor ecosystems, designed as a personalized ex vivo human cancer platform for the evaluation of the clinical response to the anticancer treatment—the CANScript and OncoCilAir—are a highly promising methodology that includes cell heterogenicity and tumor environment [17, 18]. The latter platform is new in vitro model of nonsmall cell lung cancer which combines a reconstituted human airway epithelium, human lung fibroblasts, and lung adenocarcinoma cell lines. These two are complex and expensive technologies and can emerge as a powerful platform for tailored cancer therapy. However, they do not evaluate the response of phenotypically different groups of cells to the treatment.

Until now, cellular in vitro technology has not been used in a clinic, but it is already in commercial use. According to BBC market research report, the global cell-based assays market was $ 15 billion in 2015 and is expected to reach over $ 28 billion by 2021. In the treatment of cancer, researchers return to individual, disease-determining cell research models ("Back-to-the-Future with Tumor Cell-Based Avatars"). There is no doubt that in the near future ex vivo models of tumor cells will be used in the clinic, and this would be an important step toward even more personalized cancer therapy. These approaches can be used to create tools for doctors to identify the best therapies for individual cancer patients.

Among these are the ex vivo models of the patient's tumor cells having a different phenotype. With the help of new models, we hope the importance of tumor cell subpopulations will be justified in predicting the response to the treatment for a particular patient and, in a specific case, to identify possible therapeutic efficacy.

Optimization of these tests, verification, and evaluation of the costs of the most effective therapeutic solutions are necessary.

In this review, we will present the current ex vivo tumor cell models and clinically relevant platforms to functionally test predicted drugs/drug combinations for individual patients.

2. Cancer genomics

Today, in the epoch of innovative technologies, a breakthrough in replacing conventional molecular diagnostics technologies with new ones such as next-generation sequencing (NGS), has led to higher content analyses of cancer disease with improved cost-effectiveness and speed, higher sensitivity, and specificity [19]. It has enabled cancer biologists and clinicians to obtain valuable data of complex molecular alterations from clinical cancer patient samples rapidly. Based on this, The Cancer Genome Atlas (TCGA) (a collaboration between the National Cancer Institute and the National Human Genome Research Institute) has characterized diverse genomic alterations underlying individual human cancers by using over 11,000 tumors from 33 cancer types. Multidimensional maps of key genomic changes in those tumors were generated, and systematic studies of these genetic changes were performed. Based on sequence and structure, 299 driver genes with >3400 putative missense driver mutations were identified with implications regarding their anatomical sites and cancer/cell types [20]. In addition, comprehensive characterization of 10 selected signaling pathways was performed across the 33 cancer types analyzed by TCGA. Alterations in those signaling pathways across 9125 samples from 33 cancer types were determined. RTK/RAS/MAP-kinase and PI3K/Akt signaling pathways, among others, were frequently found to be genetically altered in cancer [21]. Results from TCGA Pan Cancer Atlas project greatly deepened the current understanding in various fields of oncogenesis such as somatic driver mutations, germline pathogenic variants and their interactions in the tumor, the influence of the tumor genome and epigenome on transcriptome and proteome, and the relationship between tumor and the microenvironment, including implications of prevention and treatment [22]. Based on recent genomic cancer research, new data are currently employed in the development of novel targeted drugs focusing on genes that are mutated in a tumor, e.g., activated oncogenes and their downstream signaling components [23].

At present, in the post-genomic era of the cancer therapeutics, the shift away from the use of conventional cytotoxic drugs toward molecularly targeted agents has occurred. Conventional chemotherapy is mostly directed at the majority of proliferating cells in tumors. Cancer is a genetic disease with genotypic changes that include: mutations, insertions, gene amplifications, deletions, gene fusions, chromosomal rearrangements, transposition of the genetic elements, translocations, and microRNA alterations. Detection of genetic alterations in specific regulatory molecules that are responsible for oncogenic transformation has enabled the development of targeted therapies [24, 25]. According to Hanahan and Weinberg, six hallmarks of cancer can be highlighted: sustained proliferative signaling; evasion of growth-suppressive signaling, resistance to cell death; limitless replication;

induction of angiogenesis; invasion; and acquisition of metastatic capability. In a while, the same authors have emphasized additional cancer properties: deregulation of cellular energetics, avoidance of immune destruction, genome instability, and tumor-promoting inflammation [26]. The phenomenon of "oncogene addiction," describing a special cancer cell dependency on a particular "driver" alteration for their survival, was defined in 2002 by Weinstein. In the last decade, the strategy to eliminate acquired genetic dependencies on oncogene addiction drivers by blocking them in each patient and in each tumor cell specifically has been widely translated into the clinic. Accordingly, the major classes of current US Food and Drug Administration (FDA)-approved targeted therapies include drugs that were designed to inhibit specific oncogenic mutations and molecular alterations specific to cancer cells, or aimed to increase the antitumor immune response, or inhibiting neoangiogenesis. Additionally, beyond direct targeting of genomic defects, the process of differentiation, epigenetic alterations, and microenvironmental properties were taken into account in drug discovery. Novel treatments include advanced molecularly targeted therapies that may consist of cell-, hormone-, small molecule-, vaccine- or antibody-based therapies. They are tailored to inhibit signal transduction, regulate gene expression, induce apoptosis, diminish angiogenesis, and serve as an immunotherapeutic in specific cancers.

Individual genomic drivers are usually identified from the sequencing of the human genome. Molecular genotyping is now a customary practice applied to the cancer patients aiming to define their genetic profile. Consequently, genomic and other omics data are used to predict the drug sensitivity of an individual tumor [27, 28]. In parallel, a variety of molecularly targeted drugs are being studied in preclinical settings or clinical trials, and many targeted therapies have been approved by the FDA for treatment of different kinds of cancer. However, a range of drawbacks are monitored; for example, numerous drugs fail in early and late stages of clinical trials, partly due to insufficient drug efficacy. Before that, only 5–15% of investigational cancer drugs succeed in receiving clinical approval. Data suggest that new targeted drugs without proper stratification may reach only 10–20% efficacy. In other words, only for a small fraction of patients, the genomics-driven cancer therapy can be very effective and improve the clinical outcome. However, for the rest, such therapy will not work. It is considered that 20,000 proteins are implicated and play key roles in cancer biology; however, today, a majority of these structural and regulatory classes of proteins appear to be undruggable. Alternatively, some identified targets have no drugs developed [23, 29, 30].

Although prolonged progression-free survival is monitored after successful targeted therapy, patients with cancer usually develop resistance to the drugs within 6–12 months. As an example, in the case of lung adenocarcinoma, the initial clinical response to targeted drugs—protein kinase inhibitors—is almost always temporary due to acquired resistance [31]. In general, despite our increasing understanding of the molecular determinants of oncogenesis, many forms of the cancer remain incurable. Therefore, the complementary strategies to match their tumors to appropriate therapies are needed as genome profiling of tumors is insufficient to guide the therapy for most patients. Nowadays, molecularly guided therapy involves determination of DNA, RNA, proteins, metabolites, etc., as complementary biomarkers. Biomarker sets to detect individual and pathway drivers as molecular drug targets obtained from protein arrays, mouse avatars, and other models are also applied [24]. Among them, the application of proteomic technologies to study cell signaling networks, functionally important protein phosphorylation, and expression changes might play a key role in the discovery of both new biomarkers and new therapeutic targets [32].

Nevertheless, it should be stressed that regardless of the mechanisms of the therapies, occurring resistance is a near-universal phenomenon in patients with cancer.

It is considered that genome-based cancer therapeutic matching is limited by incomplete biological understanding of the relationship between phenotype and cancer genotype. Even more, resistance does not necessarily depend on the cancer cell genotype. Although cancer is primarily a genetic disease and genetic mutations are responsible for cancer initiation and progression, they are not necessarily responsible for the resistance to treatment and should not become the targets for therapy. In addition to more targeted agents, there is a great need for new approaches, more predictive model systems.

3. Cancer resistance

It is increasingly realized that cancer resistance occurs nearly in all patients regardless of the therapies used (targeted agents, chemotherapy or immunotherapy). Anticancer drug resistance is a complex process. The cause of tumor resistance could be both intrinsic and extrinsic and it develops through many different mechanisms.

Drug resistance can be categorized as primary (intrinsic) or secondary (acquired). Intrinsically resistant tumors do not respond to the therapy at all due to the resistance mutations which exist within cells prior to the treatment. Acquired resistance (*post-therapy resistance*) occurs due to selective propagation of pre-existing or de novo-induced molecular alterations after the anticancer therapy. Moreover, besides primary and acquired, authors name one more way for the resistance to arise. Adaptive resistance occurs due to cancer cell plasticity under the pressure of a drug, especially in the microenvironment which is throughout heterogenic. Further, acquired and adaptive resistance can also be subclassified as *on-target* or *off-target*.

Causative factors for cancer cell resistance are grouped into three categories: mutational events, non-mutational events, and changes in the surrounding microenvironment. Genetic and nongenetic resistance mechanisms can act alone or in concert, in order to confer resistance to the applied therapy [27, 33]. Genetically caused acquired resistance involves emergence of de novo mutations in cancer cells. These mutations allow escaping the oncogene-targeted therapies by many ways. *On-target* resistance (alteration of the driver oncogene) occurs when the primary target of the drug itself gets altered. In this case, resistance occurs via a second-site, or secondary, mutation in the drug target. For example, under first generation EGFR TKI treatment, appearance of EGFR-T790M mutation is known as a second-site mutation. *Off-target* resistance (activating mutations in other genes) occurs via activation of critical signaling molecules or pathways that are either parallel or downstream of the target. Upregulation of a distinct receptor tyrosine kinase is an example of such a bypass mechanism for TKI targeted therapy.

Downstream activation at the genetic level means that cancer cells can become resistant to targeted inhibitors by amplifying the target or acquiring activating mutations in signaling pathway genes downstream of the driver oncogene. In many cases, those are cell growth and survival-promoting pathways. An example of activation of downstream signaling is EGFR-driven tumors with resistant cells, which reactivate MAPK pathway at multiple downstream points by means of upregulated expression and/or enhanced activation of proteins in the EGFR/MAPK signaling pathway. Alternatively, activation of a new (parallel or surrogate) cell growth and survival-promoting signaling pathways beyond the oncogenic driver is another escape mechanism for drug resistance. It can be exemplified that the inhibition of MAPK ERK signaling pathway molecules led to the activation of a parallel PI3K/AKT/mTOR signaling pathway in lung cancer [27]. In general, various and different types of drug resistances have been shown in cancer cells. They involve activation of pro-growth and/or pro-survival signaling, cell death inhibiting pathways, altering drug targets as well as drug metabolism, enhancing DNA repair. Additional mechanisms of resistance involve alteration in epigenetically regulated drug tolerance, gene expression, epithelial-to-mesenchymal transition (EMT), phenotypic transformation, etc. [28]. Interplay between different signaling pathways, e.g., to induce adaptive activation of bypass signaling, was shown during acquired resistance.

3.1 Tumor heterogeneity

Accumulating evidence suggests that intratumoral heterogeneity plays an important role in cancer resistance to applied therapy, both conventional and targeted [9, 10]. Tumors are composed of heterogeneous cancer cell populations, either phenotypically or genetically different, and are marked by spatial and temporal heterogeneity. Even after malignant transformation, cancer cell clones remain dynamic and continue accumulating mutations. This ongoing evolution ultimately generates distinct molecular signatures in different loci of a tumor. Intratumoral heterogeneity itself may be responsible for the evolution of cancers as well as for differential levels of sensitivity to treatment. Various drug-resistant clones with different properties appear within the tumor tissue both prior and after the cancer therapy. Importantly, cellular composition of a tumor can change substantially over the time [31, 33, 34]. In that respect, the combination of different approaches—one targeting pathways and alterations implicated in resistance of different tumor composing cells and the other directed to overcome heterogeneity—is a promising strategy in cancer treatment.

Causes of intratumoral heterogeneity may be intrinsic or extrinsic and genomics or phenotypic. Among intrinsic factors, genomic instability is critical for the development of intercellular genetic heterogeneity in cancer. Genomic instability along to cell-to-cell variation leads to acquired resistance. Extrinsic factors include pH, hypoxia, paracrine signaling, interactions with stromal and other tumor cells, surrounding matrix as well as other environmental influences. Genetic alterations might be caused by exogenous mutagenic factors (UV radiation, tobacco smoke) or endogenous defective processes such as errors during DNA replication, repair, etc. Meanwhile, phenotypic diversity can reflect differences in cell cycle stage, stochastic phenotypic alterations, or hierarchical position during development. Primary genotypic or phenotypic variations prior to therapy also describe intratumoral heterogeneity in many tumors. Therefore, temporal-spatial differences between distinctive subpopulations of tumor cells within the same tumor at both genetic and epigenetic levels cause tumor heterogeneity [34].

Various models have been proposed to explain intratumoral heterogeneity.

The clonal evolution model postulates that somatic mutations stochastically occur in various clones within the tumor at different sites and different disease stages, leading to differential growth patterns and resulting in spatial-temporal tumor heterogeneity. In clonal evolution model (linear or branched) genetic mutations gained by tumor cells contribute to their altered phenotype and differences in resistance. Those differences in the biological properties are inherited by individual cancer cells clones. In this way, genomic instability leads to cell-to-cell variation as well as acquired resistance.

In the model of stem cells, clonal expansion of slow cycling cells, displaying stem cell-like behavior (self-renewal and differentiation capability), leads to tumor heterogeneity [34]. The role of cancer stem cells (CSC) in determining heterogeneity and resistance in cancer will be described below.

One more theory, the so-called phenotypic plasticity model, suggests that cancer cells are capable of switching between different transcriptional programs, and therefore, phenotypic and histological transformation occurs. In this model, unlike the clonal evolution and stem cell theories, reversible molecular changes result in tumor heterogeneity. Inconsistent drug responses between cancer cells can be a result of diversification of epigenomic, transcriptomic, proteomic, metabolic, and functional states driven by tumor cell microenvironment changes [8, 29, 35, 36]. One of the mechanisms of phenotypic change is via EMT, an evolutionarily conserved program of transdifferentiation. EMT is observed clinically in patients with acquired resistance.

Lastly, another mechanism of cancer cell evolution was described. Briefly, there are proofs that cancer cells fuse with fibroblastic or mesenchymal cells to produce genetic hybrids with enhanced malignant profile both in vivo and in vitro [37]. Taken together, all these models in concert explain all the attributes of tumor tissue heterogeneity as well as genetic cell-to-cell variation and acquired resistance. Indeed, the findings of multiple studies demonstrate that a combination of genetic, epigenetic, and functional mechanisms contributes to intratumoral heterogeneity with different levels of sensitivity to anticancer therapies. Moreover, heterogeneity is dynamically changing over time and in concert with changes in therapy [33]. Heterogeneity of cellular states in cancer has been linked to drug resistance, cancer progression, and the presence of cancer stem cells [9, 10].

3.2 Cancer stem cells

An important role in the development of cancer heterogeneity is attributed to CSCs. In this model, tumor heterogeneity is determined by CSCs existing at different levels of hierarchical tree and possessing different phenotypes. CSCs are present in almost all cancers as a small population of drug-resistant, tumor-initiating cells and make up less than 1% of the tumor cell population. Recent data show that during cancer progression, gradual loss of a differentiated phenotype and acquisition of progenitor and stem cell-like features are observed. Cells with dedifferentiated phenotype were mostly prominent in metastasis [38, 39].

Different factors are recognized as causes of CSC emergence. It can be cell fusion, horizontal gene transfer, and mutations in somatic or differentiated cancer cells, ultimately resulting in their dedifferentiation and reprogramming. Mutations leading to the aberrant regulation of a majority of stemness and proliferation pathways distinguish CSCs from non-CSCs residing within the tumor. In response to various factors such as wounding, stress, or hypoxia, a differentiated cancer cell can dedifferentiate into a CSC. Reversible transitions between CSCs and non-CSCs within the tumor contribute to intratumoral heterogeneity [40, 41].

Incidences of different oncogenic rearrangements in stem, progenitor, or mature cells can lead to the generation of CSCs too. Authors propose that breast cancer CSCs could have been generated from adult somatic cells, through acquired mutations responsible for uncontrolled reactivation of pluripotency-associated programs. Deregulated canonical and developmental signaling pathways are highly associated with CSC phenotype and regulation of CSC behavior. Alterations in proliferation, differentiation, and programmed cell death pathways have been demonstrated [42].

It is believed that CSCs are a quiescent, low-cycling cell population. Another specific property of CSCs is resistance to chemotherapeutic drugs. Self-renewal and cellular quiescence characterize both normal adult stem cells and CSCs; they also can divide asymmetrically and are able to produce progenies of multilineage differentiation. CSCs are regulated by similar cell signaling pathways and express similar cell-surface and intracellular markers as normal stem cell. Growth factor TGF-β, signaling pathways FGFR/MAPK or Akt, Wnt, Notch, and Hh, and major transcription factors Oct3/4, SOX2, and Nanog are involved in maintaining self-renewal and pluripotency of CSCs as well as of embryonic stem cells.

Many markers have been associated with the CSC phenotype; however, no universal CSCs markers were found, suggesting the existence of heterogeneous CSC populations within a heterogeneous tumor [38]. Indeed, CSCs are both genetically and phenotypically heterogeneous. CSC plasticity is the major determinant of their intratumoral heterogeneity. Dysregulation of key effectors in the above-mentioned signaling pathways modulate CSC properties [34]. Recent research has emphasized extensive metabolic variability in CSCs—each distinct CSC population possessed a unique metabolic profile. Both intrinsic factors (genetic and epigenetic alterations) and extrinsic factors (mainly tumor microenvironment) were shown to be implicated in the regulation plasticity as well as in maintaining stemness. Signaling molecules of Wnt, Hh, and Notch pathways, along with metabolic regulators such as HIF1α, maintained CSC populations within tumors [34, 38]. Even more, increasing data show that cells with self-renewal potential can be generated from terminally differentiated somatic cells, thus reverting hierarchical developmental organization. For example, there is evidence that breast CSCs have originated from non-stem cancer cells [42]. Under the regulation of multiple factors, differentiated cancer cells could regain "stemness," in this way confirming bidirectional conversion between non-stem and stem cells [34]. In that case, transformation of "non-stem cell to stem cell" contributes to the development of the heterogeneity within a tumor.

Core signaling pathways that regulate the phenotype of normal stem cells are responsible for dedifferentiation and acquisition of stem cell features in a tumor when transcriptionally and epigenetically deregulated. There are data that CSCs are maintained in the undifferentiated state through extrinsically regulated epigenetic mechanisms [39]. Therefore, CSCs may be considered as a status rather than a fixed subset of cancer cells. Transformation between modes of non-stem cells to stem cells or vice versa contributes to the development of heterogeneity within tumor.

The studies of last decades have shown a link between cancer stem cell formation and the process of epithelial-mesenchymal transition. This connection might be responsible for tumor heterogeneity, progression, and acquired resistance to therapy, followed by disease recurrence [40, 41, 43]. Namely, epithelial cells undergoing EMT acquire CSC phenotype and chemoresistance. Moreover, these cells may go back and forth along this transition. As described in a breast cancer study, two distinct populations (epithelial-to-mesenchymal and mesenchymal-to-epithelial) of CSCs were found [44]. Current data indicate that CSCs are not fixed at full epithelial or full mesenchymal cell status, but maintain plasticity between EMT and MET states [42, 45]. Consequently, tumors are supposed to consist of continuous sequence of cell states along epithelial to mesenchymal positions [46]. Also, non-stem cancer cells were shown to regain stemness through an epithelial-to-mesenchymal transition-mediated process [38].

Processes of EMT are regulated in response to the environmental changes and involve canonical and developmental signaling pathways that induce the expression of transcription factors, referred as "master regulators" of EMT, as well as epigenetic and post-translational regulators. Those include members of the Snail and ZEB transcription factor families. Different signaling pathways, e.g., Wnt/β-catenin pathway or AKT/STAT3, contribute to EMT [47–49]. Although it is widely accepted to link stemness to the EMT, there is another view proposing that these processes occur in parallel rather than through the same pathway [38]. Regardless, a wide spectrum of hybrid epithelial/mesenchymal (E/M) cellular states which combine epithelial and mesenchymal features are formed during epithelial-mesenchymal transition.

It is increasingly understood that cell plasticity in the tumor can affect treatment outcomes. EMT grants resistance to cell death induced by different agents, including conventional, targeted, and immunological, in cancer cells. Different phenotypes of cancer cells may confer changes to both sensitivity and intracellular regulation of cellular biology; different signaling may be acquired in response to one treatment. There are data about it in various cellular and preclinical models; however, more data from clinical cases are needed [50–54].

As discussed above, drug resistance is a specific property of a CSC. It involves various aspects of CSC functioning and is mediated by multiple mechanisms, such as: ATP-dependent ABC transporter-mediated drug efflux; inactivation of anticancer drugs; changing the targets of chemotherapeutic agents; slow cell cycle/quiescence; self-renewal property and stemness-regulating signaling; disrupted differentiation; metabolic modulation; antiapoptotic measures (upregulation of antiapoptotic and downregulation of proapoptotic genes); improved DNA damage response; epigenetic alterations (DNA methylation, histone alterations, microRNAs); immune escape mechanisms; etc. [34, 38].

Based on the abovenamed features and mechanisms of CSC resistance, different strategies to tackle CSC resistance were developed, mainly focusing on CSC elimination or induction of their differentiation. More than 60 CSC-targeted reagents have been registered for clinical trials (e.g., Reparixin, Demcizumab, Napabucasin, metformin, etc.) [55]. However, to our current knowledge, there are no drug discovery platforms that would include EMT reversal and overcoming its conferred resistance. Nevertheless, the results from TCGA project encourage stemness signatures were found, and certain inhibitors were proposed as potential drugs for various cancers [39].

3.3 Tumor microenvironment

Development of drug resistance in cancer, regardless of mechanism, is highly dependent on the tumor microenvironment [35]. Tumor microenvironment includes the cells composing tumor stroma (normal fibroblasts, cancer-associated fibroblasts (CAFs), vascular endothelial cells, infiltrating immune cells, etc.), soluble molecules, and the extracellular matrix (ECM). Other factors of tumor surroundings, such as availability of nutrients and oxygen, and biophysical properties of the extracellular matrix are also important factors in regulating tumor cell behavior. Cancer cell interaction with stroma cells, with other cancerous cells, and with ECM contribute to direct cell interaction-mediated drug resistance known as *tumor cell interaction-/adhesion-mediated resistance*. Probably the best-known example is the CAFs. Those specific cells are most abundant cells in the tumor stroma responsible for the buildup and remodeling of the tumor microenvironment. CAFs produce ECM components such as collagens (I, III, IV, and V), hyaluronic acid, fibronectins, and laminins; alternatively, they secrete matrix metalloproteinases. Cancer-associated fibroblasts possess high expression of α-SMA, CD44, HI-1α, MMP11, VEGF, CXCL12, TGF-β1, TGF-βRII, IL6, and TNFα biomarkers. In many studies, such cells were demonstrated to be involved in cancer progression and resistance to therapy [56–59]. As an example, it was demonstrated that functional and proliferating colon cancer stem cells that ensured tumor expansion predominantly resided at the tumor edge close to cancer-associated fibroblasts [60]. Furthermore, factors secreted by cancer cells and acting through autocrine mechanisms are involved in protection of cancer cells against treatments; that is called *soluble factor-mediated drug resistance*. Various cancer cell-released molecules are known as contributors to chemoresistance; it can be growth factors, glycoproteins, inflammatory cytokines, enzymes, chaperones, tumor-derived exosomes, etc. [61]. As an example, the recent study highlighted that cancer-associated fibroblasts induced ovarian cancer cell chemoresistance in transmanner by secretion of CCL2/CCL5 and induction of IL-6 production [62]. Microenvironment-driven dynamic heterogeneity and phenotypic plasticity was recognized as mechanisms of therapy resistance in melanoma [35]. Hence, development of drug resistance in cancer, regardless of a mechanism, is highly dependent on the tumor microenvironment. Moreover, factors secreted by tumor cells themselves or by the cells of its microenvironment play a crucial role in the development of epithelial-mesenchymal transition at the invasive front of primary tumors. Paracrine and autocrine mechanisms of EMT induction in cancer are evidenced in literature and may include exosomes or free proteins and miRNAs [63]. Consequently, distinct subpopulations of cancer cells with distinctive biological features appear in the tumor and thus respond differently to the therapy.

The critical role of tumor microenvironment, which is composed of cellular and noncellular components in cancer development and progression, is evident. As EMT is considered to be one of the key factors in progression of tumors to malignancy [64, 65], the role of ECM in this process was demonstrated. ECM composition was partially responsible for insufficient therapy and appearance of heterogenic cell populations, which were characterized by different response/susceptibility to anticancer agent [66]. Dynamic nature of ECM regulates behavior of cancer cells by triggering signaling pathways through adhesion proteins like integrins [67]. Collagen I, which is the major component of extracellular matrix, has been shown to support phenotypic changes of cancer cells [68]. Studies conducted on 3D tumor-ECM in vitro cancer models demonstrated importance of ECM composition and stiffness on this transition regulation [69, 70]. On the other hand, noncellular components of ECM, e.g., proteins, glycoproteins, and proteoglycans, form a physical barrier for penetrating drug. Numerous cell-cell and cell-ECM contacts attenuate penetration of drug molecules into different layers of tumor [71, 72].

4. Models of cancer treatment prediction

Today, a lot of conferences addressed to advancing drug discovery, cancer pharmacology, and tumor modeling are held worldwide, e.g., Predict Tumor Models (London, UK, 2017; Boston, MA, 2019), 3D-Oncology (Boston, MA, 2019), EACR Goodbye Flat Biology (Berlin, DE, 2019), and SelectBio 3D-Culture and Organoids/Organ-on-a-Chip World Congress (San Diego, CA, 2019). Realization that new approaches in oncology are necessary to improve cancer treatment is increasing. The topics in such conferences include: How to satisfy the demand for clinically relevant models for understanding disease progression; Multicellular interactions and the immune microenvironment; Advancing 3D-based models for cancer biology and drug discovery; Influence of microenvironment on stemness; Microenvironment and metabolic regulation of cancer invasion; Highlighting the pitfalls of complex approaches with regards to cost, speed and accuracy; The true utility and translatability of 3D tumor models within drug research; etc. Likewise, big pharma companies and small start-ups are offering nonconventional, patient-specific and often patent-protected cancer models, desirably reflecting the complex nature of tumor microenvironment and cell heterogeneity. For example, Champions Personalized TumorGrafts™ have offered patients and physicians using their in vivo xenograft mouse avatar-based diagnostic model at a cost of approx. $10,000 [73]. The demand for cancer models that reliably mimic the intrinsic ecosystem of a solid tumor in vivo is really high. However, to create and replicate a system consisting of malignant cells, normal and abnormal stroma, immune cells, as well as dynamic microenvironment containing gasses and nutrients, chemokines, cytokines, growth factors, together with specific extracellular matrix, is totally challenging [74, 75]. In addition, clinical application of such models may become reality only if the patient benefit justifies the cost of the methodology.

The use of reliable in vitro cell model, which precisely reflects the situation in vivo is critically important during preclinical drug studies. Due to the high mortality from cancer, the search of new and more effective anticancer agents still remains a highly challenging area of biomedical research. The principle of targeted cancer therapy is based on biochemical differences between cancer and healthy cells. In regard to low efficacy of drugs passed through Phase II and III of clinical studies and acquired resistance of tumor cells to therapy, more detailed studies of tumor structure, histology, and biology are required. These fields remain very important since a choice of inadequate in vitro drug screening system further results in low efficacy or high toxicity of anticancer agent during clinical studies [76, 77]. Advances made in cancer research in the last decades demonstrate critical role of tumor microenvironment in cancer development, progression, and response to therapy. According to different studies, potent anticancer drugs that demonstrated high efficacy in 2D cancer cell cultures had significantly reduced effectiveness during further studies in vivo [78]. In human body, tumor represents a highly complex architecture that is difficult to replicate in vitro. First of all, it is highly heterogenic multilayer structure, formed by different type of cells, e.g., cancer cells, cancer-associated fibroblasts, tumor infiltrated endothelial cells, and cells of immune system. Cellular components of tumor regulate different features of cancer cells such as proliferation, invasiveness, and susceptibility to drugs [79]. Tumor represents a mixture of genetically, epigenetically, and phenotypically different populations of transformed cells. Elimination of all viable cancer cells which are in different status makes it very challenging to target particular molecular drivers of cancer. It is known as well that cell heterogeneity is increasing with disease progression. Thus, even modern targeted therapy becomes insufficient in some cases of cancer [80–82].

Failure to advance in cancer therapy has been attributed to the complexity of the disease. A solid tumor is often called "an organ" but very heterogenic and of irregular structure with many niches and different conditions inside. Today, there is a gap between scientific understanding of tumor complexity and concrete measures to fight cancer in clinics. This gap is constantly being filled with preclinical cancer models, but up to date, no model, at the same time, is fast, accurate, affordable, and suitable for clinics.

One of the hypotheses to explain cancer resistance to therapy is cancer stem cells, or cancer-initiating cells. Although they are more recognized as a phenotypic status or mode rather than a fixed subset of cancer cells, various authors distinguish certain populations of cells within a tumor that propagate cancer [83–87]. The main trick regarding those cells is that when they are asleep, they evade chemotherapy; when they wake up, they cause cancer recurrence. Killing those cells selectively is a priority [9]. Other authors propose that cancer genome undergoes clonal evolution under the pressure of constant stress and after cancer therapy. One study compared the genomes of 100 early stage resected lung tumors and found driver mutations in EGFR, MET, BRAF, and TP53 are almost always clonal; moreover, cells from different parts of the same tumor had very heterogenic genomes [88]. Accordingly, every single case of cancer is very individual and may be genetically and in other ways substantially different. Noncellular components of tumor environment such as secreted grow factors, RNA and DNA molecules, metabolites, and extracellular matrix proteins regulate various biological functions of cancer cells [71]. Therefore, commonly used purified cancer cell lines in vitro do not possess the heterogeneity, nor genetic nor phenotypic, and thus may represent only a small fraction of this multiplexed pathology [89]. Even when heterogenic and in an enriched medium, 2D cell cultures lack the architecture and complexity of a real tumor and thus are not suitable for cancer biology and immunology studies [90]. However, ordinary cancer cell cultures on flat plastic are successfully used in fundamental research.

Trying to describe cancer cells in molecular signature led to the emergence of "biomarkers"—certain molecules that are specific to cancer cells. Although this goal is not ultimately achieved yet, many cancer biomarkers are used in cell profiling, cancer research, and targeted drug development. For example, in a search for cancer stem cells in lung cancer, CD44, CD133, and CD90 had been considered as potential biomarkers, but CD44 showed the best specificity in one study [91], and CD133+CXCR4 in another study [92]. In pancreatic cancer, co-expression of CD24, CD44, EpCAM, and CD133 corresponded to more aggressive cell behavior [93]. As we have described above, an initiative called The Cancer Genome Atlas (TCGA) has generated comprehensive, multidimensional maps of key genomic changes in 33 types of cancer in order to investigate somatic driver mutations, germline pathogenic variants, and their interactions in the tumor, the influence of the tumor genome and epigenome on transcriptome and proteome, and the relationship between tumor and the microenvironment, including implications of prevention and treatment [22]. On its basis, other authors have performed analysis by using 26 computational tools and identified 299 driver genes [20] as well as alterations in signal transduction [21]. It is worth mentioning that DNA sequencing is becoming part of routine clinical care that may result in rapid and high-throughput analysis of complex germline and somatic alterations from clinical cancer patient samples [19].

Probably more complex and more ambitious project has been started in 2017—The Human Cell Atlas. Such atlas is believed not only to append new cell types of a human body to the known ones but also to help scientists to track cell lineage, dynamic states, and stemness of cells as well as communication between cells. This database may include not only genomic and transcriptomic data from a single cell, but also profiling the accessibility of the chromatin [94]. It is really important to investigate cells one by one for many reasons when talking about cancer. For example, conversion to stem-cell state in response to microenvironmental cues was regulated by balance between epithelial and mesenchymal regulators (described by expression of CDH1 and SNAI2, respectively) in lung cancer cells [95].

4.1 In vivo models

Human tumors can be grafted into immunodeficient mice to generate so-called patient-derived xenograft (PDX) mice. PDX is a powerful tool aiming to test multiple drugs or drug regimens. It is considered as a preferred option in cancer research as it mimics the native features of tumors more closely compared to conventional cell culture drug screening platforms. With its drawbacks as a system, it is still important, widely used, and remains a gold standard for preclinical development and individual drug discovery.

Different PDX repositories exist that represent models of various tumors. Conte and colleagues try to accumulate the data into one comprehensive open global catalog of PDX models and their associated datasets that would ease the identification of PDX models relevant to specific cancer research questions [96]. The standard was also developed to unify generation, quality assurance, and use of PDX models, because the processes of creation and characterization of PDX models considerably differed among institutions [97].

Beyond PDX mouse model libraries, now patients can be offered individualized mice, which is a platform used for the measurement of efficacy of experimental treatments exploiting patient's own malignant cells. The aim is to have a model with experimental data as close as possible to human disease situation. Individual approach is vital here as cancer is the most genetically diverse and unique disease with different genetic alterations existing between individual patients, individual tumors, and even within a single tumor.

In PDX model, a patient tumor specimen is directly transplanted into immunocompromised mice. This allows representing critical molecular and biological properties of the original tumor, and immunodeficient mice prevent graft rejection. Several types of such mice are used for PDX generation. Currently, the most commonly used types of immunodeficient mice are nude, severe combined immunodeficiency (SCID), and nonobese diabetic (NOD) SCID γ (NSG). The latter is the most severely immunodeficient due to the lack of T, B, and NK cells [98]. NSG engrafting success rate is higher compared with that of in nude and NOD/SCID mice; therefore, NSG mice are considered the most suitable ones for the efficient engraftment of human tumor.

Tumor tissue fragments or single-cell suspension is used for PDX establishment, and both have their advantages and disadvantages. Tumor fragments preserve cell-cell interactions and tissue architecture of the tumor, and all this mirrors the tumor microenvironment. However, a fragment does not represent the whole tumor, unlike single-cell suspension that helps to avoid tumor subclones. One can distinguish an additional PDX model that also recapitulates the molecular heterogeneity of the corresponding tumor and can be used to study cancer biology—circulating tumor cells (CTCs). These are released from cancerous lesion into peripheral blood and may infiltrate distant tissues inducing metastasis. CTCs represent a method for liquid biopsy which is used to generate various CTC-derived preclinical models.

Tumor fragment can be implanted heterotopically, that is, into the area unrelated to the original tumor site (usually subcutaneously). A major disadvantage of heterotopic implantation is that microenvironment of the subcutaneous space differs greatly from that of the original organ. Thus, orthotopic transplant models have been developed in which tumor fragment is directly implanted into the corresponding anatomical organ. Orthotopic PDX is considered an exemplary one as unlike subcutaneous model it mimics primary tumor's natural environment that enables relevant tissue-related gene expression. In some cases, it reflects responses to therapy more closely than heterotopic PDX. Consequently, orthotopic models may be better predictors of therapeutic response [99]. Besides, subcutaneous model rarely produce metastasis [100], while orthotopic PDX is more likely to metastasize [101]. However, orthotopic PDX generation is technically demanding and tumor changes have to be monitored via expensive and laborious imaging process. Therefore, subcutaneous models are currently preferred for preclinical studies.

Tumor engraftment is a critical milestone in PDX generation. Time from tumor sample implantation to progressive growth may range greatly. Authors provide different timeframes for PDX generation or tumor graft latency ranging from 2 to 12 months [102–104]. The differences in time and engraftment rate are determined by tumor characteristics, like aggressiveness, histological type, and tumor cell percentage in the tissue [105]. Prasetyanti and colleagues showed that tumor cell proliferation was associated with successful PDX establishment and as one would expect this allowed to distinguish patients with poor clinical outcomes [106]. The others report the ability of NSCLC to grow as xenograft in mice as an accurate indicator of poor prognosis for patient survival [107, 108]. Similar data were received with breast cancer [109] and head and neck squamous cell carcinoma (HNSCC) models [110]. Here, authors claimed that the clinical application of rapid engraftment as a biomarker for risk stratification could potentially improve the outcome of patients. Despite the wide array of PDXs generated for different tumors, some cancers, e.g., prostate, luminal ER+ breast, and neuroendocrine, remain underrepresented [111].

Tumor implant location is another important factor for successful engraftment. It was shown that tumors had higher success rates grafted in subrenal capsular sites [107, 112] due to better blood supply. The strain of immunodeficient mice used for engraftment also plays its role. Not surprisingly, engrafting success rate in NSG mice is increased compared to other strains.

After harvesting the tumor, it can be cryopreserved, characterized, or dissected again for reimplantation and propagation into other mice. This allows to expand PDX from one biopsy into multiple mice and to receive numerous data points from the same original tumor.

PDX retains tumor architecture and microenvironment with physiological conditions reflecting original tumor. Grafted tumor tissue maintains the genetic and epigenetic changes found in the patient, and also it retains patient's stroma [113, 114]. PDX mice models can preserve tumor heterogeneity at least in early passages. They retain heterogenous molecular pathways of drug resistance that exist in tumor or in the cells comprising tumor environment [115]. As these models retain the biological characteristics of the donor tumors, they become indispensable for drug safety and efficacy research in preclinical studies as well as in co-clinical trials. These models are also exploited to examine personalized treatment strategies—response to antitumor therapeutics and identification of the mechanisms of resistance that can be primary or acquired [116–118]. PDXs may represent intratumoral and intrametastatic heterogeneity and, therefore, more accurately predict mechanisms of resistance to clinical treatments [119].

Mice PDX models from various kinds of tumors have been established to study tumor biology, drug screening, and biomarker discovery. Authors report PDX generated for nonsmall cell lung carcinoma closely mimics the characteristics of patient primary tumors [120, 121], lung squamous cell carcinoma [122], and colorectal cancer [123]. Data are also available for renal cell carcinoma [124], melanoma [125], gastric [126], breast [127], and other cancers.

Data show that PDXs have a predictive power in clinical therapy outcomes since drug activity in PDXs phenomenally correlates with patient's clinical outcome. In 112 out of 129 therapeutic outcomes, a remarkable correlation was observed between drug responses in patients and the corresponding PDX models of various solid tumors. Data showed that PDXs reproduced patients' clinical outcomes, even in cases when patients underwent several additional cycles of therapy over the time. This indicates the potential of these models to provide the guidance on treatments [128]. More data with PDX models of breast cancer and lung adenocarcinoma origin confirmed high rate of consistency in patient and relevant PDXs [129, 130]. In addition to that, PDX models of colorectal cancers treated with EGFR inhibitor showed response rates like those of the patient [131]. Gu et al. evaluated the correlations between PDX model-based mouse trials and cancer patient-based clinical trials. Results disclosed a high correlation in the rates of RECIST criteria between mouse trials and Phase II and III studies [132]. Research with pancreatic cancer PDX revealed that metformin treatment did not inhibit the growth of pancreatic cancer; clinical trial echoed PDX data—there was no benefit of adding metformin to combination therapy [133]. Eventually, in renal cell cancer model, correlation was noticed between PDX and clinical results in responses to Sirolimus, Sunitinib, and Dovitinib, but not Erlotinib [134].

Correlation between PDX models and clinical trials also allowed discovery of biomarkers for drug susceptibility and resistance. Vemurafenib-resistant melanoma model was generated using PDX. Resistant tumors showed reliance on BRAF signaling due to the elevated BRAF (V600E) expression [135]. Accordingly, elevated BRAF expression could be a potential biomarker for Vemurafenib resistance. The other data showed relationship between Gemcitabine resistance and survival of pancreatic cells with deoxycytidine kinase activity [136].

Co-clinical trials are parallel studies with mouse PDX models and patients. PDX model is established from the patient participating in a study, and the same treatment is applied to patient and PDX [116]. On the other hand, PDX model can be treated not only with the same drug that is used in the donor patient, but also with other drugs or drug combinations. This concept integrates preclinical and clinical data and facilitates the selection of an individual treatment to the patient. In addition, screening for prognostic biomarkers can be conducted, and drug response as well as resistance mechanisms can be investigated [137]. Usually, with the progression of cancer, the drug becomes less effective partially due to appearance of resistance mechanisms. During a clinical study, it is not possible to reveal timing and mechanism of resistance. Here, PDXs are also of use allowing to predict both the development of resistance to the first-line therapy as well as the response to second-line therapy before this is observed in the donor patient, and to adjust further treatment accordingly [138]. Authors report correlation between clinical results and PDX models. Kim et al. conducted co-clinical trial to identify predictive biomarkers for the multikinase inhibitor Dovitinib in lung squamous cell carcinoma (LSCC) and revealed that FGFR gene expression signatures were predictors for the response to Dovitinib in LSCC [139]. Stebbing et al. provided data that supported the use of the personalized TumorGraft model as an investigational platform for therapeutic decision-making that could guide treatment for rare tumors such as sarcomas [140]. Others showed that PDXs reliably replicated clinical outcome in a Phase II co-clinical study of arsenic trioxide in relapsed small-cell lung cancer [141].

Currently, there are no much data, however co-clinical trials should find their place in the future as they give possibility to evaluate the efficacies of several drugs or drug combinations, save time, and reflect personalized medicine. However, while aforementioned advancements have been made in PDX applications, these models still retain some important limitations that should be noted.

Several practical challenges are related to PDX models. First of all, it is important to transplant the representative tissue, which is a matter of concern when it comes to larger tumors. Those tumors that have genetic heterogeneity cannot always be recapitulated in serial passages if the genetic heterogeneity is not all represented in the dissected tumor that is passaged [142]. Also, the best transplantation strategy should be chosen for specific tumor type. Orthotopic transplantation is considered more suitable; however, it is more complex and special surgical technique is necessary. Consequently, more time and labor are required for model establishment. Engraftment failures are also to be discussed as percentage is still low in some tumor types. It is known that clinically aggressive tumors with many proliferative cancer cells have the highest engraftment rate [143]. Studies in which PDX models had been created simultaneously from primary and metastatic tumors proposed that metastases had a higher engraftment rate [144].

The other limitation of PDX system is the substitution of human stroma with murine components that occurs over the time with repeated passages. Human stromal elements are maintained for only 2–3 passages [111]. Later, the interaction of human cells with the murine microenvironment changes cell functioning and characteristics due to interspecies incompatibility, and the heterogeneity of exact human tumor microenvironment might not be retained. Therefore, therapeutic studies are more representative in low-passage models. To reduce the influence of murine stroma on the PDX model, co-engraftment of human mesenchymal stem cells or cancer-associated fibroblast cell lines in PDXs is explored. One promising approach is the isolation and co-engraftment of patient-derived fibroblasts [145].

How cancer emerges and develops depends on its interaction with the host immune system. In addition, cancer response to therapy is also determined by pre-existing immune phenotype; it also depends on immune system responses caused by drug introduction [146]. Lately, several cancer immunotherapies have been evaluated in preclinical and clinical studies. However, standard PDX models were inconvenient for the analysis of tumor immunology and immuno-oncology drugs (e.g., immune checkpoint inhibitors) as the immunodeficient mice had no cytotoxic T cells. To overcome this problem, humanized PDX models have been developed using injection of peripheral blood lymphocytes or tumor-infiltrating lymphocytes into NSG mice [138]. But this did not resolve the issue in general, as after several weeks severe graft-versus-host reaction appeared [147]. Therefore, such mice can be used only for short-term experiments. Other model system exploited transplantation of CD34-positive human hematopoietic stem cells into NSG mice and demonstrated the establishment of a humanized PDX model with hematopoietic restoration [148]. In addition, Morton and colleagues demonstrated that CD34-positive cells isolated from patient and injected into mouse blood successfully restored a functional immune system mimicking that of the patient [149]. Such PDX are invaluable for cancer immunology and immuno-oncology drug research. Nevertheless, the time required generating enough tumor material in sufficient number of mice, as well as patient survival, is of utmost importance for personalized medicine application. Time is the main obstacle impeding the extensive use of mouse PDX models, because right drug for the right patient must be given at a right time. Development of an individualized PDX takes anywhere from 3 to 6 or even 12 months, and in many instances, this time is too long, as in the case of metastases, patients may not even survive PDX creation time. Therefore, this method is restricted to patients with a less aggressive disease development.

In addition to that, long time needed to generate sufficient number of mice with the same tumor brings another problem—clonogenicity. Research showed that all PDX models studied experienced moderate drifts or even dramatic clonal selections even within the first mouse passage [150]. Due to selection of preexisting minor clones, authors observed rapid accumulation of copy number alterations (CNAs) during PDX passaging. Particular CNAs acquired during PDX passaging differed from those obtained during tumor development in patients. Some CNAs observed in primary tumors later disappeared in PDXs [151]. The results showed that PDXs were not static and underwent mouse-specific tumor development: PDX that originally had mirrored particular disease after some time changed into the form that did not anymore.

Financial aspects are also to be assessed. PDX models are costly as it takes much time to create PDX, while immunodeficient mice in addition are expensive. Furthermore, PDXs may have limited use in diagnostics due to their low-throughput character: they are restricted to test a few agents due to insufficient number of animal colonies with individual patient's tumor. However, it is still important for drug validation, biomarker development, and drug resistance analysis.

Other animal models exist; however, those may not meet the requirements for personalized medicine and will not be reviewed in detail here. Among others, cell line-derived xenografts did not reflect the complexity of tumor heterogeneity and displayed pronounce genomic differences compared to relevant tumor [152, 153]. Genetically engineered mouse models (GEMMs) carry mutations in genes of interest; however, generation of mutant mice carrying several genetic alterations is time-consuming, and complex activation of genetic alterations reduces the attractiveness of the method [154]. Besides, GEMMs may not be able to mirror the personalized therapy as they have less heterogeneity due to only a few genes modified.

4.2 2D in vitro models

Many reviewers have argued that conventional cancer cell lines in a usual 2D culture were an oversimplified model to study cancer. Various studies have demonstrated that both molecular and functional parameters were different depending on cell culture conditions, including substrate dimensionality as well as the method by which it was created, leading to inconsistent data [155]. Alternatively, primary cell-derived 3D spheroids demonstrated different response to therapeutic drugs when compared to spheroids from long ago established breast cancer cell lines [156]. Growing body of evidence demonstrated that cancer cells growing in 3D or 2D environment possessed different susceptibility to anticancer treatment, showing either increased or decreased sensitivity to apoptosis-inducing agents [157, 158]. Therefore, the natural question which models for cancer research should be abandoned is very relevant [159]. Regarding cancer cell lines, in general, it is well known that they are unstable and possess genetic drift. Long-term cultivation causes other problems resulting in poor reproducibility of the results [160–162]. For example, a widely used glioblastoma cell line U87MG was found to be completely different from the original donor, as DNA profiling revealed [163], many other cell lines were misidentified or contaminated [164]. Due to such obstacles, cell line stability and bioproduction are the headache for pharmaceutical companies which try to comply with strict regulations of healthcare manufacturing.

Nevertheless, these cell lines proved to be useful in basic and fundamental molecular biology research, e.g., in studying molecular action mechanisms of anticancer drugs, as reviewed many times elsewhere. Easy handling, homogeneous character, limitless growth, and high-throughput made it the model of choice for many years. After a lot of criticism from more advanced cancer modeling experts, surprisingly, they suddenly appeared to be equally valuable for translational cancer research. For example, in a large-scale study summarizing data from the analysis of 1000 cancer cell lines, their response to 265 anticancer drugs, and 11,000 patient samples of 29 different tumor types, authors concluded that a majority of molecular abnormalities found in tumors including driver mutations were also found in cancer cell lines. Furthermore, the results suggested that cell lines could predict drug response of a tumor [12]. Earlier, by application of computational methods, cell line gene expression profiling and annealing with known pharmacological profiles of anticancer drugs successfully predicted unknown drug sensitivities [165]. Such methodology may be compared to target-based drug discovery approach. However, an alternative approach—agnostic phenotypic screening—has resulted in the discovery of majority of first-in-line drugs, and authors noticed the resurgence of sophisticated, high-content phenotypic screening. By testing the unlimited number of ex vivo cancer cell lines with large libraries of chemicals or biologicals, there is a chance of having a significant hit [166, 167]. The NCI-60 panel was the first widely used cancer cell line panel in drug discovery. By demand, their genomes have been sequenced in 2012 [168]. Today, there is a Human Glioblastoma Cell Culture (HGCC) resource that consists of a biobank of 48 cell lines representing all molecular subtypes of the disease, with an associated database containing high-resolution molecular data [169]. Similar work was done with 100 ovarian cancer cell lines to make an OCCP panel where the cells were described [170]. Cancer Cell Line Encyclopedia (CCLE) and the Cancer Genome Project (CGP) have served well in identifying novel biomarkers in drug response. Recently, large collaboration efforts expanded the characterizations of CCLE to include genetic, RNA splicing, DNA methylation, histone H3 modification, microRNA expression, and reverse phase protein array data. These data were collected for 1072 cell lines of various lineages from individuals of different ethnicities to improve the understanding of the molecular features that contribute to cancer phenotypes, including drug responses. Computational integration of these data with functional characterization such as drug sensitivity, short hairpin RNA knockdown, and CRISPR-Cas9 knockout data revealed potential targets and associated biomarkers for further analysis. This information is publicly available [171]. Similarly, immortalized cell line models such as EBV-transformed lymphoblastoid cell lines (LCLs) from the International HapMap Project, Human Variation Panel, and 1000 Genomes Project with multiomics data became available for fundamental cancer research [172].

Various specific cell lines are created for scientific research. HAP1 is a semi-haploid human adherent cell line derived from the male chronic myelogenous leukemia cell line KBM-7, with a single copy of almost every human chromosome. These cells are easy to culture, and authors assert that such cell line is an invaluable tool for gene functional testing and drug discovery by facilitating gene-editing techniques [173]. The well-known resources of cell lines for research and commercial applications include ATCC, JCRB, and other cell culture biobanks with many species covered. The European Collection of Cell Cultures ECACC (UK) offers more than 1500 human iPSC lines, 450 monoclonal antibody-producing clones, and many normal tissue and cancer cell lines for disease modeling or bioproduction [174].

The first attempt to solve the disadvantage of cell line "purity" as well as personalization of the treatment approach was the introduction of primary ex vivo cancer cell lines into the cancer research, including drug testing, discovery and therapy response prediction, with improving methodologies and optimizations for cell culturing [175–178]. Heterogeneity found in cell cultures was suggested to be coded by biological mechanisms from the primary tumors, and it was acknowledged as an instrument for clinical implications. Some authors denied the global inadequacy of translating pharmacogenomic data from 2D to clinical settings suggesting that drug resistance was mainly intrinsic and did not depend on cell culturing conditions [179]. However, this question is controversial, as other authors demonstrated that DNA methylation profile rapidly changed when cells had been plated in vitro, namely there was a global loss of 5hmC modification in vitro [180]. In addition, there are also challenges at cellular level. In many reports, ex vivo cancer cell line generation often was not 100% effective, meaning that obtained cells did not proliferate sufficiently or at all. Too long time frame from biopsy to sufficient cell number (2–6 months in lung cancer) [7, 15] is not applicable in clinics as well as there is a risk to select only the fast-growing cells, the subclones that do not resemble the original tumor; moreover, in many cases, patient survival may not be that long. Nevertheless, authors suggested that drug screening may be done using fresh cells, or primary cultures, within days while still in the presence of stroma cells [73]. Additionally, the issue of cell line generation and expansion could be solved by advances in culture medium composition, cell isolation, passaging, and associated techniques, or by means of assisted cell expansion described in [181] which is favorable in the aspect that it also worked with normal cells from the same tissue. Briefly, they used human mammary and prostate epithelial cells from fresh and even frozen biospecimen using an irradiated feeder cell layer and a Rho kinase inhibitor Y-27632 in the culture medium and expanded the culture to 1 million cells in 7 days. In this way, both drug screening and toxicity studies can be carried out for the patient simultaneously in several weeks. Alternatively, recent advance in cell imaging (next-generation phenotypic screening) may enable fast, miniaturized, and physiologically relevant analysis of fresh ex vivo cells in suspension within hours after sample acquisition (e.g., IntelliCyt iQue Screener). For adherent cells, various automated, high-throughput imaging platforms, such as Cellinsight, ImageXpress Micro, Celldicoverer, MACSima, IncuCyte, etc., are available.

Additional pro for ex vivo cell cultures is the evidence of cancer stem-like cells in such cultures [91, 182, 183] and similar molecular profiles to those of in vivo cancer cells [184]. The latter study suggested that only several existing breast cancer cell lines, namely BT483, T47D and MDAMB453, had satisfactory similarity to molecular pattern of tumors. Another report supplemented the study by stating that primary ovarian cancer cells also differed from the established cell lines in tumor-associated antigen expression (namely BIRC5, CA125, CEA, DDX43, EPCAM, FOLR1, Her-2/neu, MAGE-A1, MAGE-A2, MAGE-A3, MAGE-A4, MAGE-A6, MAGE-A10, MAGE-A12, MUC-1, NY-ESO-1, PRAME, p53, TPBG, TRT, and WT1 mRNAs), but one cell line—OVCAR-3—was quite representative [185]. On the other hand, there is evidence that even in common commercial cancer cell lines established long time ago and being deposited in biobanks such as ATCC, putative cancer stem cells are present [186].

Up to this paragraph, the cell line model has been discussed. However, cells growing in monolayer lack typical interactions that are present in tumors. It was shown that cell cultivation in 2D and 3D cultures results in different cell morphology, intracellular signaling, proliferation rate, differentiation capacity, and thus different response to treatment. For example, PDGFR activity was significantly lower in three sarcoma cell lines grown in 2D than in spheroids; in addition, stem cell markers Nanog, Oct4, and Slug as well as EMT proteins Snail, Slug, and Zeb1 were significantly higher in spheroids [187]. Another study showed that different cytotoxic compounds retained their ranking both in 2D and 3D cultures; however, all the IC50 values were smaller in 3D spheroids [188]. As described by an example of anti-HER2 targeted drug trastuzumab in a beautiful review by Sokolova et al., HER2 formed heterodimers with HER3 in a monolayer culture, but in spheroids, HER2 homodimers prevailed; therefore, a greater antiproliferative effect of this antibody against spheroids in comparison to a monolayer was observed. Importantly, HER2/HER2 receptor led to activation of MAPK signal transduction pathway, whereas HER2/HER3 receptor activated alternative PI3K pathway. Another effect of dimensionality was changes in expression and the basal phosphorylation level of cell-surface receptors. It could be either higher or lower in 3D than in 2D [189]. Similarly, remarkable differences were observed in pancreatic cancer cell lines HPAF-II, HPAC and PL45 when cultivated on 2D or 3D [190]. 3D hepatocyte spheroids (named as human liver microtissues) have demonstrated better prediction of liver toxicity than two-dimensional primary human hepatocytes model [191]. Similarly, large-scale pharmacological profiling of PANC1 human pancreatic cancer and SN12C human kidney carcinoma cell lines in both 2D and 3D was performed, analyzing a collection of 1912 chemotherapeutic agents. Interestingly, comparison of pharmacological responses of cells cultured in traditional 2D monolayer conditions as well as responses obtained from cells forming spheres versus cells already in 3D spheres enabled the identification of those key signaling pathways and cellular processes that when modulated by drugs were able to reduce cancer cell viability in all growth conditions or, to our particular interest, selectively in the different cell growth modes [192]. Thus, 3D culture systems comparing to 2D cultures have more advantages for using them for drug investigation studies. Some of the disadvantages of 2D models were reduced by introducing 3D substrates, scaffolds, and extracellular matrix components, including well-known Matrigel. Such models may be placed between 2D and 3D, sometimes called

2.5D. Consequently, commercial cell lines or cells isolated from donor tissue can be used in cancer research.

Dimensionality alters cellular surface area for a drug to penetrate. On a porous scaffold, surface area of a cell may increase; however, in a compact spheroid, surface area may decrease when compared to that of a planar 2D adherent cell. One study described generation and properties of multicellular tumor spheroids from different pancreatic cancer cell lines. Briefly, large and dense spheroids represented type I, lose and of different sizes—type II, and floating monolayer films—type III. The three types displayed different expression of adhesion molecules E-cadherin, DSC, and DSG proteins; in addition, type I spheroids had higher resistance to doxorubicin and gemcitabine [155]. More importantly, cell-cell and cell-surface contacts generate intracellular signaling that has been reviewed elsewhere.

Despite the abovementioned in defense of cell cultures, other authors argue that in principle the approach is defective in one additional aspect—enzymatic digestion of a solid tissue/tumor. This procedure is almost absolutely necessary in generating cell cultures. However, the proteolytic enzymes (trypsin, collagenase, dispase, accutase, etc.) cleave both proteins of the extracellular matrix and cell-surface receptors. By doing that, digestion irreversibly changes cellular signaling [193]. However, comparison of different cell-dissociating agents for stem cell isolation from glioma tumorspheres revealed that there was a difference in CD133 antigen retention: the worst result was obtained for nonenzymatic dissociation solution NECDS, while the minimal impact was observed in Libertase-TL-treated cells [194]. On the other hand, disruption of cell-cell contacts during the initial steps of cell culture establishment favors the outgrowth of specific cells, the composition of which do not recapitulate the original heterogeneity of a tumor [177]. Therefore, organotypic tumor slices without application of proteolysis would be the best model for drug selection in the individualized cancer treatment, and it will be discussed here below. In addition, tissue slice generation time can be fast enough to receive the results in days.

4.3 3D in vitro models

Phenotypic screening-based drug discovery should rely on 3D models because monolayer culture cell concentration is strikingly low (10^5–10^6 in mL) when compared to in vivo tissue (40–50 million cells in a mL) [195]. However, this recommendation is not attributable to leukemia cell cultures where physiologically relevant concentration of the cells can be obtained in vitro for the research. Advances in cancer modeling were nicely reviewed in publications [25, 30, 89, 145, 177, 189, 196, 197]. In our previous publication [198], 3D drug testing models with end-point viability-measuring methods were presented, including scaffold-based 3D culture systems, tissue slices, cellular spheroids, organoids, and organs-on-chips. Having both models for normal tissues and a tumor from a single patient would improve the prediction of systemic toxicities to healthy stem cells. As covered by other authors, self-organized and stem cell-derived three-dimensional human organoids give promise to be applied in disease modeling, drug screening, regeneration therapy, and even for host-microbe interaction studies [199]. These models can be patient-specific and thus are suitable for personalized medicine. When generated from cancer patient cells, such organoids have the value in anticancer drug screening [200]. More frequently used 3D culture models of cancer include: tumor mono-cell spheroids, hetero-spheroids (tumoroids), tumor tissue explants, and tumor-on-a-chip. 3D printing, to our opinion, is more relevant to nongenetic pathologies where normal organ-like structures have to be replicated. Tumor, as known, is of irregular, chaotic structure; thus, there is nothing to reconstruct with a precision of a 3D printer. One more three-dimensional approach is the application of decellularized cadaver organs. For example, rat lungs have been used to determine human adenocarcinoma cell lines H358, PC9, and SW1573 proliferation on the scaffold, cell viability over the culture period and in response to treatment with cisplatin or Erlotinib. A resazurin-based reagent was perfused through the scaffold to evaluate cell number [201].

Multicellular tumor spheroids represent aggregates of cells formed in conditions where cell-cell interactions predominate over cell-substrate interactions. Spheroids closely resemble avascular primary tumors and metastases with respect to their architecture, gradient of oxygen, nutrients and metabolites distribution, distinct proliferation rates as well as microenvironment and drug penetration [202, 203]. One-cell-type spheroids are cellular aggregate formed by one type of cells, in this case cancer cells. In principal, this type of spheroids can be used as a model system for primary avascular tumor or metastasis [204]. Enhanced expression of stem cell markers and drug resistance in sphere-forming nonsmall cell lung cancer cells were reported: tumor sphere-derived cells expressed stem cell markers CD44, CD133, Sox2, and Oct4. Moreover, expression of lung resistance-related protein (LRP), glutathione-S-transferase-π (GST-π), and multidrug resistance proteins-1 (MRP1) were all significantly enhanced in sphere-derived cells [205]. In addition to spheroid formed by one type of cells, more complex multicellular spheroids are used in drug studies. This type of spheroids contains not only cancer but also other tumor-constituting cells, such as fibroblasts, endothelial cell, and immune cell, and thus is closer to situation in vivo due to additional cancer-normal cell contacts.

Various techniques can be used to obtain spheroids: plastic culture dishes with ultra-low attachment surfaces, spontaneous aggregation under free-floating conditions, liquid overlay on agarose, hanging drop cultures, spinner-flask cultures, and micro-fabricated scaffolds [204]. Simplicity in production and use of spheroids has led to widespread use of these techniques. Cancer organoids may be created from CTCs, as nicely reviewed in [206], highlighting the techniques for CTC isolation from patient blood, cell culture enrichment, culture medium supplementation, as well as CTC-derived organoid application in disease modeling, genetic instability studies, drug discovery, and precision medicine. Interestingly, authors have demonstrated that replacing fetal bovine serum with human serum could enhance spheroid formation and increase the invasiveness of cancer cells in vitro [207]. However, not all techniques provide uniform-sized spheroids, resulting in poor reproducibility of experimental data. Cell biological functionality and sensitivity to drugs have a strong correlation with the size of spheroids [208, 209]. The methods of hanging drop and microfabricated microstructures enable researches to modulate spheroid dimensions but have a limitation for mass production potential and cause difficulties for effective harvesting of spheroids. Recently, a number of optimized spheroid production protocols were developed with various robust and effective platforms for high-throughput drug screening. Opera Phenix High Content Screening System with Synchrony Optics and automated image analysis were reported to be well suitable for microtissue spheroid analysis; ImageXpressMicro Confocal automatic imaging system with MetaXpress6 software was used for similar purpose.

In a strict sense, the term "organoid" means that the microtissue has originated from stem cells that had differentiated in tissue-specific manner and formed a mini-organ or organ-like structure. Such models of other than oncologic disease research have been nicely reviewed elsewhere. However, when microtissue is formed from primary cancer cells, some authors call it organoid, and some as spheroid. In either way, cancer cells propagated in three-dimensional (3D) culture systems exhibit physiologically relevant cell-cell and cell-matrix interactions, gene expression and signaling pathway profiles, and heterogeneity and structural complexity that reflect in vivo tumors. In one study, three lines of ex vivo established colorectal tumor spheroids were analyzed. All three lines expressed EpCAM, CD133, CD44, CD24, ALDH1, and LGR5 biomarkers and maintained them stably for months in vitro. STR phenotyping and mutation profile for APC, KRAS, MLH1, serine-threonine kinase 11, and TP53 coincided with original tumors from which they had been derived [210].

Cancer modeling using organoids was nicely reviewed in [211, 212]; larger view on tumoroid application in cancer research was extensively discussed in [213]. Patient-derived tumor organoids were suggested as the best model enabling high-throughput drug testing in a clinically relevant time frame at the same time being cost-effective [23]. Although multicellular spheroids exhibit physiologically relevant structural complexity of tumor as well as cell-cell and cell-matrix interactions, smaller than 200 μm spheroids do not reflect the in vivo characteristics of tumor cell proliferation, metabolite, and oxygen gradient resulting in necrotic core formation. Authors developed an optimized protocol allowing production of large spheroids that mimic some of the complex tumor microenvironment, including hypoxia. However, in this model, spheroids were unable to develop tumor specific vascular architecture, which was achieved by transplanting of spheroids to immunosuppressed mouse .

Another study described a 3D cell culture system to study tumor-stroma interactions in nonsmall cell lung cancer cells by creating mono and co-culture spheroids of two NSCLC cell lines A549 and Colo699, and lung fibroblasts. The viability of tumor spheroids was determined after 5 and 10 days by using Annexin V/Propidium Iodide flow cytometry. Lower viability was observed in A549 monocultures compared to co-cultures, whereas Colo699 monocultures showed better viability compared to co-cultures. Additionally, tumor-fibroblast spheroid formation was characterized by scanning electron microscope, semi-thin sections, fluorescence, and immunohistochemistry of E-Cadherin, vimentin, Ki67, fibronectin, cytokeratin 7, and a-smooth muscle actin in addition to conventional histology [214].

It is rather difficult to consider which spheroid production method would be most suitable for potential drug studies. The main requirement for high-throughput analysis is reproducibility of uniform spheroids, as cell susceptibility to therapy depends on the spheroid size. It was demonstrated that the size of spheroid may depend on production method used, as growing of squamous carcinoma cells on ultralow attachment plates resulted in higher proliferation rates and increased spheroid size compared to Hanging drop production method. Despite numerous spheroid studies, it is not still clear which time point would be ideal to start treatments and evaluate drug response. Typical spheroid structure consisting of an outer layer of proliferating cells and inner layer of quiescent cells is detected in spheroids larger than 500 μm in diameter. Several agents have been found to be less effective in 3D models than in 2D cell cultures due to the drug concentration gradient in different layers of spheroid which is relative to drug delivery within solid tumor in vivo. Moreover, cell growing in 3D environment showed expression of different genes associated with resistance to therapy [205, 215].

Limited drug penetration to the tumor mass is one of the mechanisms which determines tumor resistance to applied therapy. This critical parameter is not reproduced in monolayer 2D cultures. Meanwhile, spheroids formed from cancer cells mimic both the heterogenic multilayer tumor structure and gradient drug penetration thus providing more physiologically relevant results as compared to monolayer cultures. Cells in the center of spheroid are exposed to nonoptimal drug concentrations; thus, increased drug doses or drug combinations are needed to provide antitumor effectiveness. Recent studies demonstrated the advantage of spheroid model in evaluating activity of drug combinations and treatment schedules in order to promote drug delivery and accumulation inside a tumor. Therefore, spheroid models can be used to assess penetration of different drug formulations.

In drug development, potential agents are further progressed to antitumor activity screening in vivo where syngeneic mice model, genetically engineered mice models, or xenograft models are used. All these models have some significant limitations leading to inadequate results. First of all, tumors are often implanted subcutaneously—to the site which does not reflect their original in vivo location. Due to the compromised mouse immune system, xenografts are usually characterized by higher proliferation rates compared to primary human tumor [115, 216]. Moreover, transplanted tumor interacts with stromal components which are not of human origin, thus can behave in different manner. Strategy that could significantly increase the rate of success would be more complex, physiologically relevant cellular models used in early lead discovery. For solid tumors, this would include development of 3D in vitro tumor models which recapitulate human tumor architecture and biology, thus providing greater translational potential [217, 218].

4.4 Complex 3D models

Solid tumors consist of cancer and stromal cells surrounded by extracellular matrix. All these cellular and noncellular tumor components co-exist in highly interactive 3D environment. Gradient of nutrients, soluble factors, oxygen and metabolites occurring in different layers of tumor as well as different type of interactions such as cell-cell and cell-ECM regulate cell function and behavior. Cancer cells cultivated in 3D environment, if compared to cells growing as a monolayer, are exposed to different signals that modify their response to various stimuli [158, 219]. For example, cells growing in 3D cultures experience different mechanical forces compared to cells growing in 2D. It was demonstrated that mechanical properties can regulate cellular response to therapy and angiogenesis [220]. Additionally, various interactions occurring in multilayer tumor create physical barrier attenuating drug penetration. Recent studies demonstrated that 3D microenvironment had effect on numerous cellular functions including cell morphology, viability, proliferation, differentiation, and migration potential, as well as cell signaling, gene and protein expression following response to the applied therapy. Taken together, these results indicate that 3D models of cancer provide more physiologically relevant results and have greater translational potential to successful clinical studies.

There are several artificially engineered 3D cancer models that are close to natural tissues and thus partially recapitulate the environment into which a tumor cell may invade; for example, three-dimensional organotypic microfluidic model to study the phenotype and invasion of glioma stem cells [221]. Artificial skin was built of stratified terminally differentiated epidermal compartment of keratinocytes and melanocytes, a dermal compartment of fibroblasts embedded in collagen, and a basement membrane deposited by skin cells; such skin reconstruct was used for melanoma modeling [222]. Another example is a 3D bone marrow model derived from endothelial progenitor cells and multipotent mesenchymal stromal cells embedded in alginate and Matrigel. It was used to study immunotherapy on primary multiple myeloma [223]. More advanced bone marrow models are described in [224] and may involve various soluble factors, osteoblasts and the flow of nutrients. Similarly, a lung cancer model named OncoCilAir has almost everything that is available in vivo, except immune system of a patient. Briefly, OncoCilAir was developed by plating lung fibroblasts and bronchial epithelial cells on different sides of a porous membrane. Later, nonsmall cell lung cancer cells were added to the fibroblastic side, and air-liquid interface was introduced to mimic the conditions in normal lungs [18]. In that way, OncoCilAir includes both healthy and cancerous cells; thus, it can be used to test both tumor-killing activity and the adverse effects of anticancer drugs. Moreover, the model could be maintained for up to 3 months, which theoretically enables studies of such long-term effects as air pollution toxicity, drug resistance, and tumor recurrence.

Organotypic 3D in vitro models are very close to realistic representation of a tumor. When a reasonably thin slice of a real tumor is carefully plated on a porous surface to ensure better diffusion of nutrients and metabolites, both cancerous and stroma cells are present in such a model, including the unchanged intratumoral tissue architecture with ECM and cellular contacts as well as immune cells with natural cytokines. Such a system is well suited to perform drug selection in personalized medicine as it captures the heterogeneity of a tumor, can be multiplexed for various biochemical applications, and also is transparent for optical microscopy. Probably one of the most advanced commercial systems available today is CANScript from Mitra Biotech (India). This platform is intended for prediction of clinical responses to anticancer treatment of a certain patient and is applicable in almost all types of cancer, including bladder, prostate, HCC, cervical, urogenital, NHL, and GBM. In contrast to other similar preclinical models, CANScript and its prediction algorithm has been tested in clinical settings for H&N, CRC, breast, pancreas, stomach, esophageal, lung, ovarian, AML, and CML cancers [ClinicalTrials.gov identifier (NCT number) NCT03253575]. The technology has been validated in mouse xenografts and extremely well correlated with the clinical outcome. Currently, the system is being adapted to become an automated platform available to hospitals. Briefly, the tumor sample from a patient is cut using a tissue chopper into 200–400 μm thick slices that are placed into 48-well cell culture plates with RPMI-1640 medium with supplements including patient blood serum (2%). Importantly, the cell culture plate itself is coated with tumor-grade-matched matrix. Tumor-stroma matrix proteins (TMPs) are analyzed from the same specimen by mass spectrometry after sample processing, selecting certain proteins to further constitute the protein cocktail for plate coating. It ensures the conservation of the tumor microenvironment in addition to the 3D structure of a tissue slice and native patient-specific ligands from their blood serum. It was demonstrated many times that the mentioned factors determine the fate of tumors in terms of integrity, survival, metastasis, and response to chemotherapy. In addition, the CANScript developers have demonstrated that explants in noncoated wells lost tumor architecture and exhibited decreased viability, proliferation, and activation of oncogenic pathways compared with the initial baseline [225]. The method utilizes both morphological and biochemical criteria, including measurement of cell viability, ATP utilization, proliferation status, changes in tumor area and nuclear fragmentation, activation and expression of various signaling proteins by reverse phase phosphoproteomic array, immunohistochemistry and qRT-PCR methods for molecular profiling, and quantification of biomarkers [17].

However, tissue slicing has some minor limitations. For example, when a tumor is larger than the well of a plate into which it has to be positioned, only a portion of a slice would be examined. In such a case, the unexamined part of a tumor and its response to the suggested treatment could be lost. There are data that drug sensitivity and biomarker expression vary considerably within individual samples [77, 226]; hence, multiple-site samples should be taken, making it difficult for the specialist to decide which sites to include in the sampling. Furthermore, cellular signaling and hence the drug response in slices may be altered due to suffered mechanical stress during the precision cutting and cellular necrosis signaling at the incision planes. In addition, it is characteristic to a solid tumor to maintain high interstitial fluid pressure that limits the absorption, e.g., of a drug, and this pressure is not preserved in the current models. As noticed by PREDECT team, the ultimate goal—clinical application of this method—requires standardization which is impossible in obtaining the samples manually due to different intraoperative manipulation and pathology processing even with the same type of cancer [89]. Additionally, for CANScript technology, identification and individual plate coating with required TMPs appear to be the limiting (expensive and labor consuming) steps, as for these purposes, the biopsies firstly have to be analyzed by liquid chromatography-mass spectrometry (LCMS/MS), followed by Venn diagrams and heatmaps to select the proteins to be mixed in a cocktail for the plate coating.

Another and probably the most straight-forward approach in trying to understand the nature of cancer was the initiative The Cancer Genome Atlas (TCGA), as already described above in this review. Starting from 2006, 20,000 primary cancer and matched normal samples spanning 33 cancer types have been molecularly characterized, yielding over 2.5 petabytes of genomic, epigenomic, transcriptomic, and proteomic data that will remain publicly available at portal.gdc.cancer.gov for the research community to use [227]. Comparatively similar problem in data processing is already arising from the next step in cancer modeling that included real-time monitoring and gave the fourth dimension for in vitro cancer studies. Apparently, it is not applicable in vivo, but definitely it is the future of oncology.

4.5 Single-cell approach

When talking about cancer heterogeneity, we usually think about a complex organ-like tumor. That is correct, because human body is mainly solid, and almost all cell types form solid tissues. However, blood is liquid and it contains many types of different cells; thus, it is also heterogenic. When analyzing blood, we are familiar with flow cytometry and discrimination of cells by their physical parameters and CD antigens. The same is for blood cancer: flow cytometry can discriminate various subpopulations of abnormal blood cells. Additionally, mass cytometry has emerged as a method to evaluate cellular biomarkers on a single cell. Importantly, this method has enabled studying the antibody-based cancer therapies as well as metal containing chemotherapeutic agents at one-cell resolution [228]. Similarly, Western blot method has been miniaturized even to subcellular level [229]. As mentioned previously, blood cancer is quite well treated just because there is no need for a complex model to study the cell response or resistance to a certain drug or combinations. Cells in suspension and can be readily analyzed in vitro not only for the antigens, but also for cellular signaling. For example, phospho-flow cytometry was applied in the search for B-cell precursor acute lymphoblastic leukemia individualized therapy and enabled to screen for small molecule kinase inhibitors that induced cancer cell death [230]. Functional analysis of single-cell mass accumulation rate became available by means of microchannel resonance [231]. Recent technologies have enabled single-cell RNA sequencing thus providing the power to dissect intratumoral heterogeneity and to suggest combination therapies [232]. Today, a Phase II clinical trial (NCT01620216) started in 2012 is still recruiting leukemia patients for ex vivo drug response prediction. However, even here, the microenvironment plays a role. As reported previously, the responses of leukemia cells to chemotherapy in vivo, compared to in vitro, were partly related to the interactions of leukemic cells and the three-dimensional bone marrow/stromal microenvironment. To investigate this phenomenon, leukemic cell lines were co-cultured with human bone marrow mesenchymal stem cell (hu-BM-MSC) in 3D and compared to leukemic cells treated in suspension or grown on a hu-BM-MSC monolayer (2D conditions) [233]. The authors concluded that cultures in 3D were more resistant to drug-induced apoptosis compared to cells cultured in 2D or in suspension.

Further, the modeling becomes complicated when it comes to circulating tumor cells (CTCs). During cancer progression, invasive cells evade the primary tumor and enter the vascular systems in search for better environment. Such CTCs are important in many aspects; the ability to target such cells and to eliminate them before the formation of metastasis is of high priority. CTCs are valuable for assessing the profile and heterogeneity of tumor-evading cancer cells. However, their direct use as a single-cell model in predicting tumor response to the treatment is disputable; therefore, researchers usually create CTC culture models as well as mouse xenografts [234]. However, to retrieve CTCs and later to expand their culture in vitro is challenging. One study compared three methods (RT-qPCR for cytokeratin 19, double immunofluorescence with A45-B/B3 and CD45 antibodies, and CellSearch system with CTC kit) to search for and count circulating tumor cells in breast cancer patient blood. Interestingly, there was virtually no agreement between the methods, including the cancer marker CK19 mRNA-positive cells that were also present in 26 healthy female donors [235]. This study demonstrated the limitations of biomarker-based cell characterization as well as weakness of technical standardization procedures. However, authors described that they have succeeded (16.5% success rate) to establish long-term cell cultures from breast cancer CTCs, growing them in serum free media supplemented with epidermal growth factor and basic fibroblast growth factor under nonadherent, hypoxic conditions [236]. Other reports demonstrated that in the case of colorectal cancer, CTC cell line generation was possible only from the patients with stage IV cancer and was not successful in earlier stages, and the cell cultures demonstrated all the attributes of cancer stem cells [182].

In general, pharmacologic response of every single cell from the heterogenic cancer tissue should be analyzed whenever possible. In the case of CTCs, single cell analysis is very helpful in defining their response to the drugs when cells have already escaped from their niche in the tumor tissue, i.e. when cancer cells are circulating in pre-metastatic fashion. However, their behavior does not necessarily correspond to the response of cells in solid tumor from which they have originated. Various microscopy imaging techniques that distinguish individual cells should be preferred over pan analysis methods both in vitro and in vivo [237, 238].

5. Upcoming technologies and perspectives

As of particular interest, there are several reports of drug response analysis in situ by microinjections into the intact solid tumor, as reviewed in "In situ functional diagnostics" [30]. Briefly, the drugs were delivered into the xenograft tumors either as a monotherapy compound or up to 16 slowly releasing drug reservoirs, and the response was evaluated by retrieving the whole tumor for analysis. Alternative approach was used to design acoustofluidic 3D tumor platform to investigate the localized release of temperature-sensitive liposomal doxorubicin in glioblastoma model [239]. Basically, focused ultrasound raises the temperature in the zone of the targeted several square millimeters. When directed at a tumor, such heating favors the disassembly of circulating cargo liposomes that contain toxic substances. This method shows promise in localized activation/release of chemotherapeutic drugs that are not well tolerated in organism and thus fail in dose-escalation trials. One more example is a nano device iNANIVID-assisted multiphoton microscopy of individual cells when physically inserted into a live solid tissue [240]. This short-term (up to 4 h) intravital mouse tumor monitoring was performed in order to validate the nanodevice for drug release; in this particular case, for analyzing EGF-induced chemotaxis of metastatic mammary tumor cells. Although this technology seems to us not applicable to humans, at least for long-term drug response studies, such progress may indicate the evolution of 4D cancer modeling.

Summarizing the above stated, the best cancer model is fully natural tumor in a living human. Although it might sound wired, it is true to some extent when talking about child cancer in the United States. More than 80% of children who have cancer are cured successfully in United States so they are comparatively better served by available therapies, as compared to adults. Authors postulate that mainly it was a result of incredibly effective chemotherapy combinations that were established through highly empirical and incremental clinical trials [241]. However, more technical approaches may be emerging to advance noninvasive cancer response monitoring in a patient to guide the best treatment. For example, magnetic resonance methods are able to some extent visualize tumor characteristics and its metabolic phenotypes on an anatomical, microvascular, microstructural, microenvironmental, and metabolomics scale [242]. More specifically, magnetic resonance imaging of muscle-invasive bladder cancer revealed that quantification of apparent diffusion coefficient (ADC) of water could reliably predict patient response to the neoadjuvant chemotherapy, i.e., resistant tumors were more heterogeneous in their spatial distribution of ADC values [243]. Alternatively, positron emission tomography showed promising results in molecular cancer biomarker imaging in vivo by using newly developed imaging agents for precise molecular targets. This technique can be useful in clinics for measuring early treatment response to predict therapeutic efficacy and relating tumor response to survival [244].

The next best thing to the real tumor monitoring in vivo (so-called 4D cancer model) is sophisticated 3D in vitro and in vivo mouse models. For fundamental studies, light sheet fluorescent microscopy is a new technology for rapid, low phototoxicity 3D imaging with resolution similar to that of confocal microscopy; moreover, super-resolution variations of the method are becoming available. Probably the best model in both genetic and physiological relevance, more than a humanized mouse, is the putative "patient-on-a-chip." The model would be comprised of many organ-on-a-chip building blocks that presumably would be printed from patient-derived and differentiated iPSCs, later connecting those blocks in a physiological order by microfluidic channels [245]. For example, an array of 3D bioprinted tissues (skin, bone and cartilage), microfluidics-based kidney-on-a-chip, lumen forming intestine microtissues, and heart model as a multilayer of cardiac fibroblasts alternately layered with iPSC-differentiated myocytes on an elastic silicone membrane for efficient beating, are promising components of such a system [246]. However, this kind of model is considered only in a preclinical setting for drug research. Computational time-lapse movie data analysis also will require the creation of most intelligent software [247].

Photo-degradable gelatin may be used for very specific reasons in 3D gel cellular models. Using this delicate approach, heterogenous cell cultures may be cultivated in one dish until a cell or a colony of interest has to be extracted for analysis, leaving the remaining culture intact. This method was used to separate morphologically different subpopulations from a murine breast cancer cell line [248]. No digestion, no labeling, no flow cytometry is needed.

For 2D cell cultures, noninvasive, time-lapse compatible electrical impedance may be used for phenotypic screening, target identification, compound screening, lead selection, investigating the mechanism of action, and testing drug safety and toxicity [249]. The method also requires gold-plated electrode for cell adhesion.

For single-cell approach, advanced microfluidic techniques are being developed for multiomics data acquisition in nanodroplets. Briefly, high-throughput single-cell isolation and nucleic acid barcoding methods are making it possible to measure the (epi)genomic, transcriptomic, or proteomic state of individual cells by elegant strategies and techniques described in [250]. Single-cell methods complemented with gene-editing technologies were recognized among the most perspective models for disease modeling [159]. Furthermore, a new technology directed at cellular spheroid generation using microwells that are much smaller than a well of a 1536-well plate may be paving its way. The method involves limiting dilution principle within traditional 2D cell culture plates coated with polydimethylsiloxane. The advantage of this method over traditional limiting dilution is that the small volume of a well limits diffusion of autocrine factors and improves extracellular survival signaling; at the same time, there is no danger of evaporation. Moreover, many clones (300 and more) and other types of cells from a heterogenous cancer tissue may be present in the same culture medium allowing paracrine signaling without complex microfluidic connections [251] or in a microchip format as developed earlier [252].

6. Concluding remarks

Regardless of the abundance of approaches and various models and methods developed, the question remains, which models are the best to assess cell heterogeneous response to anticancer treatment and to evaluate its clinical relevance? Recently, authors have performed SWOT (strengths, weaknesses, opportunities, and threats) analysis of 3D cell models and suggested that more transparent assessment of the value of new 3D models was needed. Currently, it looks like many popular 3D models have no standardized protocols for validation in clinics as well as they are not convenient enough, do not mimic cancer biology sufficiently, and thus are not suitable for use in clinic. As a result, early enthusiasm regarding 3D models is already followed by disillusionment and disappointing results. Development of long-term, low-throughput, inconsistent, and expensive models should be abandoned for clinical applications; however, such models may have merit in fundamental research [253].

We suggest that the best model would be simple, miniaturized, inexpensive and, at the same time, multifaceted, involving ex vivo analysis of individual cells in different states and in different conditions—suspension, 2D and 3D as well as co-cultures with stroma cells. Drug screening in such a model would require knowledge of which cellular states survive the specific treatment and, according to that, combinational therapy—not only by content but also organized in time and sequence—should be tested in the model system. The short-term cultivation in vitro should be complied for to preserve the patient-specific cellular heterogeneity, cell differentiation status, and molecular profile. For this particular reason, as well as for the ability to recheck the obtained results, patient's tumor specimen freezing protocols should be developed.

Acknowledgements

This project has received funding from the European Regional Development Fund (Project No. 01.2.2-LMT-K-718-01-0072) under grant agreement with the Research Council of Lithuania (LMTLT).

Author details

Aurimas Stulpinas, Aušra Imbrasaitė, Natalija Krestnikova
and Audronė Valerija Kalvelytė*
Institute of Biochemistry, Vilnius University Life Sciences Center, Vilnius, Lithuania

*Address all correspondence to: audrone.kalvelyte@bchi.vu.lt

References

[1] Tomasetti C, Li L, Vogelstein B. Stem cell divisions, somatic mutations, cancer etiology, and cancer prevention. Science. 2017;**355**(6331):1330-1133

[2] Song M, Vogelstein B, Giovannucci EL, Willett WC, Tomasetti C. Cancer prevention: Molecular and epidemiologic consensus. Science. 2018;**361**(6409):1317-1318

[3] Vitale I, Kroemer G. Spontaneous DNA damage propels tumorigenicity. Cell Research. 2017;**27**(6):720-721

[4] Liu X, Li F, Huang Q, Zhang Z, Zhou L, Deng Y, et al. Self-inflicted DNA double-strand breaks sustain tumorigenicity and stemness of cancer cells. Cell Research. 2017;**27**(6):764-783

[5] Prasad V. Perspective: The precision-oncology illusion. Nature. 2016;**537**(7619):S63

[6] Ferreri AJM, Illerhaus G, Zucca E, Cavalli F. Flows and flaws in primary central nervous system lymphoma. Nature Reviews. Clinical Oncology. 2010;**7**:1-2

[7] Scarborough HA, Bunn PA, DeGregori J. Personalized one-two punches for lung cancer. Cell Research. 2015;**25**(3):269-270

[8] Prasetyanti PR, Medema JP. Intra-tumor heterogeneity from a cancer stem cell perspective. Molecular Cancer. 2017;**16**(1):41

[9] Yoshida GJ, Saya H. Therapeutic strategies targeting cancer stem cells. Cancer Science. 2016;**107**(1):5-11

[10] Tammela T, Sanchez-Rivera FJ, Cetinbas NM, Wu K, Joshi NS, Helenius K, et al. A Wnt-producing niche drives proliferative potential and progression in lung adenocarcinoma. Nature. 2017;**545**(7654):355-359

[11] Rybinski B, Yun K. Addressing intra-tumoral heterogeneity and therapy resistance. Oncotarget. 2016;**7**(44):72322-72342

[12] Iorio F, Knijnenburg TA, Vis DJ, Bignell GR, Menden MP, Schubert M, et al. A landscape of pharmacogenomic interactions in Cancer. Cell. 2016;**166**(3):740-754

[13] Garralda E, Paz K, López-Casas PP, Jones S, Katz A, Kann LM, et al. Integrated next-generation sequencing and avatar mouse models for personalized cancer treatment. Clinical Cancer Research. 2014;**20**(9):2476-2484

[14] Heath JR, Ribas A, Mischel PS. Single-cell analysis tools for drug discovery and development. Nature Reviews. Drug Discovery. 2016;**15**:204-216

[15] Crystal AS, Shaw AT, Sequist LV, Friboulet L, Niederst MJ, Lockerman EL, et al. Patient-derived models of acquired resistance can identify effective drug combinations for cancer. Science. 2014;**346**(6216):1480-1486

[16] Blom K, Nygren P, Alvarsson J, Larsson R, Andersson CR. Ex vivo assessment of drug activity in patient tumor cells as a basis for tailored cancer therapy. Journal of Laboratory Automation. 2016;**21**(1):178-187

[17] Brijwani N, Jain M, Dhandapani M, Zahed F, Mukhopadhyay P, Biswas M, et al. Rationally co-targeting divergent pathways in KRAS wild-type colorectal cancers by CANscript technology reveals tumor dependence on Notch and Erbb2. Scientific Reports. 2017;**7**(1):1502

[18] Mas C, Boda B, CaulFuty M, Huang S, Wiszniewski L, Constant S. Antitumour efficacy of the selumetinib

and trametinib MEK inhibitors in a combined human airway-tumour-stroma lung cancer model. Journal of Biotechnology. 2015;**205**:111-119

[19] Marino P, Touzani R, Perrier L, Rouleau E, Kossi DS, Zhaomin Z, et al. Cost of cancer diagnosis using next-generation sequencing targeted gene panels in routine practice: A nationwide French study. European Journal of Human Genetics. 2018;**26**(3):314-323

[20] Bailey MH, Tokheim C, Porta-Pardo E, Sengupta S, Bertrand D, Weerasinghe A, et al. Comprehensive characterization of cancer driver genes and mutations. Cell. 2018;**173**(2):371.e18-385.e18

[21] Sanchez-Vega F, Mina M, Armenia J, Chatila WK, Luna A, La KC, et al. Oncogenic signaling pathways in the cancer genome atlas. Cell. 2018;**173**(2):321.e10-337.e10

[22] Ding L, Bailey MH, Porta-Pardo E, Thorsson V, Colaprico A, Bertrand D, et al. Perspective on oncogenic processes at the end of the beginning of cancer genomics. Cell. 2018;**173**(2):305.e10-320.e10

[23] Grandori C, Kemp CJ. Personalized cancer models for target discovery and precision medicine. Trends in Cancer. 2018;**4**(9):634-642

[24] Senft D, Leiserson MDM, Ruppin E, Ronai ZA. Precision oncology: The road ahead. Trends in Molecular Medicine. 2017;**23**(10):874-898

[25] Constant S, Huang S, Wisniewski L, Mas C. Advanced human in vitro models for the discovery and development of lung cancer therapies. In: Vallisuta O, Olimat S, editors. Open Access Book: Drug Discovery and Development—From Molecules to Medicine. Rijeka, Croatia: IntechOpen; 2015. Available from: https://www.intechopen.com/books/drug-discovery-and-development-from-molecules-to-medicine/advanced-human-in-vitro-models-for-the-discovery-and-development-of-lung-cancer-therapies

[26] Hanahan D, Weinberg RA. Hallmarks of cancer: The next generation. Cell. 2011;**144**(5):646-674

[27] Lin JJ, Shaw AT. Resisting resistance: Targeted therapies in lung cancer. Trends in Cancer. 2016;**2**(7):350-336

[28] Mansoori B, Mohammadi A, Davudian S, Shirjang S, Baradaran B. The different mechanisms of cancer drug resistance: A brief review. Advanced Pharmaceutical Bulletin. 2017;**7**(3):339-348

[29] Goto T, Hirotsu Y, Amemiya K, Mochizuki H, Omata M. Understanding intratumor heterogeneity and evolution in NSCLC and potential new therapeutic approach. Cancers. 2018;**10**(7):pii: E212

[30] Friedman AA, Letai A, Fisher DE, Flaherty KT. Precision medicine for cancer with next-generation functional diagnostics. Nature Reviews. Cancer. 2015;**15**(12):747-756

[31] Neel DS, Bivona TG. Resistance is futile: Overcoming resistance to targeted therapies in lung adenocarcinoma. npj Precision Oncology. 2017;**1**:pii: 3

[32] Dias MH, Kitano ES, Zelanis A, Iwai LK. Proteomics and drug discovery in cancer. Drug Discovery Today. 2016;**21**(2):264-277

[33] Dagogo-Jack I, Shaw AT. Tumour heterogeneity and resistance to cancer therapies. Nature Reviews. Clinical Oncology. 2018;**15**(2):81-94

[34] Gao JP, Xu W, Liu WT, Yan M, Zhu ZG. Tumor heterogeneity of gastric cancer: From the perspective of tumor-initiating cell. World

Journal of Gastroenterology. 2018;**24**(24):2567-2581

[35] Ahmed F, Haass NK. Microenvironment-driven dynamic heterogeneity and phenotypic plasticity as a mechanism of melanoma therapy resistance. Frontiers in Oncology. 2018;**8**:173

[36] Roerink SF, Sasaki N, Lee-Six H, Young MD, Alexandrov LB, Behjati S, et al. Intra-tumour diversification in colorectal cancer at the single-cell level. Nature. 2018;**556**(7702):457-462

[37] Gast CE, Silk AD, Zarour L, Riegler L, Burkhart JG, Gustafson KT, et al. Cell fusion potentiates tumor heterogeneity and reveals circulating hybrid cells that correlate with stage and survival. Science Advances. 2018;**4**(9):eaat7828

[38] Nimmakayala RK, Batra SK, Ponnusamy MP. Unraveling the journey of cancer stem cells from origin to metastasis. Biochimica et Biophysica Acta, Reviews on Cancer. 2019;**1871**(1):50-63

[39] Malta TM, Sokolov A, Gentles AJ, Burzykowski T, Poisson L, Weinstein JN, et al. Machine learning identifies stemness features associated with oncogenic dedifferentiation. Cell. 2018;**173**(2):338.e15-354.e15

[40] Eun K, Ham SW, Kim H. Cancer stem cell heterogeneity: Origin and new perspectives on CSC targeting. BMB Reports. 2017;**50**(3):117-125

[41] Bocci F, Gearhart-Serna L, Boareto M, Ribeiro M, Ben-Jacob E, Devi GR, et al. Toward understanding cancer stem cell heterogeneity in the tumor microenvironment. Proceedings of the National Academy of Sciences of the United States of America. 2019;**116**(1):148-157

[42] Fonseca NA, Cruz AF, Moura V, Simões S, Moreira JN. The cancer stem cell phenotype as a determinant factor of the heterotypic nature of breast tumors. Critical Reviews in Oncology/Hematology. 2017;**113**:111-121

[43] Pietras A. Cancer stem cells in tumor heterogeneity. Advances in Cancer Research. 2011;**112**:255-281. DOI: 10.1016/B978-0-12-387688-1.00009-0

[44] Liu S, Cong Y, Wang D, Sun Y, Deng L, Liu Y, et al. Breast cancer stem cells transition between epithelial and mesenchymal states reflective of their normal counterparts. Stem Cell Reports. 2014;**2**(1):78-91

[45] Luo M, Brooks M, Wicha M. Epithelial-mesenchymal plasticity of breast cancer stem cells: Implications for metastasis and therapeutic resistance. Current Pharmaceutical Design. 2015;**21**(10):1301-1310

[46] Wahl GM, Spike BT. Cell state plasticity, stem cells, EMT, and the generation of intra-tumoral heterogeneity. npj Breast Cancer. 2017;**3**:14

[47] Lourenço AR, Coffer PJ. SOX4: Joining the master regulators of epithelial-to-mesenchymal transition? Trends in Cancer. 2017;**3**(8):571-582

[48] Kim S, Han Y, Kim SI, Kim H-S, Kim SJ, Song YS. Tumor evolution and chemoresistance in ovarian cancer. npj Precision Oncology. 2018;**2**:20

[49] Nieto MA, Huang RYYJ, Jackson RAA, Thiery JPP. EMT: 2016. Cell. 2016;**166**(1):21-45

[50] Dongre A, Weinberg RA. New insights into the mechanisms of epithelial–mesenchymal transition and implications for cancer. Nature Reviews. Molecular Cell Biology. 2019;**20**(2):69-84

[51] Santamaría PG, Moreno-Bueno G, Cano A. Contribution of epithelial plasticity to therapy resistance. Journal of Clinical Medicine. 2019;**8**(5):676

[52] Tulchinsky E, Demidov O, Kriajevska M, Barlev NA, Imyanitov E. EMT: A mechanism for escape from EGFR-targeted therapy in lung cancer. Biochimica et Biophysica Acta, Reviews on Cancer. 2019;**1871**(1):29-39

[53] Vad-Nielsen J, Gammelgaard KR, Daugaard TF, Nielsen AL. Cause-and-effect relationship between FGFR1 expression and epithelial-mesenchymal transition in EGFR-mutated non-small cell lung cancer cells. Lung Cancer. 2019;**132**:132-140

[54] Poh M-E, Liam C-K, Rajadurai P, Chai C-S. Epithelial-to-mesenchymal transition (EMT) causing acquired resistance to afatinib in a patient with epidermal growth factor receptor (EGFR)-mutant lung adenocarcinoma. Journal of Thoracic Disease. 2018;**10**(7):E560-E563

[55] Kaiser J. The cancer stem cell gamble. Science. 2015;**347**(6219):226-229

[56] Arena S, Salati M, Sorgentoni G, Barbisan F, Orciani M. Characterization of tumor-derived mesenchymal stem cells potentially differentiating into cancer-associated fibroblasts in lung cancer. Clinical & Translational Oncology. 2018;**20**(12):1582-1591

[57] Kinugasa Y, Matsui T, Takakura N. CD44 expressed on cancer-associated fibroblasts is a functional molecule supporting the stemness and drug resistance of malignant cancer cells in the tumor microenvironment. Stem Cells. 2014;**32**(1):145-156

[58] Su S, Chen J, Yao H, Liu J, Yu S, Lao L, et al. CD10 + GPR77 + cancer-associated fibroblasts promote cancer formation and chemoresistance by sustaining cancer stemness. Cell. 2018;**172**(4):841.e16-856.e16

[59] Chen X, Song E. Turning foes to friends: Targeting cancer-associated fibroblasts. Nature Reviews. Drug Discovery. 2019;**18**(2):99-115

[60] Lenos KJ, Miedema DM, Lodestijn SC, Nijman LE, van den Bosch T, Romero Ros X, et al. Stem cell functionality is microenvironmentally defined during tumour expansion and therapy response in colon cancer. Nature Cell Biology. 2018;**20**(10):1193-1202

[61] Butera G, Pacchiana R, Donadelli M. Autocrine mechanisms of cancer chemoresistance. Seminars in Cell and Developmental Biology. 2018;**78**:3-12

[62] Pasquier J, Gosset M, Geyl C, Hoarau-Véchot J, Chevrot A, Pocard M, et al. CCL2/CCL5 secreted by the stroma induce IL-6/PYK2 dependent chemoresistance in ovarian cancer. Molecular Cancer. 2018;**17**(1):47

[63] Dalla Pozza E, Forciniti S, Palmieri M, Dando I. Secreted molecules inducing epithelial-to-mesenchymal transition in cancer development. Seminars in Cell and Developmental Biology. 2018;**78**:62-72

[64] Van Zijl F, Mair M, Csiszar A, Schneller D, Zulehner G, Huber H, et al. Hepatic tumor-stroma crosstalk guides epithelial to mesenchymal transition at the tumor edge. Oncogene. 2009;**28**(45):4022-4033

[65] Polyak K, Weinberg RA. Transitions between epithelial and mesenchymal states: Acquisition of malignant and stem cell traits. Nature Reviews. Cancer. 2009;**9**(4):265-273

[66] Mani SA, Guo W, Liao M-J, Eaton EN, Ayyanan A, Zhou AY, et al. The epithelial-mesenchymal transition generates cells with properties of stem cells. Cell. 2008;**133**(4):704-715

[67] Fiorilli P, Partridge D, Staniszewska I, Wang JY, Grabacka M, So K, et al. Integrins mediate adhesion

of medulloblastoma cells to tenascin and activate pathways associated with survival and proliferation. Laboratory Investigation. 2008;**88**(11):1143-1156

[68] Kirkland SC. Type i collagen inhibits differentiation and promotes a stem cell-like phenotype in human colorectal carcinoma cells. British Journal of Cancer. 2009;**101**(2):320-326

[69] Rice AJ, Cortes E, Lachowski D, Cheung BCH, Karim SA, Morton JP, et al. Matrix stiffness induces epithelial-mesenchymal transition and promotes chemoresistance in pancreatic cancer cells. Oncogene. 2017;**6**(7):e352

[70] Puls TJ, Tan X, Whittington CF, Voytik-Harbin SL. 3D collagen fibrillar microstructure guides pancreatic cancer cell phenotype and serves as a critical design parameter for phenotypic models of EMT. PLoS One. 2017;**12**(11):e0188870

[71] Patel H, Nilendu P, Jahagirdar D, Pal JK, Sharma NK. Modulating secreted componentsoftumormicroenvironment: A masterstroke in tumor therapeutics. Cancer Biology & Therapy. 2018;**19**(1):3-12

[72] Minchinton AI, Tannock IF. Drug penetration in solid tumours. Nature Reviews. Cancer. 2006;**6**(8):583-592

[73] Back-to-the-Future with Tumor Cell-Based Avatars [Online]. Available from: https://www.genengnews.com/insights/back-to-the-future-with-tumor-cell-based-avatars/ [Accessed: 08 April 2019]

[74] Dhandapani M, Goldman A. Preclinical cancer models and biomarkers for drug development: New technologies and emerging tools. Journal of Molecular Biomarkers and Diagnosis. 2017;**8**(5):pii: 356

[75] Zhang YS, Zhang YN, Zhang W. Cancer-on-a-chip systems at the frontier of nanomedicine. Drug Discovery Today. 2017;**22**(9):1392-1399

[76] Aggarwal BB, Danda D, Gupta S, Gehlot P. Models for prevention and treatment of cancer: Problems vs promises. Biochemical Pharmacology. 2009;**78**(9):1083-1094

[77] Weigelt B, Ghajar CM, Bissell MJ. The need for complex 3D culture models to unravel novel pathways and identify accurate biomarkers in breast cancer. Advanced Drug Delivery Reviews. 2014;**69-70**:42-51

[78] Birgersdotter A, Sandberg R, Ernberg I. Gene expression perturbation in vitro—A growing case for three-dimensional (3D) culture systems. Seminars in Cancer Biology. 2005;**15**(5):405-412

[79] Fedorenko IV, Smalley KSM. The complexity of microenvironment-mediated drug resistance. Genes & Cancer. 2015;**6**(9-10):367-368

[80] Gay L, Baker A-M, Graham TA. Tumour cell heterogeneity. F1000Research. 2016;**5**:pii: F1000 Faculty Rev-238

[81] Gross K, Wronski A, Skibinski A, Phillips S, Kuperwasser C. Cell fate decisions during breast cancer development. Journal of Developmental Biology. 2016;**4**(1):4

[82] Fisher R, Pusztai L, Swanton C. Cancer heterogeneity: Implications for targeted therapeutics. British Journal of Cancer. 2013;**108**(3):479-485

[83] Chen J, Li Y, Yu T-S, McKay RM, Burns D, Kernie SG, et al. A restricted cell population propagates glioblastoma growth following chemotherapy Jian. Nature. 2012;**488**(7412):522-526

[84] Jahchan NS, Lim JS, Bola B, Morris K, Seitz G, Tran KQ, et al. Identification and targeting of

long-term tumor-propagating cells in small cell lung cancer. Cell Reports. 2016;**16**(3):644-656

[85] Marx V. How to pull the blanket off dormant cancer cells. Nature Methods. 2018;**15**(4):249-252

[86] Chen L, Long C, Tran KAM, Lee J. A synthetic binder of breast cancer stem cells. Chemistry - A European Journal. 2018;**24**(15):3694-3698

[87] Ponti D, Costa A, Zaffaroni N, Pratesi G, Petrangolini G, Coradini D, et al. Isolation and In vitro propagation of tumorigenic breast cancer cells with stem/progenitor cell properties. Cancer Research. 2005;**13**:5506-5511

[88] Jamal-Hanjani M, Wilson GA, McGranahan N, Birkbak NJ, Watkins TBK, Veeriah S, et al. Tracking the evolution of non–small-cell lung cancer. The New England Journal of Medicine. 2017;**376**(22):2109-2121

[89] Hickman JA, Graeser R, de Hoogt R, Vidic S, Brito C, Gutekunst M, et al. Three-dimensional models of cancer for pharmacology and cancer cell biology: Capturing tumor complexity in vitro/ex vivo. Biotechnology Journal. 2014;**9**(9):1115-1128

[90] De Hoogt R, Estrada MF, Vidic S, Davies EJ, Osswald A, Barbier M, et al. Data descriptor: Protocols and characterization data for 2d, 3d, and slice-based tumor models from the predect project. Scientific Data. 2017;**4**:1-23

[91] Wang P, Gao Q, Suo Z, Munthe E, Solberg S, Ma L, et al. Identification and characterization of cells with cancer stem cell properties in human primary lung cancer cell lines. PLoS One. 2013;**8**(3):e57020

[92] Moro M, Bertolini G, Pastorino U, Roz L, Sozzi G. Combination treatment with all-trans retinoic acid prevents cisplatin-induced enrichment of CD133+ tumor-initiating cells and reveals heterogeneity of cancer stem cell compartment in lung cancer. Journal of Thoracic Oncology. 2015;**10**(7):1027-1036

[93] Skoda J, Hermanova M, Loja T, Nemec P, Neradil J, Karasek P, et al. Co-expression of cancer stem cell markers corresponds to a pro-tumorigenic expression profile in pancreatic adenocarcinoma. PLoS One. 2016;**11**(7):e0159255

[94] Rozenblatt-Rosen O, Stubbington MJT, Regev A, Teichmann SA. The human cell atlas: From vision to reality. Nature. 2017;**550**(7677):451-453

[95] Andriani F, Bertolini G, Facchinetti F, Baldoli E, Moro M, Casalini P, et al. Conversion to stem-cell state in response to microenvironmental cues is regulated by balance between epithelial and mesenchymal features in lung cancer cells. Molecular Oncology. 2016;**10**(2):253-271

[96] Conte N, Mason JC, Halmagyi C, Neuhauser S, Mosaku A, Yordanova G, et al. PDX Finder: A portal for patient-derived tumor xenograft model discovery. Nucleic Acids Research. 2019;**47**(D1):D1073-D1079

[97] Meehan TF, Conte N, Goldstein T, Inghirami G, Murakami MA, Brabetz S, et al. PDX-MI: Minimal information for patient-derived tumor xenograft models. Cancer Research. 2017;**77**(21):e62-e66

[98] Shultz LD, Lyons BL, Burzenski LM, Gott B, Chen X, Chaleff S, et al. Human lymphoid and myeloid cell development in NOD/LtSz-scid IL2R gamma null mice engrafted with mobilized human hemopoietic stem cells. Journal of Immunology. 2005;**174**(10):6477-6489

[99] Garrido-Laguna I, Uson M, Rajeshkumar NV, Tan AC, De Oliveira E, Karikari C, et al. Tumor engraftment in nude mice and enrichment in stroma-related gene pathways predict poor survival and resistance to gemcitabine in patients with pancreatic cancer. Clinical Cancer Research. 2011;**17**(17):5793-5800

[100] Jin K, Teng L, Shen Y, He K, Xu Z, Li G. Patient-derived human tumour tissue xenografts in immunodeficient mice: A systematic review. Clinical and Translational Oncology. 2010;**12**(7):473-480

[101] Fu X, Theodorescu D, Kerbel RS, Hoffman RM. Extensive multi-organ metastasis following orthotopic onplantation of histologically-intact human bladder carcinoma tissue in nude mice. International Journal of Cancer. 1991;**49**:938-939

[102] Morton CL, Houghton PJ. Establishment of human tumor xenografts in immunodeficient mice. Nature Protocols. 2007;**2**(2):247-250

[103] Bergamaschi A, Hjortland GO, Triulzi T, Sørlie T, Johnsen H, Ree AH, et al. Molecular profiling and characterization of luminal-like and basal-like in vivo breast cancer xenograft models. Molecular Oncology. 2009;**3**(5-6):469-482

[104] Dangles-Marie V, Pocard M, Richon S, Weiswald LB, Assayag F, Saulnier P, et al. Establishment of human colon cancer cell lines from fresh tumors versus xenografts: Comparison of success rate and cell line features. Cancer Research. 2007;**67**(1):398-407

[105] Jung J, Seol HS, Chang S. The generation and application of patient-derived xenograft model for cancer research. Cancer Research and Treatment. 2018;**50**(1):1-10

[106] Prasetyanti PR, van Hooff SR, van Herwaarden T, de Vries N, Kalloe K, Rodermond H, et al. Capturing colorectal cancer inter-tumor heterogeneity in patient-derived xenograft (PDX) models. International Journal of Cancer. 2019;**144**(2):366-371

[107] Wang Y, Wang JX, Xue H, Lin D, Dong X, Gout PW, et al. Subrenal capsule grafting technology in human cancer modeling and translational cancer research. Differentiation. 2016;**91**(4-5):15-19

[108] John T, Kohler D, Pintilie M, Yanagawa N, Pham NA, Li M, et al. The ability to form primary tumor xenografts is predictive of increased risk of disease recurrence in early-stage non-small cell lung cancer. Clinical Cancer Research. 2011;**17**(1):134-141

[109] McAuliffe PF, Evans KW, Akcakanat A, Chen K, Zheng X, Zhao H, et al. Ability to generate patient-derived breast cancer xenografts is enhanced in chemoresistant disease and predicts poor patient outcomes. PLoS One. 2015;**10**(9):e0136851

[110] Karamboulas C, Bruce JP, Hope AJ, Meens J, Huang SH, Erdmann N, et al. Patient-derived xenografts for prognostication and personalized treatment for head and neck squamous cell carcinoma. Cell Reports. 2018;**25**(5):1318-1331.e4

[111] Rosfjord E, Lucas J, Li G, Gerber HP. Advances in patient-derived tumor xenografts: From target identification to predicting clinical response rates in oncology. Biochemical Pharmacology. 2014;**91**(2):135-143

[112] Heo EJ, Cho YJ, Cho WC, Hong JE, Jeon HK, Oh DY, et al. Patient-derived xenograft models of epithelial ovarian cancer for preclinical studies. Cancer Research and Treatment. 2017;**49**(4):915-926

[113] Tentler JJ, Tan AC, Weekes CD, Jimeno A, Leong S, Pitts TM, et al. Patient-derived tumour xenografts as models for oncology drug development. Nature Reviews. Clinical Oncology. 2012;**9**(6):338-350

[114] Richmond A, Su Y. Mouse xenograft models vs GEM models for human cancer therapeutics. Disease Models & Mechanisms. 2008;**1**(2-3):78-82

[115] Hutchinson L, Kirk R. High drug attrition rates—Where are we going wrong? Nature Reviews. Clinical Oncology. 2011;**8**(4):189-190

[116] Hidalgo M, Amant F, Biankin AV, Budinská E, Byrne AT, Caldas C, et al. Patient-derived Xenograft models: An emerging platform for translational cancer research. Cancer Discovery. 2014;**4**(9):998-1013

[117] Malaney P, Nicosia SV, Davé V. One mouse, one patient paradigm: New avatars of personalized cancer therapy. Cancer Letters. 2014;**344**(1):1-12

[118] Garraway LA, Jänne PA. Circumventing cancer drug resistance in the era of personalized medicine. Cancer Discovery. 2012;**2**(3):214-226

[119] Xu C, Li X, Liu P, Li M, Luo F. Patient-derived xenograft mouse models: A high fidelity tool for individualized medicine (review). Oncology Letters. 2019;**17**(1):3-10

[120] Wang D, Pham N-A, Tong J, Sakashita S, Allo G, Kim L, et al. Molecular heterogeneity of non-small cell lung carcinoma patient-derived xenografts closely reflect their primary tumors. International Journal of Cancer. 2017;**140**(3):662-673

[121] Cutz JC, Guan J, Bayani J, Yoshimoto M, Xue H, Sutcliffe M, et al. Establishment in severe combined immunodeficiency mice of subrenal capsule xenografts and transplantable tumor lines from a variety of primary human lung cancers: Potential models for studying tumor progression-related changes. Clinical Cancer Research. 2006;**12**(13):4043-4054

[122] Lu D, Luo P, Zhang J, Ye Y, Wang Q, Li M, et al. Patient-derived tumor xenografts of lung squamous cell carcinoma alter long non-coding RNA profile but not responsiveness to cisplatin. Oncology Letters. 2018;**15**(6):8589-8603

[123] Spreafico A, Tentler JJ, Pitts TM, Tan AC, Gregory MA, Arcaroli JJ, et al. Rational combination of a MEK inhibitor, selumetinib, and the wnt/calcium pathway modulator, cyclosporin a, in preclinical models of colorectal cancer. Clinical Cancer Research. 2013;**19**(15):4149-4162

[124] Jiménez-Valerio G, Martínez-Lozano M, Bassani N, Vidal A, Ochoa-de-Olza M, Suárez C, et al. Resistance to antiangiogenic therapies by metabolic symbiosis in renal cell carcinoma PDX models and patients. Cell Reports. 2016;**15**(6):1134-1143

[125] Harris AL, Joseph RW, Copland JA. Patient-derived tumor xenograft models for melanoma drug discovery. Expert Opinion on Drug Discovery. 2016;**11**(9):895-906

[126] Zhu Y, Tian T, Li Z, Tang Z, Wang L, Wu J, et al. Establishment and characterization of patient-derived tumor xenograft using gastroscopic biopsies in gastric cancer. Scientific Reports. 2015;**5**:8542

[127] Derose YS, Wang G, Lin YC, Bernard PS, Buys SS, Ebbert MTW, et al. Tumor grafts derived from women with breast cancer authentically reflect tumor pathology, growth, metastasis and disease outcomes. Nature Medicine. 2011;**17**(11):1514-1520

[128] Izumchenko E, Paz K, Ciznadija D, Sloma I, Katz A, Vasquez-Dunddel D, et al. Patient-derived xenografts effectively capture responses to oncology therapy in a heterogeneous cohort of patients with solid tumors. Annals of Oncology. 2017;**28**(10):2595-2605

[129] Zhang X, Claerhout S, Prat A, Dobrolecki LE, Petrovic I, Lai Q, et al. A renewable tissue resource of phenotypically stable, biologically and ethnically diverse, patient-derived human breast cancer xenograft models. Cancer Research. 2013;**73**(15):4885-4897

[130] Stewart EL, Mascaux C, Pham NA, Sakashita S, Sykes J, Kim L, et al. Clinical utility of patient-derived xenografts to determine biomarkers of prognosis and map resistance pathways in EGFR-mutant lung adenocarcinoma. Journal of Clinical Oncology. 2015;**33**(22):2472-2480

[131] Bertotti A, Migliardi G, Galimi F, Sassi F, Torti D, Isella C, et al. A molecularly annotated platform of patient- derived xenografts ('xenopatients') identifies HER2 as an effective therapeutic target in cetuximab-resistant colorectal cancer. Cancer Discovery. 2011;**1**(6):508-523

[132] Gu Z, Jiang J, Yan Y, Tan T, Yu T, Liu Z, et al. Evaluation of the correlations between patient-derived xenograft (PDX) model-based mouse trials and cancer patient-based clinical trials. Journal of Clinical Oncology. 2017;**35**(15_suppl):e23140

[133] Lipner MB, Marayati R, Deng Y, Wang X, Raftery L, O'Neil BH, et al. Metformin treatment does not inhibit growth of pancreatic cancer patient-derived xenografts. PLoS One. 2016;**11**(1):e0147113

[134] Sivanand S, Peña-Llopis S, Zhao H, Kucejova B, Spence P, Pavia-Jimenez A, et al. A validated tumorgraft model reveals activity of dovitinib against renal cell carcinoma. Science Translational Medicine. 2012;**4**(137):137ra75

[135] Das Thakur M, Salangsang F, Landman AS, Sellers WR, Pryer NK, Levesque MP, et al. Modelling vemurafenib resistance in melanoma reveals a strategy to forestall drug resistance. Nature. 2013;**494**(7436):251-255

[136] Sebastiani V, Ricci F, Rubio-Viqueira B, Kulesza P, Yeo CJ, Hidalgo M, et al. Immunohistochemical and genetic evaluation of deoxycytidine kinase in pancreatic cancer: relationship to molecular mechanisms of gemcitabine resistance and survival. Clinical Cancer Research. 2006;**12**(8):2492-2497

[137] Clohessy JG, Pandolfi PP. Mouse hospital and co-clinical trial project-from bench to bedside. Nature Reviews. Clinical Oncology. 2015;**12**(8):491-498

[138] Vargas R, Gopal P, Kuzmishin GB, DeBernardo R, Koyfman SA, Jha BK, et al. Case study: Patient-derived clear cell adenocarcinoma xenograft model longitudinally predicts treatment response. npj Precision Oncology. 2018;**2**:14

[139] Kim HR, Kang HN, Shim HS, Kim EY, Kim J, Kim DJ, et al. Co-clinical trials demonstrate predictive biomarkers for dovitinib, an FGFR inhibitor, in lung squamous cell carcinoma. Annals of Oncology. 2017;**28**(6):1250-1259

[140] Stebbing J, Paz K, Schwartz GK, Wexler LH, Maki R, Pollock RE, et al. Patient-derived xenografts for individualized care in advanced sarcoma. Cancer. 2014;**120**(13):2006-2015

[141] Owonikoko TK, Zhang G, Kim HS, Stinson RM, Bechara R, Zhang C, et al. Patient-derived xenografts faithfully replicated clinical outcome in a phase

II co-clinical trial of arsenic trioxide in relapsed small cell lung cancer. Journal of Translational Medicine. 2016;**14**(1):111

[142] Choi Y, Lee S, Kim K, Kim SH, Chung YJ, Lee C. Studying cancer immunotherapy using patient-derived xenografts (PDXs) in humanized mice. Experimental and Molecular Medicine. 2018;**50**(8):99

[143] Russell PJ, Russell P, Rudduck C, Tse BWC, Williams ED, Raghavan D. Establishing prostate cancer patient derived xenografts: Lessons learned from older studies. Prostate. 2015;**75**(6):628-636

[144] Némati F, Sastre-Garau X, Laurent C, Couturier J, Mariani P, Desjardins L, et al. Establishment and characterization of a panel of human uveal melanoma xenografts derived from primary and/or metastatic tumors. Clinical Cancer Research. 2010;**16**(8):2352-2362

[145] Gambar G, Gaeble M, Keilhol U, Regenbrecht CRA, Silvestri A. From chemotherapy to combined targeted therapeutics: In vitro and in vivo models to decipher intra-tumor heterogeneity. Frontiers in Pharmacology. 2018;**9**(FEB):1-18

[146] Zitvogel L, Apetoh L, Ghiringhelli F, Kroemer G. Immunological aspects of cancer chemotherapy. Nature Reviews. Immunology. 2008;**8**(1):59-73

[147] Shultz LD, Brehm MA, Garcia-Martinez JV, Greiner DL. Humanized mice for immune system investigation: Progress, promise and challenges. Nature Reviews. Immunology. 2012;**12**(11):786-798

[148] Wiekmeijer A-S, Pike-Overzet K, Brugman MH, Salvatori DCF, Egeler RM, Bredius RGM, et al. Sustained engraftment of cryopreserved human bone marrow CD34 + cells in young adult NSG mice. BioResearch Open Access. 2014;**3**:110-116

[149] Morton JJ, Bird G, Keysar SB, Astling DP, Lyons TR, Anderson RT, et al. XactMice: Humanizing mouse bone marrow enables microenvironment reconstitution in a patient-derived xenograft model of head and neck cancer. Oncogene. 2016;**35**(3):290-300

[150] Eirew P, Steif A, Khattra J, Ha G, Yap D, Farahani H, et al. Dynamics of genomic clones in breast cancer patient xenografts at single-cell resolution. Nature. 2015;**518**(7539):422-426

[151] Ben-David U, Ha G, Tseng YY, Greenwald NF, Oh C, Shih J, et al. Patient-derived xenografts undergo mouse-specific tumor evolution. Nature Genetics. 2017;**49**(11):1567-1575

[152] Gillet J-P, Calcagno AM, Varma S, Marino M, Green LJ, Vora MI, et al. Redefining the relevance of established cancer cell lines to the study of mechanisms of clinical anti-cancer drug resistance. Proceedings of the National Academy of Sciences. 2011;**108**(46):18708-18713

[153] Ertel A, Verghese A, Byers SW, Ochs M, Tozeren A. Pathway-specific differences between tumor cell lines and normal and tumor tissue cells. Molecular Cancer. 2006;**5**(1):55

[154] Guerra C, Barbacid M. Genetically engineered mouse models of pancreatic adenocarcinoma. Molecular Oncology. 2013;**7**(2):232-247

[155] Svirshchevskaya E, Doronina E, Grechikhina M, Matushevskaya E, Kotsareva O, Fattakhova G, et al. Characteristics of multicellular tumor spheroids formed by pancreatic cells expressing different adhesion molecules. Life Sciences. 2019;**219**:343-352

[156] Halfter K, Hoffmann O, Ditsch N, Ahne M, Arnold F, Paepke S, et al. Testing chemotherapy efficacy in HER2 negative breast cancer using patient-derived spheroids. Journal of Translational Medicine. 2016;**14**(1):112

[157] Hongisto V, Jernström S, Fey V, Mpindi JP, Kleivi Sahlberg K, Kallioniemi O, et al. High-throughput 3D screening reveals differences in drug sensitivities between culture models of JIMT1 breast cancer cells. PLoS One. 2013;**8**(10):e77232

[158] Ekert JE, Johnson K, Strake B, Pardinas J, Jarantow S, Perkinson R, et al. Three-dimensional lung tumor microenvironment modulates therapeutic compound responsiveness in vitro—Implication for drug development. PLoS One. 2014;**9**(3):e92248

[159] Horvath P, Aulner N, Bickle M, Davies AM, Del Nery E, Ebner D, et al. Screening out irrelevant cell-based models of disease. Nature Reviews. Drug Discovery. 2016;**15**(11):751-769

[160] Torsvik A, Stieber D, Enger PØ, Golebiewska A, Molven A, Svendsen A, et al. U-251 revisited: Genetic drift and phenotypic consequences of long-term cultures of glioblastoma cells. Cancer Medicine. 2014;**3**(4):812-824

[161] Hughes P, Marshall D, Reid Y, Parkes H, Gelber C. The costs of using unauthenticated, over-passaged cell lines: How much more data do we need? BioTechniques. 2007;**43**(5):575, 577-578, 581-582

[162] Freedman LP, Gibson MC, Ethier SP, Soule HR, Neve RM, Reid YA. Reproducibility: Changing the policies and culture of cell line authentication. Nature Methods. 2015;**12**(6):493-497

[163] Allen M, Bjerke M, Edlund H, Nelander S, Westermark B. Origin of the U87MG glioma cell line: Good news and bad news. Science Translational Medicine. 2016;**8**(354):354re3

[164] Drexler HG, Dirks WG, Matsuo Y, MacLeod RAF. False leukemia-lymphoma cell lines: An update on over 500 cell lines. Leukemia. 2003;**17**(2):416-426

[165] Barretina J, Caponigro G, Stransky N, Venkatesan K, Margolin AA, Kim S, et al. The cancer cell line encyclopedia enables predictive modelling of anticancer drug sensitivity. Nature. 2012;**483**(7391):603-607

[166] Wagner BK, Schreiber SL. The power of sophisticated phenotypic screening and modern mechanism-of-action methods. Cell Chemical Biology. 2016;**23**(1):3-9

[167] Schirle M, Jenkins JL. Identifying compound efficacy targets in phenotypic drug discovery. Drug Discovery Today. 2016;**21**(1):82-89

[168] Abaan OD, Polley EC, Davis SR, Zhu YJ, Bilke S, Walker RL, et al. The exomes of the NCI-60 panel: A genomic resource for cancer biology and systems pharmacology. Cancer Research. 2013;**73**(14):4372-4382

[169] Xie Y, Bergström T, Jiang Y, Johansson P, Marinescu VD, Lindberg N, et al. The human glioblastoma cell culture resource: Validated cell models representing all molecular subtypes. eBioMedicine. 2015;**2**(10):1351-1363

[170] Beaufort CM, Helmijr JCA, Piskorz AM, Hoogstraat M, Ruigrok-Ritstier K, Besselink N, et al. Ovarian cancer cell line panel (OCCP): Clinical importance of in vitro morphological subtypes. PLoS One. 2014;**9**(9):e103988

[171] Ghandi M, Huang FW, Jané-Valbuena J, Kryukov GV, Lo CC,

McDonald ER, et al. Next-generation characterization of the cancer cell line encyclopedia. Nature. 2019;**569**(7757):503-508

[172] Niu N, Wang L. In vitro human cell line models to predict clinical response to anticancer drugs. Pharmacogenomics. 2015;**16**(3):273-285

[173] Zou X, Owusu M, Harris R, Jackson SP, Loizou JI, Nik-Zainal S. Validating the concept of mutational signatures with isogenic cell models. Nature Communications. 2018;**9**(1):1744

[174] ECACC: A Dynamic Culture Collection for Disease Research [Online]. Available from: https://www.phe-culturecollections.org.uk/news/ecacc-news/ecacc-a-dynamic-culture-collection-for-disease-research.aspx [Accessed: 20 May 2019]

[175] Seo J, Park SJ, Kim J, Choi SJ, Moon SH, Chung HM. Effective method for the isolation and proliferation of primary lung cancer cells from patient lung tissues. Biotechnology Letters. 2013;**35**(8):1165-1174

[176] Kodack DP, Farago AF, Dastur A, Held MA, Dardaei L, Friboulet L, et al. Primary patient-derived cancer cells and their potential for personalized cancer patient care. Cell Reports. 2017;**21**(11):3298-3309

[177] Meijer TG, Naipal KA, Jager A, van Gent DC. Ex vivo tumor culture systems for functional drug testing and therapy response prediction. Future Science OA. 2017;**3**(2):FSO190

[178] Hynds RE, Ben Aissa A, Gowers KHC, Watkins TBK, Bosshard-Carter L, Rowan AJ, et al. Expansion of airway basal epithelial cells from primary human non-small cell lung cancer tumors. International Journal of Cancer. 2018;**143**(1):160-166

[179] Goodspeed A, Heiser LM, Gray JW, Costello JC. Tumor-derived cell lines as molecular models of cancer pharmacogenomics. Molecular Cancer Research. 2015;**14**(1):3-13

[180] Nestor CE, Ottaviano R, Reinhardt D, Cruickshanks HA, Mjoseng HK, McPherson RC, et al. Rapid reprogramming of epigenetic and transcriptional profiles in mammalian culture systems. Genome Biology. 2015;**16**:11

[181] Liu X, Krawczyk E, Suprynowicz FA, Palechor-Ceron N, Yuan H, Dakic A, et al. Conditional reprogramming and long-term expansion of normal and tumor cells from human biospecimens. Nature Protocols. 2017;**12**(2):439-451

[182] Grillet F, Bayet E, Villeronce O, Zappia L, Lagerqvist EL, Lunke S, et al. Circulating tumour cells from patients with colorectal cancer have cancer stem cell hallmarks in ex vivo culture. Gut. 2017;**66**(10):1802-1810

[183] De Angelis ML, Zeuner A, Policicchio E, Russo G, Bruselles A, Signore M, et al. Cancer stem cell-based models of colorectal cancer reveal molecular determinants of therapy resistance. Stem Cells Translational Medicine. 2016;**5**(4):511-523

[184] Jiang G, Zhang S, Yazdanparast A, Li M, Pawar AV, Liu Y, et al. Comprehensive comparison of molecular portraits between cell lines and tumors in breast cancer. BMC Genomics. 2016;**17**(Suppl 7):525

[185] Kloudová K, Hromádková H, Partlová S, Brtnický T, Rob L, Bartůňková J, et al. Expression of tumor antigens on primary ovarian cancer cells compared to established ovarian cancer cell lines. Oncotarget. 2016;**7**(29):46120-46126

[186] Telang N. Putative cancer-initiating stem cells in cell culture

models for molecular subtypes of clinical breast cancer. Oncology Letters. 2015;**10**(6):3840-3846

[187] Chang KK, Yoon C, Yi BC, Tap WD, Simon MC, Yoon SS. Platelet-derived growth factor receptor-α and -β promote cancer stem cell phenotypes in sarcomas. Oncogene. 2018;**7**(6):47

[188] Sirenko O, Mitlo T, Hesley J, Luke S, Owens W, Cromwell EF. High-content assays for characterizing the viability and morphology of 3D cancer spheroid cultures. Assay and Drug Development Technologies. 2015;**13**(7):402-414

[189] Sokolova EA, Vodeneev VA, Deyev SM, Balalaeva IV. 3D in vitro models of tumors expressing EGFR family receptors: A potent tool for studying receptor biology and targeted drug development. Drug Discovery Today. 2019;**24**(1):99-111

[190] Gagliano N, Sforza C, Sommariva M, Menon A, Conte V, Sartori P, et al. 3D-spheroids: What can they tell us about pancreatic ductal adenocarcinoma cell phenotype? Experimental Cell Research. 2017;**357**(2):299-309

[191] Proctor WR, Foster AJ, Vogt J, Summers C, Middleton B, Pilling MA, et al. Utility of spherical human liver microtissues for prediction of clinical drug-induced liver injury. Archives of Toxicology. 2017;**91**(8):2849-2863

[192] Griner LAM, Zhang X, Guha R, Mcknight C, Goldlust IS, Lal-nag M, et al. Large-scale pharmacological profiling of 3D tumor models of cancer cells. Cell Death & Disease. 2016;**7**(12):e2492

[193] Shologu N, Szegezdi E, Lowery A, Kerin M, Pandit A, Zeugolis DI. Recreating complex pathophysiologies in vitro with extracellular matrix surrogates for anticancer therapeutics screening. Drug Discovery Today. 2016;**21**(9):1521-1531

[194] Lv D, hua Ma Q, jie Duan J, bo Wu H, long Zhao X, cang Yu S, et al. Optimized dissociation protocol for isolating human glioma stem cells from tumorspheres via fluorescence-activated cell sorting. Cancer Letters. 2016;**377**(1):105-115

[195] Sender R, Fuchs S, Milo R. Revised estimates for the number of human and bacteria cells in the body. PLoS Biology. 2016;**14**(8):e1002533

[196] Gorshkov K, Chen CZ, Marshall RE, Mihatov N, Choi Y, Nguyen DT, et al. Advancing precision medicine with personalized drug screening. Drug Discovery Today. 2019;**24**(1):272-278

[197] Kelm JM, Lal-Nag M, Sittampalam GS, Ferrer M. Translational in vitro research: Integrating 3D drug discovery and development processes into the drug development pipeline. Drug Discovery Today. 2019;**24**(1):26-30

[198] Kalvelytė AV, Imbrasaitė A, Krestnikova N, Stulpinas A. Adult stem cells and anticancer therapy. In: Fishbein J, Heilman J, editors. Advances in Molecular Toxicology. Vol. 11. Academic Press; 2017. pp. 123-202

[199] Dutta D, Heo I, Clevers H. Disease modeling in stem cell-derived 3D organoid systems. Trends in Molecular Medicine. 2017;**23**(5):393-410

[200] Mebarki M, Bennaceur A, Bonhomme-faivre L. Human-cell-derived organoids as a new ex vivo model for drug assays in oncology. Drug Discovery Today. 2018;**23**(4):857-863

[201] Tapias LF, Gilpin SE, Ren X, Wei L, Fuchs BC, Tanabe KK, et al. Assessment of proliferation and cytotoxicity in a biomimetic three-dimensional model

of lung cancer. The Annals of Thoracic Surgery. 2015;**100**(2):414-421

[202] Lovitt C, Shelper T, Avery V. Advanced cell culture techniques for cancer drug discovery. Biology (Basel). 2014;**3**(2):345-367

[203] Wang C, Tang Z, Zhao Y, Yao R, Li L, Sun W. Three-dimensional in vitro cancer models: A short review. Biofabrication. Apr. 2014;**6**(2):022001

[204] Sant S, Johnston PA. The production of 3D tumor spheroids for cancer drug discovery. Drug Discovery Today: Technologies. 2017;**23**:27-36

[205] Sun F, Hu Y, Xiong L, Tu X, Zhao J, Chen S, et al. Enhanced expression of stem cell markers and drug resistance in sphere-forming non-small cell lung cancer cells. International Journal of Clinical and Experimental Pathology. 2015;**8**(6):6287-6300

[206] Praharaj PP, Bhutia SK, Nagrath S, Bitting RL, Deep G. Circulating tumor cell-derived organoids: Current challenges and promises in medical research and precision medicine. Biochimica et Biophysica Acta, Reviews on Cancer. 2018;**1869**(2):117-127

[207] Heger JI, Froehlich K, Pastuschek J, Schmidt A, Baer C, Mrowka R, et al. Human serum alters cell culture behavior and improves spheroid formation in comparison to fetal bovine serum. Experimental Cell Research. 2018;**365**(1):57-65

[208] Jung HR, Kang HM, Ryu JW, Kim DS, Noh KH, Kim ES, et al. Cell spheroids with enhanced aggressiveness to mimic human liver cancer in vitro and in vivo. Scientific Reports. 2017;**7**(1):10499

[209] Gong X, Lin C, Cheng J, Su J, Zhao H, Liu T, et al. Generation of multicellular tumor spheroids with microwell-based agarose scaffolds for drug testing. PLoS One. 2015;**10**(6):e0130348

[210] Lee S, Hwa J, Ki H, Seok J, Kim B, Lee J, et al. Colorectal cancer-derived tumor spheroids retain the characteristics of original tumors. Cancer Letters. 2015;**367**(1):34-42

[211] Baker LA, Tiriac H, Clevers H, Tuveson DA. Modeling pancreatic cancer with organoids. Trends in Cancer. 2016;**2**(4):176-190

[212] Jin M, Han R, Qiu G, Ju X, Lou G, Jin W. Organoids: An intermediate modeling platform in precision oncology. Cancer Letters. 2018;**414**:174-180

[213] Xu H, Lyu X, Yi M, Zhao W, Song Y, Wu K. Organoid technology and applications in cancer research. Journal of Hematology & Oncology. 2018;**11**(1):116

[214] Amann A, Zwierzina M, Gamerith G, Bitsche M, Huber JM, Vogel GF, et al. Development of an innovative 3D cell culture system to study tumour–Stroma interactions in non-small cell lung cancer cells. PLoS One. 2014;**9**(3):e92511

[215] Perche F, Torchilin VP. Cancer cell spheroids as a model to evaluate chemotherapy protocols. Cancer Biology & Therapy. 2012;**13**(12):1205-1213

[216] Ocana A, Pandiella A, Siu LL, Tannock IF. Preclinical development of molecular-targeted agents for cancer. Nature Reviews. Clinical Oncology. 2011;**8**(4):200-209

[217] Pampaloni F, Reynaud EG, Stelzer EHK. The third dimension bridges the gap between cell culture and live tissue. Nature Reviews. Molecular Cell Biology. 2007;**8**(10):839-845

[218] Ryan S-L, Baird A-M, Vaz G, Urquhart AJ, Senge M, Richard DJ, et al.

Drug discovery approaches utilizing three-dimensional cell culture. Assay and Drug Development Technologies. 2016;**14**(1):19-28

[219] Shin CS, Kwak B, Han B, Park K. Development of an in vitro 3D tumor model to study therapeutic efficiency of an anticancer drug. Molecular Pharmaceutics. 2013;**10**(6):2167-2175

[220] Fischbach C, Chen R, Matsumoto T, Schmelzle T, Brugge JS, Polverini PJ, et al. Engineering tumors with 3D scaffolds. Nature Methods. 2007;**4**(10):855-860

[221] Truong D, Fiorelli R, Barrientos ES, Luna E, Sanai N, Mehta S, et al. A three-dimensional (3D) organotypic micro fl uidic model for glioma stem cells–vascular interactions. Biomaterials. 2019;**198**:63-77

[222] Beaumont K, Mohana-Kumaran N, Haass N. Modeling melanoma in vitro and in vivo. Healthcare (Basel). 2013;**2**(1):27-46

[223] Braham MVJ, Minnema MC, Aarts T, Sebestyen Z, Straetemans T, Vyborova A, et al. Cellular immunotherapy on primary multiple myeloma expanded in a 3D bone marrow niche model. OncoImmunology. 2018;**7**(6):e1434465

[224] Naolou T, Chatterjee C, Raic A, Lee-Thedieck C, Mohra A. 3D models of the bone marrow in health and disease: Yesterday, today, and tomorrow. MRS Communications. 2018;**9**(1):37-52

[225] Majumder B, Baraneedharan U, Thiyagarajan S, Radhakrishnan P, Narasimhan H, Dhandapani M, et al. Predicting clinical response to anticancer drugs using an ex vivo platform that captures tumour heterogeneity. Nature Communications. 2015;**6**:1-14

[226] Li L, Knutsdottir H, Hui K, Weiss MJ, He J, Philosophe B, et al. Human primary liver cancer organoids reveal intratumor and interpatient drug response heterogeneity. JCI Insight. 2019;**4**(2):pii: 121490

[227] The Cancer Genome Atlas Program - National Cancer Institute [Online]. Available from: https://www.cancer.gov/about-nci/organization/ccg/research/structural-genomics/tcga [Accessed: 20 May 2019]

[228] Single Cell ICP-MS for Cancer Research | Chemotherapy Resistance | PerkinElmer [Online]. Available from: https://www.perkinelmer.com/category/single-cell-icp-ms-for-cancer-research [Accessed: 31 May 2019]

[229] Yamauchi KA, Herr AE. Subcellular western blotting of single cells. Microsystems & Nanoengineering. 2017;**3**:16079

[230] George AA, Paz H, Fei F, Kirzner J, Kim YM, Heisterkamp N, et al. Phosphoflow-based evaluation of Mek inhibitors as small-molecule therapeutics for B-cell precursor acute lymphoblastic leukemia. PLoS One. 2015;**10**(9):e0137917

[231] Stevens MM, Maire CL, Chou N, Murakami MA, Knoff DS, Kikuchi Y, et al. Drug sensitivity of single cancer cells is predicted by changes in mass accumulation rate. Nature Biotechnology. 2016;**34**(11):1161-1167

[232] Levitin HM, Yuan J, Sims PA. Single-cell transcriptomic analysis of tumor heterogeneity. Trends in Cancer. 2018;**4**(4):264-268

[233] Aljitawi OS, Li D, Xiao Y, Zhang D, Ramachandran K, Stehno-Bittel L, et al. A novel three-dimensional stromal-based model for in vitro chemotherapy sensitivity testing of leukemia cells. Leukemia & Lymphoma. 2014;**55**(2):378-391

[234] Hodgkinson CL, Morrow CJ, Li Y, Metcalf RL, Rothwell DG, Trapani F,

et al. Tumorigenicity and genetic profiling of circulating tumor cells in small-cell lung cancer. Nature Medicine. 2014;**20**(8):897-903

[235] Politaki E, Agelaki S, Apostolaki S, Hatzidaki D, Strati A, Koinis F, et al. A comparison of three methods for the detection of circulating tumor cells in patients with early and metastatic breast cancer. Cellular Physiology and Biochemistry. 2017;**44**(2):594-606

[236] Maheswaran S, Haber DA. Ex vivo culture of CTCs: An emerging resource to guide cancer therapy. Cancer Research. 2015;**75**(12):2411-2415

[237] Chan LLY, Smith T, Kumph KA, Kuksin D, Kessel S, Déry O, et al. A high-throughput AO/PI-based cell concentration and viability detection method using the Celigo image cytometry. Cytotechnology. 2016;**68**(5):2015-2025

[238] Vinegoni C, Dubach JM, Thurber GM, Miller MA, Mazitschek R, Weissleder R. Advances in measuring single-cell pharmacology in vivo. Drug Discovery Today. 2015;**20**(9):1087-1092

[239] Zervantonakis IK, Arvanitis CD. Controlled drug release and chemotherapy response in a novel acoustofluidic 3D tumor platform. Small. 2016;**12**(19):2616-2626

[240] Williams JK, Entenberg D, Wang Y, Avivar-Valderas A, Padgen M, Clark A, et al. Validation of a device for the active manipulation of the tumor microenvironment during intravital imaging. IntraVital. 2016;**5**(2):e1182271

[241] Murakami MA, Weinstock DM. Cancer models: The next best thing. Nature. 2017;**549**(7670):39-41

[242] Lin G, Keshari KR, Park JM. Cancer metabolism and tumor heterogeneity: Imaging perspectives using MR imaging and spectroscopy. Contrast Media & Molecular Imaging. 2017;**2017**:6053879

[243] Nguyen HT, Mortazavi A, Pohar KS, Zynger DL, Wei L, Shah ZK, et al. Quantitative assessment of heterogeneity in bladder tumor MRI diffusivity: Can response be predicted prior to neoadjuvant chemotherapy? Bladder Cancer. 2017;**3**(4):237-244

[244] Pantel AR, Mankoff DA. Molecular imaging to guide systemic cancer therapy: Illustrative examples of PET imaging cancer biomarkers. Cancer Letters. 2017;**387**:25-31

[245] Menshykau D. Emerging technologies for prediction of drug candidate efficacy in the preclinical pipeline. Drug Discovery Today. 2017;**22**(11):1598-1603

[246] 3D Cell Culture Draws Drug Developers' Interest [Online]. Available from: https://www.genengnews.com/magazine/3d-cell-culture-draws-drug-developers-interest/ [Accessed: 23 May 2019]

[247] Bhadriraju K, Halter M, Amelot J, Bajcsy P, Chalfoun J, Vandecreme A, et al. Large-scale time-lapse microscopy of Oct4 expression in human embryonic stem cell colonies. Stem Cell Research. 2016;**17**(1):122-129

[248] Tamura M, Sugiura S, Takagi T, Satoh T, Sumaru K, Kanamori T, et al. Morphology-based optical separation of subpopulations from a heterogeneous murine breast cancer cell line. PLoS One. 2017;**12**(6):1-13

[249] Hillger JM, Lieuw WL, Heitman LH, IJzerman AP. Label-free technology and patient cells: From early drug development to precision medicine. Drug Discovery Today. 2017;**22**(12):1808-1815

[250] Leonavicius K, Nainys J, Kuciauskas D, Mazutis L. Multi-omics

at single-cell resolution: Comparison of experimental and data fusion approaches. Current Opinion in Biotechnology. 2019;**55**:159-166

[251] Lee JW, Sung JS, Park YS, Chung S, Kim YH. Isolation of spheroid-forming single cells from gastric cancer cell lines: Enrichment of cancer stem-like cells. BioTechniques. 2018;**65**(4):197-203

[252] Chen Y, Gao D, Liu H, Lin S, Jiang Y. Drug cytotoxicity and signaling pathway analysis with three-dimensional tumor spheroids in a microwell-based microfluidic chip for drug screening. Analytica Chimica Acta. 2015;**898**:85-92

[253] Carragher N, Piccinini F, Tesei A, Trask OJ Jr, Bickle M, Horvath P. Concerns, challenges and promises of high-content analysis of 3D cellular models. Nature Reviews Drug Discovery. 2018;**17**(8):606

Chapter 8

The Principles behind Targeted Therapy for Cancer Treatment

Wabel AL-Busairi and Maitham Khajah

Abstract

The advent of molecular and genetic advancement in the field of oncology research has led to a shift in the treatment of various forms of cancer from traditional chemotherapeutics to targeted therapy. The principle behind targeted therapy is utilizing therapeutics designed to interfere with specific molecules that have a relatively specific or higher expression profile in cancer cells and are critical for cancer growth and progression. These were designed as mechanistic therapeutics in the form of small molecules and monoclonal antibodies. Currently, they have been modified to incorporate passive or active targeting delivery systems to improve their specific distribution and enhance cytotoxicity towards cancer cells while simultaneously reducing their systemic toxicity profile. Passive targeting employs encapsulated delivery systems to take advantage of the enhanced permeation and retention effect of the tumor microenvironment, while active targeting relies on receptor mediated interactions, such as cell surface ligands conjugated to the therapeutic moiety. A synergistic strategy for cancer therapy is evolving, where precision medicine acts as a diagnostic prerequisite for targeted therapy via prognostic biomarkers and tumor genotyping. Despite the plethora of research undertaken in targeted therapy, limited numbers were approved for clinical use, and significant challenges remain to be addressed.

Keywords: targeted therapy, cancer, chemotherapy, resistance, toxicity

1. Introduction

Various forms of cancers remain to be the leading cause of mortality worldwide. A recent article estimated the incidence and mortality of cancer in 20 world regions (using the GLOBOCAN 2018 estimates), and suggested approximately 18 million new cases and 9.6 million deaths in the year of 2018. Lung cancer was most commonly diagnosed, and the leading cause of cancer-related death followed by breast, prostate, colorectal, stomach, and liver cancer [1]. Although surgery and radiation therapy are considered the primary treatment for localized forms of cancers, chemotherapeutic agents must be used when cancer cells metastasize to the regional lymphatic vessels and bloodstream. This placed more emphasis on the development of drugs and biological molecules as chemotherapeutic agents to minimize the risk of cancer metastasis to other organs, which will lead to organ failure and death [2, 3].

2. Traditional chemotherapeutic agents

The era of cancer drug development was pioneered in the 1940s after using nitrogen mustard as a toxic treatment for cancer [2]. Traditional chemotherapeutic agents

IntechOpen

mediate cytotoxicity by interrupting processes or inhibiting molecules required for rapid cellular division and DNA synthesis at the cell cycle level. They are categorized as either cell cycle specific (they target a specific phase in the cell cycle) or cell cycle non-specific (they target all cell cycle phases) agents [4]. Their main disadvantage relies on their relative non-selectivity in targeting rapidly dividing non-cancerous cells such as hair follicles, bone marrow and gastrointestinal epithelial cells. This commonly manifests as serious adverse effects on patients such as hair loss, anemia, infections (due to low white blood cell count), infertility, nausea and vomiting. As a result, the effective therapeutic dose is unattained and the efficacy of conventional chemotherapeutic agents is compromised. This is commonly experienced in the clinic, when a chemotherapy regimen is administered for a delimited period, but the dose has to be reduced or treatment is postponed as a safety precaution despite tumor responsiveness [5, 6]. Furthermore, many conventional chemotherapeutics do not accumulate in the tumor mass at effective therapeutic concentrations, thereby cannot effectively inhibit their proliferation and metastasis. This is particularly true at the core micro-regions of tumors; due to the disorganized intratumoral vasculature and high interstitial fluid pressure as a consequence of aberrant angiogenesis and poor lymphatic drainage. Some types of cancers such as brain gliomas, are also difficult to reach with traditional chemotherapeutics, as they are unable to penetrate the blood brain barrier. These factors play a paramount role in drug resistance [7]. Chemotherapeutic agents with inadequate bioavailability and pharmacokinetic profiles are more inclined to metabolism and excretion before reaching cancerous cells [8]. Cancerous cells not killed during treatment are likely to acquire resistance and eventually lead to a more aggressive form of tumors with high probability of organ damage and death [4]. In addition, various oncogenes and oncoproteins in a variety of cancers are able to inactivate chemotherapeutic agents and/or eliminate them from tumor cells (e.g., through the activity of multi-drug resistance; MDR) [7, 8].

Mechanisms that mediate resistance have been studied abundantly, and many are attributed to mutations of various oncogenes. They include altered transport of chemotherapeutics across the plasma membrane by ATP-dependent multidrug transporters or upregulation of multidrug resistant gene, which encodes P-glycoprotein responsible for xenobiotic efflux out of cells [7]. Another example are defects in the apoptotic pathways leading to a loss of function in the tumor suppressor gene p53, allowing cells with damaged DNA to continue replicating and hence be unresponsive to DNA damaging effects of chemotherapeutics such as pyrimidine antagonist 5-fluorouracil and the mitotic spindle inhibitor paclitaxel [7, 8]. Enhanced action of DNA repair proteins in cancer cells also contributes to acquired forms of chemoresistance. This phenomenon has been observed with chemotherapeutics causing direct damage to the structural integrity of DNA such as intercalating agents like cisplatin and alkylating agents [7, 8]. While chemotherapeutics that mediate their action by binding to the topoisomerase-DNA complex to prevent DNA synthesis, such as doxorubicin, etoposide and camptothecin are rendered inactive by the altered activity of topoisomerase I and II, hence resistance facilitates the repair of topoisomerase-DNA complex [7, 8].

The design and development of conventional chemotherapeutics is prehistoric relative to recent findings in the complex cancer pathophysiology and tumor microenvironment. Recently, the heterogeneity of tumors is widely established as a challenge for traditional forms of cancer therapy. It is recognized to result from the higher genetic instability of uncontrolled cell division; increasing the likelihood of multiple mutations and replications errors. Ultimately it manifests as phenotypic and functional tumor heterogeneity that can occur within and between tumors [9]. Dynamic and regional variations in the tumor microenvironment in blood, lymphatic vasculature, extracellular matrix metalloproteases and cellular secretions in the tumor stroma may greatly influence the diverse development of cancer cells. Furthermore, a distinct population of cells within tumors termed cancer stem cells with a capacity for self-renewal and differentiation are recognized to be responsible for cancer relapse, also contributing to this factor [9]. The heterogeneity of tumors has proved to be a limitation to treatment with traditional chemotherapeutics and restricts their use for a variety of cancer types, it also supports intrinsic resistance to cancer therapy. In order to combat these limitations which ultimately lead to cancer progression and reduces the survival rates of patients, more selective/targeted/efficient therapies are required. This lead to the discovery of new agents which are based on the investigation of molecular behavior, biomarkers, oncogenes and biological pathways used by cancer cells to determine specific key distinctions between them and normal cells, that are responsible for tumor cell proliferation, survival and progression. Once identified these distinctions are targeted "with precision" while sparing normal cells. This concept has been renowned the "magic bullet" of cancer therapy and is the fundamental principle behind targeted cancer therapy [10].

The advent of targeted cancer therapy was established by the development of molecular targeted therapeutics, also recognized as mechanistic or direct-targeted cancer therapy [11]. This strategy utilizes small molecules or monoclonal antibodies (MAb) designed to interfere with specific molecular targets that have a relatively specific or higher expression profile in cancer cells and are critical for their growth and metastasis [11, 12]. Small molecule targeted therapies are usually low molecular weight organic compounds (<800 Daltons), that have a higher rate of cell entry relative to MAb, and so are designed to interfere with the expression/activity of intracellular signaling molecules [4]. On the other hand, MAbs generally have high binding affinities to extracellular domains expressed on cancer cells and are commonly designed to target the extracellular surface of cancerous cells; they mediate their mode of action through receptor ligand interactions [4].

3. Types of targeted therapies

Various types of molecular target mechanisms have been identified for cancer therapy; these include signal transduction inhibitors, hormone therapies, gene expression modulators, apoptosis inducers, angiogenesis inhibitors, immunotherapies and toxin delivery molecules. Many of these mechanisms overlap and with the advancement in cancer research a single anticancer therapeutic agent can encompass multiple molecular mechanisms. This is further elaborated in the subsequent paragraphs of this chapter.

3.1 Signal transduction inhibitors

Signal transduction is considered the link between a ligand mediated activation of a receptor to the resultant cellular responses such as metabolism, gene expression, cell division and apoptosis, and motility/migration, etc. [13]. Hence it is a vital route to explore for molecular-targeted therapies. Many remarkably successful agents have been developed under this category, owning to the understanding of signal transduction pathways in cancer cells. Genetic and epigenetic changes that occur in cancer cells lead to uncontrolled cellular functions (such as proliferation) in part through aberrant/modulated activity of various signaling and metabolic networks [13]. While normal cells have redundant overlapping pathways that allow for alternative signal transduction when one is inhibited, cancer cells have placed more emphasis on distinct signaling pathways owning to various mutations [13]. As a result, they have a diminished signaling network with "hyper-active" pathways to sustain cell proliferation and survival [13]. These "hyper-active" pathways are reflected in the overexpression of certain proteins in cancer cells. Together, these characteristics make cancerous cells more sensitive to stress and mutagens [13]. This forms the basis of signal transduction targeted molecular therapy. Therefore, theoretically depriving cancer cells from essential signaling elements needed for survival will lead to apoptosis and growth arrest [13]. Furthermore, some cancer cells are "addicted" to specific signaling proteins, as they are dependent on their activity for survival; a prime example is in chronic myeloid leukemia (CML) cancer. CML cells particularly in the early stage of cancer have absolute dependency on the kinase activity of Bcr-Abl fusion protein [13]. Bcr-Abl fusion protein results from an abnormal translocation in the Philadelphia chromosome (Ph) in 95% of CML patients. Fusion of Bcr and Abl genes leads to constitutive activation of Bcr-Abl tyrosine kinase, causing CML cells to grow and divide excessively [13]. Protein kinases are enzymes that regulate the biological activity of proteins by phosphorylation of specific amino acids with adenosine triphosphate (ATP) to induce conformational changes from the inactive to the active form [14]. Protein Kinases have been implicated in cell proliferation and many have transforming capacity making them oncoproteins [14]. Consequently, protein kinases have been extensively studied as a signal transduction inhibitor pathway in targeted drug therapy [13–15].

One of the most successful molecular targets of anticancer agents is the protein tyrosine kinase inhibitor imatinib (Gleevec®), for the treatment of Ph positive CML [4, 9, 10, 12–15]. Its success is based on the extreme "addiction" of CML cells to Bcr-Abl fusion pathway. Imatinib is designed as an ATP mimic which acts by blocking tyrosine phosphorylation, it competitively binds to the ATP binding site on Bcr-Abl fusion protein to disrupt tyrosine kinase activity [14]. It is reported to have up to 80% response rate in Ph positive CML patients [14]. This protein kinase inhibitor is also indicated for a subset of patients with gastrointestinal stromal (GIST) tumors, which have activated point mutations in the c-Kit proto-oncogene or platelet derived growth factor receptor (PDGFR)-α kinase [4, 12, 13]. Constitutive activation of kinase, as in the Bcr-Abl fusion protein, inhibits apoptosis and stimulates cell proliferation [3, 12, 13]. Although imatinib is a highly selective agent, it has been responsive for the inhibition of Bcr-Abl, PDGFR, cKit and FIt3 protein kinases [13]. Unfortunately, long term use of imatinib in some late stage GIST or CML patients may cause drug resistance leading to therapeutic failure. The dynamically complex oncogenic signaling network of cancer cells is able to "escape the addiction" of the Bcr-Abl oncogene as it becomes mutated. Furthermore, tyrosine kinase inhibitors cannot completely eradicate leukemic stem cells; both of these factors facilitate the progression of tumors [13]. Luckily, next generation tyrosine kinase inhibitors are available for imatinib resistant patients [13]. The broad-spectrum protein tyrosine kinase inhibitor Dasatinib (Sprycel®) not only binds to the mutated Brc-Abl kinase but also to Src tyrosine kinase. Despite the reduced selectivity of this inhibitor, the Src kinase family is also responsible for tumor progression, and their overexpression has been linked to several malignancies [13]. Nilotinib (Tasigna®) is another tyrosine kinase inhibitor, which shares imatinib's narrow tyrosine kinase selectivity profile, it inhibits the mutated Brc-Abl kinase activity, and is more efficient when compared to imatinib [13, 16]. Although lifelong therapy is expected with these next generation tyrosine kinase inhibitors, they are reported to achieve longer response rates [13, 16]. The FDA has approved both agents for first line use in patients with Ph positive CML in the chronic phase and for patients with resistance to imatinib [17]. Another dual Src and Bcr-Abl tyrosine kinase inhibitor called bosutinib (Bosulif®) has also been approved by the FDA for patients with Ph positive CML that have been treated with both imatinib and next generation tyrosine kinase inhibitors. It has been reported to have a superior molecular response profile relative to imatinib in terms of inhibition potency to Bcr-Abl mutated tyrosine kinase and more selectivity, thereby decreasing its toxicity profile [18]. Imatinib indicated for GIST patients has partial response rates and differs between subset populations depending on the cKit point mutation. Imatinib is able to extend patient life but resistance usually emerges due to modified point mutations in the cKit gene on GIST stem cells, or mutations in other oncogenes and enhanced drug efflux transporters. A second line broad-spectrum tyrosine kinase inhibitor Sunitinib (Sutent®) is indicated for imatinib resistant GIST patients. This is a multi-target inhibitor that affects vascular endothelial growth factor receptor (VEGFR) and PDGFR protein tyrosine kinases; it has also been approved for the treatment of advanced renal cell carcinoma [13].

Most cell surface growth factor receptors have tyrosine kinase activity, and play an important role in cancer pathogenesis. One of the most notable for molecular targeted signal transduction cancer therapy is epidermal growth factor receptor (EGFR/ ErbB1/ HER1). It is a member of the epidermal growth factor receptors family (ErbB) of protein tyrosine kinases, which also include ErbB2/HER2, ErbB3/ Her3, and ErbB4/ Her4. Binding of a complementary ligand to these receptors induces receptor homo/hetero dimerization and subsequent tyrosine auto-phosphorylation, leading to activation of various downstream signaling molecules. In various types of cancers, the expression/activity profile of these receptors is increased leading to enhanced cell proliferation. Oncogenic mutations within the receptor kinases of this family have also been found in epithelial tumors, breast carcinomas, gliomas (glioblastoma multiforme) and in the case of EGFR in 10% of patients with non-small cell lung carcinoma (NSCLC) [13]. Currently, there are two FDA approved selective EGFR tyrosine kinase inhibitors gefitinib (Iressa®) and erlotinib (Tarceva®) and are indicated as first line therapy for NSCLC patients [13]. Initially, the response rates in patients after administration were not as efficient as expected, and it was later determined that the presence of EGFR overexpression alone does not predict effective therapy [13]. Instead, patients with particular types of EGFR substitution mutation, such as L858R mutation in the kinase domain are more likely to benefit from anti-EGFR therapy [13]. This was concluded from several clinical trials carried out on NSCLC patients comparing the administration of gefitinib to docetaxel in patients pretreated with platinum-based chemotherapy [19, 20]. Results of the trial concluded that gefitinib was either equally effective [19] or more effective [20] than docetaxel. A latter trial was conducted on patients of non-smoker Asian origin, and it was determined that they had a higher incidence of harboring the specific activating mutations in the EGFR kinase domain [13, 20]. Docetaxel is a well-established conventional chemotherapeutic agent which reversibly binds to microtubules with high affinity leading to inhibition of mitotic cell division. It is administered intravenously, and has been reported to cause dose-limiting toxicity and adverse effects of grade 3 and 4 neutropenia in 30% of patients, as well as edema and other common side effects shared by conventional chemotherapies [21]. Gefitinib, on the other hand, is administered orally, with reported adverse effects of grade 1 and 2 diarrhea and skin rash [22]. Therefore, in terms of patient compliance, therapy with gefitinib has greater efficiency than chemotherapy with docetaxel even if they provide the same therapeutic efficacy, since there is a lower incidence of severe adverse effects and oral administration is preferred over intravenous administration. Another important aspect is that not all EGFR mutations in the kinase domain are sufficient to determine patient response and instead only patients with specific EGFR mutations can benefit from certain molecular targeted treatments. In the case of gefitinib, the use of genetic screening is required prior to treatment. This prerequisite highlights the application of precision medicine in targeted cancer therapy and the need for diagnostic strategies involving prognostic biomarkers and tumor genotyping to determine the choice of targeted therapeutic. Manufacturer AstraZeneca, of gefitinib as Iressa® had partnered with Qiagen to provide FDA-approved Therascreen® EGFR companion diagnostic test to identify eligible patients for this treatment, once they test positive for the specific EGFR substitution mutations [22].

Another member of the ErbB receptor family, HER2, has received wide recognition as a target for breast carcinoma, since it has been found to be upregulated in 20–30% of breast cancers [23]. HER2 tyrosine kinase activation is initiated by homo or hetero dimerization with other ErbB receptors, in turn phosphorylation leads to signaling through two main downstream cascades, phosphatidylinositol 3 kinase (PI3K)/Akt and mitogen- activated protein kinase (MAPK); both predominantly involved in promoting cell growth and survival [13, 23]. The first FDA approved targeted monoclonal antibody (Mab) for cancer was transtuzumab (Herceptin®), which interacts with the extracellular domain of HER2 (with high affinity) and is known to be one of the most successful recombinant humanized anti-ErbB- receptor family antibodies [13]. The advantage of transtuzumab as an antibody, over previously mentioned small molecular targeted therapies, is that it exerts its cytotoxicity by several mechanisms as well as binding to the extracellular domain of HER2 on cancer cells with high affinity. Antibodies generally bind to their complementary receptor with higher selectivity or even specificity compared to small molecule therapeutics. Transtuzumab binds HER2 on the surface of cancer cells with high affinity to hinder HER2 dimerization. This also leads to degradation of the receptor and prevents HER2 recycling. As a result, downstream signaling cascades of PI3K and MAPK are diminished, promoting cell-cycle arrest and apoptosis. Furthermore, transtuzumab is able to modulate the immune system by inducing antibody-dependent cellular cytotoxicity (ADCC) through its Fc domain [13]. It can also bind to Fc receptors on various immune cells, markedly natural killer cells, but also neutrophils, mononuclear phagocytes, macrophages and dendritic cells leading to immune cell recruitment to the tumor tissue. Cytotoxicity is mediated in various ways, natural killer cells inhibit cell proliferation and intratumoral angiogenesis by the secretion of cytokines and chemokines, and they also promote tumor immunogenicity by inducing the expression of major histocompatibility antigen on cancer cells [13]. Macrophages and phagocytes carry out phagocytosis by engulfing and eliminating tumor cells [13]. Complement dependent cytotoxicity is mediated after an antibody bound to the surface of a tumor cell also binds to a nearby complement protein C1q. This activates a series of enzymatic cascades in the classical complement pathway, ultimately facilitating the formation of a cytolytic membrane attack complex on the surface of tumor cells in the form of pores that generate an influx of ions and water molecules leading to tumor cell lysis [13]. Transtuzumab has also been identified to play a role in the inhibition of angiogenesis by interfering with pro-angiogenic and anti-angiogenic factors, and reverting tumor vasculature back into normal vasculature [13]. This is supported by the enhanced localization of paclitaxel in tumors during combination therapy with transtuzumab [24]. Unfortunately, one of the limitations of transtuzumab is that it is only able to block the dimerization of HER2 with unbound HER3. Consequently, dimerization of HER2 with EGFR and ligand-bound HER3 proceeds despite transtuzumab therapy, serving as one of the reasons of acquired resistance to transtuzumab. Concurrent therapy with another Mab pertuzumab (Perjeta®) is sometimes administered as it targets dimerization of HER2 with neuregulin ligand bound HER3 [13]. Resistance may also develop by mutations that prevent the complementary binding of transtuzumab to the HER2 extracellular domain. For instance, proteolysis leading to mutated isoforms of HER2 kinases, or elevation in the expression of Mucin-4 an O-glycosylated membrane protein that dimerizes with HER2 [23]. Overexpression of other ErbB members such as EGFR that are able to dimerize with HER2 is also common, in this case a small molecule tyrosine kinase inhibitor lapatinib (Tykerb®), with dual action against HER2 and EGFR has been used [13, 23]. This further reinforces the challenges to treat patients with different molecular subtypes of breast carcinoma. As a result, transtuzumab is indicated for women that have been diagnostically found to strongly overexpress HER2 on their tumor cells and successful treatment response is more likely with early therapy. Transtuzumab has also been indicated as an adjuvant therapeutic particularly after surgery in order to eliminate micrometastases. It is also used in combination with various anticancer agents [13, 23, 24].

3.2 Hormone-based therapies

Various hormones are implicated in the pathogenesis of many forms of tumors such as breast, ovarian, and prostate. Hyperplasia and neoplasia can develop from excessive hormonal stimulation or loss of tumor suppressor genes that dictate hormonal secretions as they have a proliferating effect on target cells. Steroid hormone such as estrogen binds to estrogen receptors (ER) that belong to a superfamily of nuclear receptors. Upon binding, the receptor complex homo-dimerizes and interacts with sequence specific estrogen response elements in corresponding genes, leading to the activation of nuclear transcription factors that produce complementary mRNA. Elevated mRNA levels increase protein production in the endoplasmic reticulum, which ultimately result in various effector responses such as enhanced cell proliferation [25, 26]. While estrogen activity mainly regulates growth, development and physiology of reproductive systems in both sexes, ERs are also found in neuroendocrine, skeletal, adipose and cardiovascular systems [25]. Estrogen signaling pathways are complex due to its nuclear and non-genomic influences, and downstream transcriptional activities affect the biological function of different tissues expressing ERs [25]. Two types of ER have been identified ERα and ERβ, where ERα expression is considered the hallmark of hormone dependent tumor growth [25–27]. About 70% of breast cancer patients express the hormone receptors ER and/ or progesterone, making them susceptible to endocrine therapy [25–27]. These receptors have categorized breast cancer as intrinsic and molecular subtypes based on the genes the cancer cell expresses, and act as a blueprint for targeted breast cancer therapy [27]. The aim of hormone-receptor positive breast cancer therapy is to reduce the growth stimulatory effects of estrogen on breast cancer cells. A primary way to do this is by interfering with the ability of estrogen to bind to its receptor, via targeting estrogen receptors on breast cancer tumors that overexpress ER and competitively binding ERs to reduce the capacity for estradiol to bind. This concept actually paved the way for targeted cancer therapy, and was first demonstrated by the renowned non-steroidal derivative tamoxifen (Nolvadex®) [25–28]. After FDA approval in the 1970s, tamoxifen became one of the world's best-selling hormonal cancer drugs largely relating to its efficacy and short-term safety profile relative to traditional chemotherapeutics at the time [28].

Tamoxifen is non-steroidal triphenylethylene derivative; it is classified as a prodrug, since its metabolites have a more pronounced effect on ERs [25, 28]. Tamoxifen and its metabolites act as selective estrogen receptor modulators (SERM) since they have both anti-estrogenic and pro-estrogenic activity contingents on the target tissue [25, 28]. On mammary epithelia, tamoxifen is able to bind competitively to ERα thereby disrupting the binding of estrogen and inhibiting the transcription of estrogen responsive genes that ultimately antagonize hormone dependent breast cancer cell proliferation and tumor development [25, 28]. Tamoxifen is metabolized hepatically by cytochrome P450 (CYP450) isoforms into pharmacologically active metabolites 4-hydroxytamoxifen (4-OHT), N-desmethyl tamoxifen and endoxifen. These metabolites have a higher affinity for ERs. 4-OHT binds to ERs in breast tissue with an affinity similar to that of estradiol and inhibits ER-mediated gene transcription by recruiting co-repressors that modulate gene expression [29]. Their anti-tumorigenic activity is attributed to induction of apoptosis by downstream ER signaling pathways, inhibition of mitogenic growth factors activity and reduction of angiogenesis [30, 31]. Literature has demonstrated the complex mechanisms of action for tamoxifen and its metabolites and the difficulty in determining the molecule responsible for each mechanism, it is also hypothesized that the response to tamoxifen therapy is an aggregate of the parent and metabolites actions [29]. Pro-estrogenic activities of tamoxifen and its metabolites are demonstrated on bone density, as it decreases bone loss and inhibits osteoclasts in post-menopausal women but causes deleterious effects on bone density in healthy pre-menopausal women [32]. Another pro-estrogenic activity of tamoxifen and its metabolites is found in uterine epithelia, and it has been linked to endometrial cancer in some women restricting its use to 5 years and labeling tamoxifen as a carcinogen [25, 28]. Tamoxifen has been indicated for pre- and post-menopausal women and men diagnosed with hormone-responsive ER positive early stage breast cancer after surgery and as a chemopreventative for high-risk women [25, 27, 28].

Alternatives to SERMs exist, particularly for patients with advanced breast cancer or as a second line therapy to tamoxifen resistant tumors. These include selective estrogen receptor down regulators such as Fluvestrant (Faslodex®) [33]. Their molecular activity is also mediated by binding to ER, however, they function entirely as ER antagonists, causing downregulation and degradation of ER and ultimately inhibiting proliferation of estrogen dependent breast cancer cells. An advantage to the use of fluvestrant over tamoxifen as it is devoid of ER endometrial adverse effects [33]. It has been used in combination with docetaxel as it enhances the sensitization of breast cancer cells to chemotherapy [33].

Another group of endocrine therapy that has been indicated for postmenopausal women with hormone responsive ER breast cancer is aromatase inhibitor (AI) [26]. Their principle mode of action is to decrease circulating levels of estrogen and function by targeting and interfering with the enzyme responsible for the conversion of androgens to estradiol. CYP450 enzyme complex aromatase is responsible for catalyzing the final step in the biosynthesis of estradiol in both pre and post-menopausal women. In premenopausal women, the primary source of estrogen is from the ovaries, while in post-menopausal women adrenal and ovarian androgens are converted to estrogen by enzyme aromatase in peripheral tissues [26, 33, 34]. AIs have been categorized into two main groups, Type I and Type II inhibitors. Type I AIs are irreversible inhibitors of aromatase, they are also known as mechanism based inactivators [26, 34]. These AIs are designed to mimic the substrate of aromatase androstenedione and are recognized by the enzyme as alternate substrates. Hence they undergo irreversible chemical reactions and are converted into intermediates during catalysis; the intermediate however, is reactive and causes inactivation of the enzyme [26, 33, 34]. A successful example of a steroidal AI inhibitor is exemestane (Aromasin) [26, 33, 34]. It is an inhibitor of human placental aromatase and has shown relatively prolonged reduction of estrogen levels (4-5 days) in postmenopausal women with breast cancer due to irreversible binding to aromatase [34]. Exemestane has been found to decrease hormone dependent mammary tumors in hormone receptor positive metastatic breast cancer [34]. Type II inhibitors act by non-covalent competitive binding to the active site of aromatase to decrease the amount of estrogen formed. These inhibitors are designed to target aromatase selectively in order to avoid binding to other CYP450 enzymes [26, 34]. They contain a triazole ring, which aids in their selective binding to the haeme iron of aromatase [26]. As the binding is non-covalent it is reversible, hence therapy with these inhibitors must be continued [26, 34]. Non-steroidal examples of these AI include anastrazole (Arimidex®) and letrozole (Femara®), they are found to inhibit more than 95% of estrogen biosynthesis in post-menopausal women with advanced breast cancer [26, 34]. The FDA has approved the use of AI for postmenopausal women diagnosed with hormone receptor positive breast cancer in the early stage as adjuvant therapy and for advanced and metastatic stages after tamoxifen treatment [26, 34].

3.3 Anti angiogenic therapies

Angiogenesis is a physiological process where new blood vessels are formed from preexisting mature vasculature [35]. This process allows the surrounding tissues to be supplied with nutrients and oxygen and simultaneously gets rid of metabolic waste products and carbon dioxide. In healthy tissue, angiogenesis is a temporary process and occurs during mensuration and embryogenesis, it is also an attribute of wound healing [35]. Prolonged angiogenesis however, is usually an indication of a pathogenic state such as cancer [35, 36]. The aberrant proliferation of cells during tumor formation in many types of cancers requires an extensive capacity of vasculature to manage the high demand in oxygen and nutrients and eliminate accumulated metabolic waste for tumor cells to grow and survive. Hypoxia in the tumor microenvironment leads to the production of hypoxia-inducible factor 1α; a stimulus for angiogenic switch, inducing the overexpression of pro-angiogenic factors mainly vascular endothelial growth factor (VEGF)- A, as well as fibroblast growth factor (FGF), placental growth factor (PlGF) and platelet derived growth factor (PDGF) by tumor and host cells [13, 35, 36]. Subsequently, proliferation of endothelial cells is stimulated and chemotaxis to tumor tissue facilitates the formation of the vascular lumen architecture and simultaneous disruption of surrounding vascular membrane structure [13, 36]. These factors contribute to the defective heterogeneous vasculature surrounding and within the tumor microenvironment, differentiating it from normal vasculature [35, 36]. Tumor vasculature has fenestrated blood vessels, with diminished pericyte coverage, and intratumoral blood vessels resemble immature perforated capillaries. As a result, vasculature is highly permeable, leaky, has poor blood perfusion and interrupted blood flow [35, 36]. Furthermore, the enhanced microvascular permeability leads to the aggregation of fibrin and other plasma proteins in the stroma of tumors, increasing the interstitial fluid pressure within tumors particularly in the absence of adequate lymphatic drainage [35]. This dynamically chaotic tumor microenvironment favors tumor progression in multiple ways. The high interstitial fluid pressure prompts the dissemination of tumor cells into intratumoral capillaries and neo-vessels providing a route for metastasis [36]. Elevated pressure in the tumor core resists the delivery of chemotherapeutics into these micro-regions of the tumor [35, 36]. The heterogeneous vascularization of the tumor microenvironment is dependent on the degree of angiogenesis inflected by tumor cells, so it can be different within and between tumor tissues, and obviously for different types of cancers [36]. These variations are amplified because intratumoral neo-vessel formation is mediated when pro-angiogenic factors outweigh anti-angiogenic factors within the tumor microenvironment. Luckily, the differential activation of angiogenesis in normal tissue compared to tumor tissue provides a means of targeting this pathophysiology selectively, based on the phenotypic and functional differences between intratumoral vasculature and normal vasculature. Therefore, anti-angiogenic strategies serve as attractive cancer therapy; with the aim of terminating the blood supply to tumor tissues and micro-regions in order to impose widespread hypoxia and necrosis selectively within solid tumors while sparing normal cells.

The most extensively studied target to inhibit the angiogenesis process is the VEGF and its receptor (VEGFR). VEGF is a soluble glycoprotein with pro-angiogenic activity, which is overexpressed in tumor tissue, and also by host fibroblasts and inflammatory cells. It is a ligand for the soluble and membrane bound tyrosine kinase VEGFR expressed on endothelial cells. Upon binding, a signaling cascade is activated leading to endothelial cell proliferation, maturation and migration to tumor tissue and neo-vessel formation. Different isoforms of VEGFR and ligands of VEGF exist; the most influential interaction for intratumoral angiogenesis is VEGF-A/VEGFR-2. The first and currently most successful anti-angiogenic cancer therapeutic approved by the FDA is the humanized monoclonal anti-VEGF-A antibody bevacizumab (Avastin®). It contains complimentary-determining regions of a mice antibody that selectively binds to circulating VEGF-A to neutralize it and inhibit its interaction with VEGFR2 [13, 35, 36]. Hence a unique feature of bevacizumab is that unlike most antibodies that bind to receptors, it binds and traps the ligand VEGF-A, limiting its availability to bind to VEGFR2. This initially leads to vascular normalization, which involves reduction in the overall intratumoral vasculature and hence limits the blood supply to tumors. The interstitial fluid pressure is lowered, hypoxia decreases and intratumoral perfusion is enhanced in the core of tumor tissues. Combination therapy is usually administered with bevacizumab to take advantage of the localization of chemotherapeutics deep into the micro-regions of solid tumors [35, 36]. Bevacizumab has been approved for the treatment of renal cell carcinoma, metastatic colorectal cancer, advanced NSCLC and recurrent glioblastoma [35, 36].

Another anti-angiogenic agent which has a similar mode of action to bevacizumab is ziv-aflibercept (Zaltrap®), acts as a decoy receptor. It is a recombinant fusion protein designed by fusion of extracellular VEGF-A binding domain portions of two isoforms of VEGFR (VEGFR1 & VEGFR2) with Fc portion of human IgG1 immunoglobulin [37]. Incorporation of the two VEGFR isoform binding domains in aflibercept allows this angiogenesis inhibitor to trap VEGF-A, VEGF-B and PlGF [36]. Although VEGF-B is not implicated in the stimulation of angiogenesis, it is overexpressed in metastatic tumors and findings suggest it has a role tumor progression by maintaining existing vasculature, while PlGF is required for inflammation-associated angiogenesis in cancer progression. The FDA approves ziv-aflibercept for metastatic colorectal cancer in combination with chemotherapeutic agents 5-Fluorouracil, irinotecan and leucovorin.

Many receptors that mediate angiogenesis are activated by the tyrosine kinase motif attached to their intracellular domain, most prominently is VEGFR, but also FGF and PDGR. Therefore, small molecule receptor tyrosine kinase inhibitors have been utilized as angiogenesis inhibitors; these include sunitinib (mentioned previously) and sorafenib (Nexavar®). Like sunitinib, sorafenib has multiple receptor tyrosine kinase inhibition activity, so its mode of action is not limited to the inhibition of angiogenesis, which it does by binding to VEGFR-1, VEGFR-2 and PDGF-B receptors, leading to morphological vascular normalization of tumor tissue [35, 36]. It also inhibits activation of signaling pathway Raf kinase (Raf/MEK/ERK) which is found to be activated in renal cell carcinoma among other cancer types, and c-KIT and Flt-3 kinases; also implicated in different cancer types [35, 36]. Multiple receptor tyrosine kinase inhibitors can be prescribed as mono-therapy since they act on multiple targets in cancer cells. In fact, their co-administration with chemotherapeutics was not found to improve the drug accumulation in tumor tissues [35]. However, it was found less likely to develop resistance to multiple tyrosine kinase inhibitors compared to selective single targeted anti-angiogenic therapies [36]. The opposite is true for bevacizumab and is the reason why it is co-administered with chemotherapeutic agents [35, 36]. During the initial phases of anti-angiogenic therapy, the intratumoral vasculature undergoes vascular normalization. However, continuous administration of bevacizumab and several other anti-angiogenic therapies causes vascular shutdown and regional tumor tissue necrosis, leaving tumor cells adjacent to normal vasculature viable and prone to resistance [35, 36]. The turning point between vascular normalization and vascular shutdown for anti-angiogenic therapies is called the normalization window and it is this duration that is found to provide optimal intratumoral drug accumulation of chemotherapeutics [35, 36]. Therefore, several factors are taken into account to maximize cancer therapy using angiogenic inhibitors. These include the type of cancer; whether it is dependent on angiogenesis, type of angiogenic inhibitor; hypertension is a common adverse effect for bevacizumab while multi-tyrosine kinase inhibitors can cause more adverse effects. The type of chemotherapeutic agent to insure it will be effective once accumulated in tumor tissues and will not counteract the angiogenic inhibitor. In addition to their temporal sequence and the time lapse between administrations that would define the normalization window; so that the chemotherapeutic agent will be able to localized and accumulate within the tumor core after vascular normalization is induced by the angiogenic inhibitor to increase the overall tumor cell exposure to cytotoxic drugs [35, 36].

In order to define the vascular normalization window and success of anti-angiogenic therapy, predictive detection of vascular parameters is required to enable precision and personal therapy for each patient. Microvascular density analysis is significant to determine vascular integrity during patient treatment and the sensitivity of the cancer to anti-angiogenic therapy; it can be monitored *in vivo* by magnetic resonance imaging and vessel architectural imaging. These techniques have led to the finding that HER2-negative (triple negative) breast cancer patients have a variable response to bevacizumab therapy and the FDA withdrew its approval for breast cancer [35, 36]. Hypoxia detection is also a significant parameter to consider not only for angiogenesis but also since hypoxia is an indication of cancer aggressiveness, its metastatic potential and it can also contribute to tumor resistance particularly during radiotherapy. This parameter can be evaluated by monitoring oxygenation status during therapy. The use of positron emission tomography for hypoxia imaging has been implemented to select patients that will benefit from specific therapies. Tracers, biomarkers and genetically encoded fluorescent sensors have also been utilized as predictors of vascular normalization. **Table 1** summarizes examples of molecular targeted therapeutic agents and the main target they affect.

The previous sections discussed targeted therapeutics based on their molecular mechanisms of action. Although many have proved successful and more efficient than conventional chemotherapeutics, there still remained limitations in terms of toxicity and resistance. The next section addresses a new field in targeted cancer therapy that aims to improve on molecularly targeted therapies by embedding further selectivity into therapeutics. The general principle behind this new and growing field is utilizing the selective delivery of therapeutics to target tumor tissue as well as the selective molecular mechanisms observed in molecularly targeted therapeutics. Targeted delivery therapeutics can be classified into passive targeting which takes advantage of the enhanced permeation and retention effects of the tumor microenvironment or active targeting, which is based on incorporating targeting moieties that will guide the cancer agents to their targets. The following section discusses these two categories in more detail.

3.4 Passive targeting delivery therapeutics

Chemotherapeutic agents are often low molecular weight molecules, with characteristically unfavorable pharmacokinetic profiles usually having short half-lives,

• Tyrosine kinase inhibitors: o Imatinib (Bcr-Abl/c-kit/PDGFR) o Dasatinib (Bcr-Abl/Src) o Nilotinib (Bcr-Abl) o Bosutinib (Bcr-Abl) o Sunitinib (VEGFR/PDGFR) o Gefinitib (EGFR) o Erlotinib (EGFR) o Sorafenib (VEGFR-1/2.PDGF-B/Raf/MEK/ERK) o Lapatinib (HER2/EGFR)
• Monoclonal antibodies: o Transtuzumab (HER2) o Bevacizumab (VEGF-A)
• Hormonal therapies: o Tamoxifen (ER) o Fluvestrant (ER) o Exemestane (aromatase enzyme) o Anastrazole (aromatase enzyme) o Letrozole (aromatase enzyme)
• Anti-angiogenic therapies: o Ziv-aflibercept (VEGF-A)

Table 1.
Examples of molecular targeted therapeutic anticancer agents with their main target.

large volumes of distribution in healthy tissue but suboptimal biodistribution in tumors. The systemic circulation also influences their plasma protein binding strength limiting the free drug available for therapeutic action. Polar, and low molecular weight chemotherapeutic molecules (less than 30 kDa) generally have short systemic circulation exposure as they are cleared by glomerular filtration in the kidneys. On the contrary, macromolecules are commonly recognized by macrophages and cleared from the circulation by the reticuloendothelial (RES) system in the liver. Both of these mechanisms of clearance pose a threat to the drug concentration required to produce the desired therapeutic effect in tumor tissue. In turn, higher concentrations of these drugs that usually have a low therapeutic index, need to be administered making non-selective toxicity inevitable. Furthermore, the inability of conventional chemotherapeutics to sufficiently localize and accumulate in the core of tumors contributes to severe adverse effects and therapeutic resistance, rendering many incompetents for cancer therapy.

Passive targeting of cancer therapeutics aims to improve the pharmacokinetic properties of anticancer agents and tailor them to take advantage of the characteristics and architecture of the tumor microenvironment. The principle behind passively targeted chemotherapeutics is to design delivery systems with improved pharmacokinetic profiles complimentary to the tumor microenvironment. So that encapsulated chemotherapeutics can be transported in the circulation safely for longer durations with minimal toxicity to surrounding healthy tissue. Once they reach the tumor microenvironment they passively accumulate in tumor tissues and are released at therapeutic concentrations to exert their cytotoxicity against cancer cells. As mentioned previously, tumor vasculature is different from normal vasculature. These variations have a unique impact on the behavior of substances in the vicinity of the tumor microenvironment; the phenomenon is known as the enhanced permeation and retention (EPR) effect of tumors. It is attributed to the abnormal vasculature and impaired lymphatic drainage in the tumor microenvironment [37]. The imbalance in angiogenic factors and matrix metalloproteinases leads to the formation of highly disorganized dilated vessels with fenestrations, due to pores and wide gap junctions between endothelial cells that lack sufficient pericytes and a basement membrane [37]. Intratumoral vessels usually lack the smooth muscle layer surrounding endothelial cells and hence remain dilated [37]. As a result, intratumoral vasculature is leaky enough to extravasate macromolecules >600 nM in diameter into tumor tissues as opposed to normal vasculature where tight junctions restrict the permeability of molecules sized >4 nM [37]. Furthermore, the impaired lymphatic system in the tumor microenvironment retains extravasated molecules allowing them to accumulate [37]. Therefore, the enhanced permeation of macromolecules in neoplastic vasculature and their retention and accumulation into tumor tissues lead to the application of nanotherapeutics as delivery systems for targeted cancer therapy.

The design of delivery systems with improved pharmacokinetic profiles and biodistribution that complement the pathophysiology of the tumor microenvironment is made possible by utilizing nanocarriers. The field of nanomedicine, derived from nanotechnology is extremely broad with a deluge of components synthesized and investigated for various diseased states. Nanocarriers are colloidal drug delivery systems with sizes in the nanometer range (generally <500 nM) imparting a high surface to volume ratio to them and their cargo. This is a significant feature for their characteristics. Variations in size, shape, and synthetic constituents have been investigated to determine the ideal nanocarriers for enhanced bioavailability and therapeutic efficiency of anticancer agents. The principle behind nanocarriers is to allow drugs to behave as though they have a larger molecular weight. Much research has gone into determining the ideal size of nanocarriers for cancer therapy and it was found to range from 10 to 100 nM [38]. Justified as nanocarriers >10 nM are more likely to escape rapid excretion by glomerular filtration in the kidneys. While nanocarrier >100 nM are more likely to be absorbed by proteins for opsonization prior to hepatic uptake and clearance by RES [38]. Surface charge of nanocarriers is another modifiable property to manipulate the pharmacokinetic profiles of therapeutics. It is attributable to the various types of nanomaterial formulations available to synthesis these carriers. Neutral and anionic nanocarriers are favorable in evading renal elimination whereas cationic nanocarriers form better interactions with the negatively charged cell membrane and enhances their cellular uptake [38]. Another way to modify the surface of nanoparticles is by a process called PEGylation. It involves coating the surface of nanoparticles with an inert polymer polyethylene glycol (PEG) so that they are shielded from interactions during systemic circulation, particularly from protein blood components and even aggregation with one another. This imparts stealth properties to nanoparticles and has been effective in increasing circulation times of nanoparticles as they avoid surface absorption and opsonization, reducing the frequency of clearance by phagocytosis and the RES system [39].

Nanocarriers can be categorized into 3 types based on their constituents, organic, inorganic, and hybrid [40]. Organic carriers include liposomes, solid lipid nanoparticles, dendrimers, polymer nanoparticles and polymeric micelles. Inorganic nanocarriers include carbon nanotubes and mesoporous silica nanoparticles, while hybrids are a combination of both. This part of the chapter discusses the most prevalent organic nanocarriers as only two have been approved by the FDA to date for anticancer use.

4. Organic nanocarriers

4.1 Liposomes

These microscopic lipid bilayers have become very popular after the success of the reformulated anticancer drug Doxil (Caelyx®) [41]. They are spherical vesicles with an aqueous core surrounded by single or multiple lipid bilayers, composed from natural or synthetic lipids such as phospholipids and cholesterol that can enter cells by endocytosis. The structure of liposomes allows them to encapsulate both water and lipid soluble drug payloads [41]. Schematic of liposome arrangement is shown in **Figure 1**. Hence liposomes can improve the pharmacokinetic properties of a range of drugs with different solubilities. Moreover, they can be coated with polymers or PEGylated to provide stealth properties. Doxil for instance is a polyethylene glycol coated liposome with the chemotherapeutic doxorubicin as the drug payload. Currently, it is the sole liposomal cytotoxic agent approved for solid tumors, and indicated by the FDA for ovarian cancer and multiple myeloma [41]. The chemotherapeutic doxorubicin is an anthracycline, which mediates its cytotoxicity by intercalating with DNA and inhibiting topoisomerase I and II activity, leading to apoptosis induction in cancer cells [42]. However, one of its main drawbacks is cardiotoxicity which can be fatal or lead to congestive heart failure, hence patients are only permitted a limited dose in their lifetime [41, 42]. The reformulation of doxorubicin as doxil has overcome this adverse effect; in fact, it has a very different toxicity profile from doxorubicin [41, 42]. While being dose limited by mucocutaneous toxicities, its adverse effects are much less severe. Furthermore, the bioavailability of doxil is preferential to doxorubicin as it is more stable in systemic circulation, has a longer half-life and slower clearance rate [42]. It is also able to extravasate into leaky intratumoral vasculature where its concentration is low compared to normal vasculature where its concentration is higher, by passive diffusion and accumulate substantially more in solid tumors [42]. As a result, it has a better therapeutic efficacy and index compared to doxorubicin [42].

4.2 Nanoparticles

Nanoparticles have been synthesized in a variety of forms from various constituents. Solid lipid nanoparticles constitute organic solid lipids such as mono- di- and

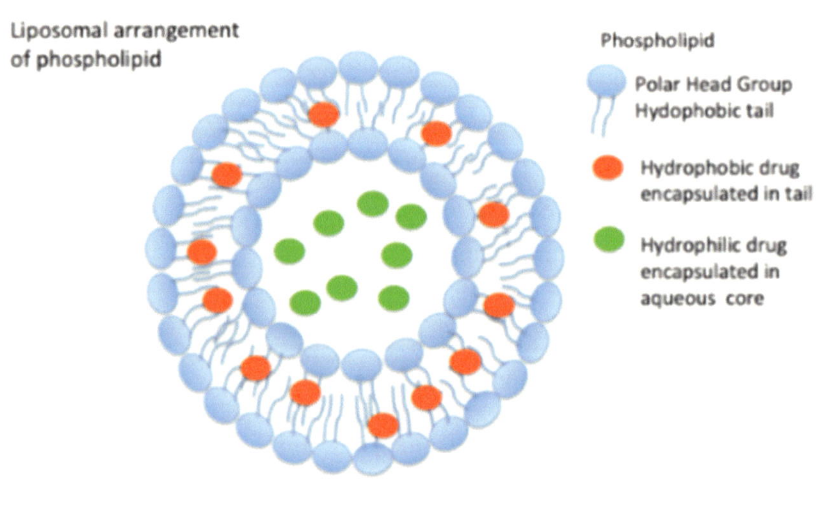

Figure 1.
Schematic diagram of liposomal arrangement of phospholipid (not to scale).

triglycerides, free fatty acids and alcohols or waxes and steroids [40]. These lipids are dispensed in water to form a nanosized colloidal dispersion with a large size range of 50–1000 nM, an emulsifier is added to stabilize the formulation [40]. Lipid constituents offer great advantages as nanocarriers for anticancer drugs classified as class II and class IV in the Biopharmaceutical classification system, where aqueous solubility is low [40]. This is because they increase the solubilization of lipophilic drugs and enhance their bioavailability. These delivery systems also provide controlled drug delivery, they are biocompatible and biodegradable and have greater drug payloads as well as improved stability and are feasible for large-scale manufacture [40]. Another type of nanoparticles is polymeric nanoparticles these are solid nanosized colloidal particles that are formulated as nanospheres or nanocapsules depending on the structural organization [40]. They are made from both synthetic biodegradable polymers such as polylactic acid, polyglycolic acid, PEG and N-(2-hydroxypropyl) methacrylamide, or natural polymers such as albumin, alginate, collagen, chitosan and heparin [40]. The advantage of using polymeric nanoparticles is that they are usually biocompatible and biodegradable, hence reduce toxicity and are degraded in the body by normal metabolic routes [40]. They also offer greater drug stability in the circulation and during storage, are formulated to be homogenous compared to liposomes and retain the enhanced bioavailability characteristic of nanocarriers [40].

A successful example of an anticancer polymeric nanoparticle that has been approved by the FDA is Abraxane®, for the treatment of metastatic breast cancer and NSCLC. It constitutes the chemotherapeutic taxane paclitaxel bound to the natural polymer albumin in a solvent free formulation, forming a colloidal suspension of 130 nM particles. This formulation has several advantages over the use of the traditional chemotherapeutic paclitaxel limited by its poor aqueous solubility. Previously, paclitaxel was administered in a formulation with Cremophor® a solubilizing agent to enhance its solubility in the systemic circulation, however, many patients suffered hypersensitivity reactions from Cremophor® and pretreatment with steroids or antihistamine is recommended for these cases [43]. Albumin acts as a carrier for hydrophobic paclitaxel without Cremophor®, and is found to accumulate in tumors along with its bound constituents [42]. It is also able to enhance the endothelial cellular uptake of paclitaxel by the formation of caveolaes during transcytosis, this is reflected in clinical trials where the permeation and antitumor activity of Abraxane® was higher compared to paclitaxel. It is also found to have a higher maximum tolerated dose and the adverse effects of Abraxane® were reported to be less severe and frequent than the general taxane associated adverse effects [41, 43].

4.3 Nanocarriers for gene therapy and smart delivery systems

The enhanced stability during systemic circulation offered by nanocarrier to their cargo has served as a key advantage to the application of targeted gene delivery for cancer therapy. Gene therapy has been implicated to replace or knock out mutations commonly detected in cancer or insert new genes into cancerous cells to induce apoptosis. Therefore, by targeting endogenous tumor gene expressions, a highly potent and specific therapeutic effect can be instigated with minimal off-target toxicity. This is widely applicable to cancer therapy due to its dependence on oncoproteins and oncogenes. Moreover, multiple genes can be targeted to inhibit tumorigenesis, recurrence and resistance [44]. However, challenges with regard to toxicity and instability have rendered gene therapeutics immature for cancer therapy. The introduction of naked genetic material such as DNA, plasmid DNA, small interfering RNA, nucleotides, and peptides in the systemic circulation is limited due to instability and degradation by serum nucleases in the plasma as well as rapid renal clearance and phagocytosis by immune cells [44].

In addition, not only is cellular uptake restricted but nuclear delivery of genes into non-dividing target cells is inefficient and discrepancies exist on long term incorporation of genetic DNA information into the host cell, as it is likely to have unforeseen implications on patient's safety and toxic immune responses have been reported [44].

Nanocarriers have the potential to be delivery vectors for genetic material as cargo to their target tissue. Their versatility allows them to be designed in a manner that allows high gene delivery efficiency and payload capacity [44]. Genetic material can be incorporated and attached into nanocarriers by electrostatic interactions or surface conjugation [44]. Cationic nanocarriers like liposomes synthesized from cationic and neutrally charged lipids are able to condense DNA, siRNA, nucleotides, peptides and proteins to form complexes of plasmid DNA lipids that self-assemble into lipoplexes. Similarly, polymer nanocarriers are able to form polyplexes with nucleic acids [44]. These complexes protect the genetic cargo from enzymatic degradation in the systemic circulation and aid in cellular interactions that facilitate endocytosis. Hence they are able to deliver their cargo intracellularly increasing the likelihood of efficient transfection.

Moreover, nanocarrier can be synthesized from polymers that are able to respond to specific stimuli based on physiochemical differences between cancer and non-cancerous cells, leading to the development of smart drug delivery systems [45]. Their aim is to reduce dosage frequency in a spatially controlled manner and facilitate the delivery and accumulation of the therapeutic system to the target tumor tissue. Followed by the release of anticancer agent at the specific location at a precise concentration based on internal or external stimuli [45]. Smart polymer nanocarriers can respond to stimuli such as changes in pH, enzyme configurations, redox reactions and light [45]. The application of passive targeted therapy in cancer has proved to dampen down adverse effects experienced with traditional chemotherapeutics. In addition, the improved pharmacokinetic profiles and enhanced efficiency of passive targeted cancer delivery systems has increased the response and survival rates of patients. However, this strategy of targeted cancer therapy is not devoid of challenges as non-selective toxicity and resistance remains to be an issue that impedes cancer therapy. Hence a further extension to passive targeted cancer therapy was explored that pioneered the birth of a different strategy for targeted delivery it is active targeted therapy and is discussed in the final section of this chapter.

4.4 Active targeting delivery therapeutics

Active targeting anticancer therapeutics aims to further increase the selectivity of chemotherapeutics to tumor tissue via delivery strategies through preferentially potentiating their affinity towards cancer cells and escalating endocytic internalization. The principle mechanism of active targeted cancer therapy is based on receptor-mediated interactions. Their framework is established through targeting moieties such as small molecule ligands or antibodies that bind to receptor of proteins, sugars or lipids on the surface of target cells. As a result, these ligands act as delivery agents for the anticancer therapeutic system, prompting its tumor accumulation and enhancing its residence time.

Many of the same receptors targeted in molecular targeted therapeutics have been utilized as active targeted delivery therapeutics, imparting a second functionality to active targeted delivery cancer therapy, whereby one part of the system acts by targeted delivery and the other part mediates molecular mechanisms of cytotoxicity. Commonly targeted cell surface receptors include EGFR and HER2. Widely explored cell surface receptors include folic acid receptor, transferrin, and prostate specific membrane antigen [11]. The scope of this targeting strategy is endless and a heterogeneous array of targeting components have been utilized and reported as drug-targeting conjugates such as antibodies in antibody drug conjugates (ADC), proteins, peptiodomimetic and small molecules.

Much of the success of active targeted delivery therapeutics for cancer therapy has been achieved with ADC. They constitute extremely potent chemotherapeutic agents that are not administered alone, due to their narrow therapeutic window and extreme non-selective toxicity, examples include maytansinoids and auristatins. Maytansinoids are second-generation microtubulin polymerization inhibitors similar to vinca-alkaloid traditional chemotherapeutics, that have been modified to bind to tubulin with >100-fold higher affinity [46]. The ADC transtuzumab emtansine (Kadcyla®/T-DM1) has been synthesized with a derivative of maytansin (DM1) conjugated to transtuzumab, previously mentioned, a MAb for breast cancer patients that overexpress HER2. This design allows targeted delivery of a highly potent cytotoxic agent to tumor cells that express HER2 with a favorable therapeutic window that would otherwise not be achieved by the cytotoxic agent alone. Many factors need to be taken into account with the design of ADC, particularly the binding affinity of the targeting ligand to the receptor after conjugation with the therapeutic agent, in the case of T-DM1, it binds to HER2 with a similar binding affinity to free transtuzumab [46]. This is not always the case as conjugation and linkers connecting the targeting moiety and therapeutic agent can cause steric hindrance or altered structural configurations, which restricts or dissolves binding. Linkers are designed to stably carry the therapeutic system in systemic circulation and insure the therapeutic agent will not dissociate until it has reached the target site. This is achieved to a higher degree with non-cleavable linkers, but cleavable linkers are utilized more commonly as complete cleavage of the therapeutic agent from the system ensures efficient cytotoxic action. Binding of the targeting moiety to the receptor usually induces cellular internalization of the therapeutic system. Targeting moieties and linkers are also designed to facilitate intracellular release of the cytotoxic agent. Transtuzumab in T-DM1 aids in the internalization of DM1 into cancer cells, it contains a non-cleavable linker that keeps the system stable in circulation but may compromise the cytotoxic activity of DM1 if proteolytic lysosomal degradation of transtuzumab is inefficient [46]. In addition to the cytotoxic action of DM1 after intracellular release, T-DM1 is also able to inflect the antitumor action of transtuzumab regarding inhibition of HER2 signaling and marking HER2 overexpressing cells for ADCC [46].

Although no small molecule active targeting delivery therapeutics for cancer therapy have been approved by the FDA to date, research in this field is growing exponentially. Many of these potential therapeutics in clinical stages of development utilize nanoparticles that are decorated with targeting ligands on their surface and encapsulate anticancer drugs as payloads [11].

5. Conclusion

The origins of targeted therapy started by challenging cytotoxic chemotherapy with an alternative approach to treatment, achieved by adopting the "magic bullet" theory of selectivity between pharmacological principles of cancer and non-cancer cells. Targeted anticancer therapy is an exponentially growing class of chemotherapeutic agents with advantages over conventional anticancer drugs. The advantage is a result of selective targeting of cytotoxic agents towards cancer cells over normal cells. Selective targeting is based on variations in genes, proteins and pathophysiology of cancer cells compared to non-cancerous cells. This has been explored and achieved in molecular mechanism therapeutics as well as passive and active targeting delivery strategies for cancer therapy. The progress in cancer therapy stems from the understanding cancer biology leading to detailed distinctions between the pathophysiology of tumors and the physiology of normal tissue.

Strategies of targeted anticancer therapy have advanced by applying meticulous selectivity to chemotherapeutic. This commenced with variations in molecular mechanisms of action in mechanistic therapeutics with much success in targeting signal transduction pathways specifically tyrosine kinase proteins. Subsequently, a greater degree of selectivity is investigated by passive targeting mechanisms, which utilizes nanocarriers to take advantage of the enhanced permeation and retention effects of the tumor microenvironment. This strategy has also shown that not only is the pharmacodynamic profile of the anticancer agents significant for the success of cancer therapy but so is their pharmacokinetic profile. Further selectivity has also been explored by active targeting delivery via receptor-mediated interactions with cancer cells. All these targeting strategies can be combined and tailored to achieve efficient response rates for patients.

The application of targeted therapeutics has shifted therapy protocols for cancer patients towards precision medicine; hence various aspects need to be considered with targeting cancer therapy. This approach involves determining diagnostic biomarkers and genotyping tumors to choose the relevant targeted therapeutic for the patient. Furthermore, treatment needs to be designed and tailored for patients in terms of duration, dose and monitoring of adverse effects. Careful selection of combination therapies and dosing regimens are also critical to the success of cancer therapy.

Targeted cancer therapy has proven more effective than conventional chemotherapeutics as the maximum tolerated dose is higher so patients are able to tolerate therapeutic doses with less severe adverse effects. This resulted in improved patient response rates and survival. Although resistance is still an issue with cancer therapy, the strategies employed by targeted therapy have widened the scope of therapeutics available if resistance occurs. Although much of this field is still under development, the progress made with targeted cancer therapy is changing the perspective of cancer from a fatal disease to a chronic one that can be managed throughout the patient's lifetime.

Author details

Wabel AL-Busairi[1] and Maitham Khajah[2*]

1 Department of Pharmaceutics, Kuwait University, Kuwait

2 Department of Pharmacology and Therapeutics, Faculty of Pharmacy, Kuwait University, Kuwait

*Address all correspondence to: maitham@hsc.edu.kw

References

[1] Bray F, Ferlay J, Soerjomataram I, Siegel RL, Torre LA, Jemal A. Global cancer statistics 2018: GLOBOCAN estimates of incidence and mortality worldwide for 36 cancers in 185 countries. CA: A Cancer Journal for Clinicians. 2018;**68**(6):394-424

[2] Chabner BA, Roberts TG Jr. Chemotherapy and the war on cancer. Nature Reviews Cancer. 2005;**65**:72-75

[3] Pérez-Herrero E, Fernández-Medarde A. Advanced targeted therapies in cancer: Drug nanocarriers, the future of chemotherapy. European Journal of Pharmaceutics and Biopharmaceutics. 2015;**93**:52-79

[4] Baudino TA. Targeted cancer therapy: The next generation of cancer treatment. Current Drug Discovery Technologies. 2015;**5**:3-20

[5] Ratain MJ, Postel-Vinay S. Advances in drug development current developments in oncology drug research redefining dose limiting toxicity. Clinical Advances in Hematology & Oncology. 2015;**13**(2):87-89

[6] Remesh A. Toxicities of anticancer drugs and its management. International Journal of Basic & Clinical Pharmacology. 2012;**1**(1):2-12

[7] Luqmani YA. Mechanisms of drug resistance in cancer therapy. Medical Principles and Practice. 2005;**14**(1):35-48

[8] Raguz S, Yague E. Resistance to chemotherapy: New treatments and novel insights into an old problem. British Journal of Cancer. 2008;**99**:387-391

[9] Huang M, Shen A, Ding J, Geng M. Molecularly targeted cancer therapy: Some lessons from the past decade. Trends in Pharmacological Sciences. 2014;**35**:41-50

[10] Joo WD, Visintin I, Mor G. Targeted cancer therapy—Are the days of systemic chemotherapy numbered? Maturitas. 2013;**76**(4):308-314

[11] Kue CS, Kamkaew A, Burgess K, Kiew LV, Chung LY, Lee HB. Small molecules for active targeting in cancer. Medicinal Research Reviews. 2016;**36**(3):494-575

[12] Sawyers C. Targeted cancer therapy. Nature. 2004;**432**:294-297

[13] Levitzki A, Klein S. Signal transduction therapy of cancer. Molecular Aspects of Medicine. 2010;**31**:287-329

[14] Avendano C, Menendez JC. Chapter 9—Drugs that inhibit signaling pathways for tumor cell growth and proliferation. In: Medicinal Chemistry of Anticancer Drugs. Elsevier; 2008. pp. 251-305. Paperback ISBN: 9780444626493, eBook ISBN: 9780444626677

[15] Zhang J, Yang PL, Gray NS. Targeting cancer with small molecule kinase inhibitors. Nature Reviews Cancer. 2009;**9**:28-39

[16] O'Hare T. A decade of Nilotinib and Dasatinib: From in vitro studies to first-line tyrosine kinase inhibitors. Canser Research. 2005;**65**:4500-4505

[17] Online FDA website

[18] Jean Khoury H, Cortes J, Kantarjian H, Gambacorti-Passerini C, Baccarani M, Kim D-W, et al. Bosutinib is active in chronic phase chronic myeloid leukemia after imatinib and dasatinib and/or nolitinib therapy failure. Blood. 2012;**119**(15):3403-3412

[19] Kim ES, Hirsh V, Mok T, Socinski MA, Gervais R, Wu Y-L, et al. Gefintinib versus docetaxel in previously treated non-small-cell ling cancer (INTREST):

A randomized phase III trial. The Lancet. 2008;**372**(9652):1809-1818

[20] Lee DH, Park K, Kim JH, Lee J-S, Shin SW, Kang J-H, et al. Randomized Phase III Trial of gefitinib versus docetaxel in non-small cell lung cancer patients who have previously received platinum based chemotherapy. Clinical Cancer Research. 2010;**16**(4):1370-1314

[21] Gubens MA, Wakelee HA. Docetaxel in the treatment of non-small cell lung carcinoma: An update and analysis. Lung Cancer: Targets and Therapy. 2010;**1**:63-76

[22] Online article: https://www.astrazeneca-us.com/media/press-releases/2015/iressa-approved-by-the-fda-20150713.html#

[23] Vu T, Claret FX. Transtuzumab: Updated mechanisms of action and resistance in breast cancer. Frontiers in Oncology. 2012;**2**(62):1-6

[24] Nahta R, Esteva FJ. Transtuzumab: Triumphs and tribulations. Oncogene. 2007;**26**:3637-3643

[25] Williams C, Lin C-Y. Oestrogen receptors in breast cancer: Basic mechanisms and clinical implications. Ecancermedicalscience. 2013;7(370):1-12

[26] Breuggemeier R, Hackett J, Cruz ED. Aromatase Inhibitors in the treatment of breast cancer. Endocrine Reviews. 2005;**26**(3):331-345

[27] Lim E, Metzger-Filho O, Winer EP. The natural history of hormone receptor positive breast cancer. Oncology. 2012;**26**(8):688-701

[28] Shagufta, Ahmad I. Tamoxifen a pioneering drug: An update on the therapeutic potential of tamoxifen derivates. European Journal of Medicinal Chemistry. 2018;**143**:515-531

[29] Johnson MD, Zuo H, et al. Pharmacological characterization of 4-hydroxy-N-desmethyl tamoxifen, a novel metabolite of tamoxifen. Breast Cancer Research and Treatment. 2004;**85**:151-159

[30] Gauduchon J, Gouilleux F, et al. 4-Hydroxytamoxifen inhibits proliferation of multiple myeloma cells in vitro through down-regulation of c-Myc, up regulation of p27Kip1, and modulation of Bcl-2 family members. Cancer Therapy. 2005;**11**:2345-2354

[31] Freiss G, Rochefort H, Vignon F. Mechanisms of 4-Hydroxytamoxifen anti-growth factor activity in breast cancer cells: Alterations of growth factor receptor binding site and tyrosine kinase activity. Biochemical and Biophysical Research Communications. 1990;**173**(3):919-926

[32] Powles TJ, Hickish T, Kanis JA, et al. Effect of tamoxifen on bone mineral density measured by dual-energy x-ray absorptiometry in healthy premenopausal and post menopausal women. Journal of Clinical Oncology. 1996;**14**:78-84

[33] Lumachi F, Santeufemia D, Basso S. Current medical treatment of oestrogen receptor-positive breast cancer. World Journal of Biological Chemistry. 2015;**6**(3):231-239

[34] Lombardi P. Exemestane, a new steroidal aromatase inhibitor of clinical relevance. Biochimica et Biophysica Acta. 2002;**1587**(2-3):326-337

[35] Ma J, Waxman DJ. Combination of Anti-angiogenesis with chemotherapy for more effective cancer treatment. Molecular Cancer. 2008;7(12):3670-3684

[36] Al-Abd A, Alamoudi A, Abdel-Naim A, Neamatalla T, Ashour O. Anti-angiogenic agents for the treatment of solid tumors: Potential pathways,

therapy and current strategies—A review. Journal of Advanced Research. 2017;**8**:591-605

[37] Bazak R, Houri M, Elachy S, Hussein W, Refaat T. Passive targeting of nanoparticles to cancer: A comprehensive review of literature. Molecular and Clinical Oncology. 2014;**2**:904-908

[38] Narayanan E, Wakaskar R. Utilization of nanoparticulate therapy in cancer targeting. Cogent Medicine. 2018;**5**(1504504):1-9

[39] Soo Suk J, Xu Q, Kim N, Hanes J, Ensign LM. PEGylation as a strategy for improving nanoparticle-based drug gene delivery. Advanced Drug Delivery Reviews. 2016;**99**:28-51

[40] Din F u, Ullah WAI, et al. Effective use of nanocarriers as drug delivery systems for the treatment of selected tumors. International Journal of Nanomedicine. 2017;**12**:7291-7309

[41] Li R, Zheng K, Yuan C, Chen Z, Huang M. Be active or Not: The relative contribution of active and passive tumor targeting of nanomaterials. Nano. 2017;**1**(4):346-357

[42] Gabizon A. Pegylated liposomal doxorubicin: Metamorphosis of an old drug into a new form of chemotherapy. Cancer Investigation. 2001;**19**(4):424-436

[43] Miele E, Spineli GP, Miele E, Tomao F, Tomao S. Albumin-bound formulation of paclitaxel (Abraxane ABI-007) in the treatment of breast cancer. International Journal of Nanomedicine. 2009;**4**:99-105

[44] Wang K, Kievit FM, Zhang M. Nanoparticles for cancer gene therapy: Recent advances, challenges and strategies. Pharmacological Research. 2016;**114**:56-66

[45] Hossen S, Khalid Hossain M, Basher MK, Mia MNH, Rahman MT, Jalal Uddin M. Smart nanocarrier-based drug delivery systems for cancer therapy and toxicity studies: A review. Journal of Advanced Research. 2019;**15**:1-18

[46] Girish S, Gupta M, Wang B, Lu D, et al. Clinical pharmacology of transtuzumab emtansine (T-DM1): An antibody drug conjugate in development of the treatment for HER2-positive cancer. Cancer Chemotherapy and Pharmacology. 2012;**69**(5):1229-1240

Section 4

New Perspectives for Cancer Diagnosis and Therapy

Chapter 9

Stereotactic Radiosurgery for Recurrent Glioblastoma Multiforme

Cheng-Ta Hsieh and Da-Tong Ju

Abstract

Glioblastoma multiforme (GBM) is the most aggressive intracranial tumor that primarily affects adults. Since the introduction of temozolomide in 2005, maximal resection surgery with concurrent chemoradiation has become the standard treatment method for patients with newly diagnosed GBM. Although newly discovered chemoagents have been demonstrated to improve the median survival time, GBM still recurs in most patients. Recurrent GBM is still a therapeutic challenge for clinical physicians. Surgical intervention and other conventional chemoagents have been applied to manage recurrent GBM. Stereotactic radiosurgery (SRS) provides a highly precise radiation dose to the tumor lesion and reduces the dose to the adjacent normal brain tissue. After standard treatment for newly diagnosed GBM is completed, conventional re-irradiation therapy is not suitable for patients with recurrent GBMs. Therefore, SRS may become an alternative option in the treatment of recurrent GBMs. In this review, we discuss the relevant literature regarding SRS for recurrent GBMs and provide treatment advice for clinical physicians.

Keywords: stereotactic radiosurgery, recurrent glioblastoma multiforme, re-irradiation, survival time, prognosis

1. Introduction

Glioblastoma multiforme (GBM) is the most common primary brain neoplasm in adults [1, 2]. There are 1.6 times more males than females who develop a GBM [1]. According to the latest statistical report of the Central Brain Tumor Registry of the USA, the annual incidence of GBM has been estimated at approximately 3.22 cases per 100,000 people, and the median age is 65 years [3]. The current standard treatment of patients with a newly diagnosed GBM was established in 2005, and it consists of maximal surgical resection of the tumor followed by chemotherapy and conventional radiotherapy [4, 5]. Despite this therapy, the median overall survival time is approximately 15–17 months [2].

GBM is a refractory malignant and infiltrating tumor that may recur any time after initial multimodal treatments are completed [6]. Managing recurrent GBM has always been challenging, and a balance has to be achieved between significant treatment toxicity and associated morbidities and mortalities [6, 7]. Reoperation with maximal resection at recurrence remains as an independent predictor to improve overall survival [8, 9]. However, repeat gross-total resection may not be

IntechOpen

easily achieved when recurrent GBM involves important eloquent brain structures, such as the brainstem or motor area. Extensive bevacizumab and temozolomide are the two main FDA-approved chemoagents used to treat patients with recurrent GBMs, but the prognosis remains poor [10].

Re-irradiation is an alternative option for managing recurrent GBMs [11]. The majority of recurrent tumors occur at the initial or adjacent regional sites [12]. Because a total dose of 60 Gy in 30 fractions has been prescribed for initial radiation therapy, re-irradiation with further dose escalation appears to produce more significant toxicity [10, 11]. Stereotactic radiosurgery (SRS) is a noninvasive treatment that provides a highly precise, targeted additional radiation boost to the tumor lesion, and it maintains an acceptable rate of adverse radiation effects while reducing the dose to adjacent normal brain tissues [13]. In this review, we searched the relevant literature and investigated the role of SRS in the management of recurrent GBMs. Our results may provide treatment information for clinical treatment.

2. Search methodology

In this study, different combinations of the keywords “recurrent glioblastoma multiple,” “high-grade glioma,” “stereotactic radiosurgery,” and “re-irradiation” were used to search the published literature in the PubMed database until October 31, 2019. The inclusion criteria of the study were (1) patients with recurrent GBMs, (2) treatment with stereotactic radiosurgery (SRS) or a fractionated radiosurgery (less than 5 fractions), and (3) outcomes with overall survival time. Tumor progression was also accepted as a recurrent disease. Potentially relevant studies were identified from the reference lists of the studies obtained from the database search. Articles excluded from the review were those written in languages other than English and those that lacked survival response data. Finally, a total of 49 studies were included in this review.

3. The summary of patients with recurrent GBMs treated with SRS

A total of 49 studies published from 1994 to 2019 were enrolled in this review, as summarized in **Table 1** [13–61]. There were 6 prospective studies and 43 retrospective studies. About 2066 patients with recurrent glioblastomas treated with SRS, including linear accelerator (LINAC) radiosurgery, Gamma Knife radiosurgery, and Cyberknife radiosurgery, are reported. In all studies, the median age of the patients who received SRS treatment for recurrent GBM ranged from 34 to 62 years. The majority of patients were males. The median prescribed dose of SRS ranged from 6 to 30 Gy. The median targeted volume for treatment ranged from 1.35 to 21.3 cc. The overall survival time from treatment for SRS ranged from 3.9 to 17.9 months, where the progression-free survival time from the treatment of SRS ranged from 2.1 to 14.9 months. In the prognostic analysis of survival time in patients with recurrent GBMs treated with SRS, a small tumor volume, younger age, higher Karnofsky performance scale (KPS) score, lower recursive partitioning analysis (RPA) class, adjuvant bevacizumab, methylated O6-methylguanine-DNA-methyltransferase (MGMT) promoter, and longer interval between the original surgery and SRS were significantly associated with patients’ survival outcomes.

3.1 The effect of LINAC radiosurgery in patients with recurrent GBMs

From 1994 to 2018, a total of 501 patients with recurrent GBMs treated with LINAC SRS were enrolled in 22 studies, including 3 prospective trials and 17

Year	Author	Study type	Enrolled year	All patients	Numbers of patients with rGBM	Gender	Age (years)			Treatment Modality of SRS	Radiation dose (Gy)			Adjuvant chemo agents	Target volume (cm3)			Median overall survival after SRS (months)	Median progressive-free survival after SRS(months)	Factors associated with favorable outcome	
						Male: Female	Mean	Median	Range		Median marginal dose	Mean marginal dose	Range		Median	Mean	Range			Univariate analysis	Multivariate analysis
1994	Chamerlain et al.[14]	Prospective phase II	NR	20	5			34[a]	8-62a	LINAC	13.4[a]		12-15.7[a]		17[a]		3-53.5[a]	8[a]	4[a]		
1995	Shrieve et al.[16]	Retrospective	1985-1993	118	72			46[a]	9-77[a]	LINAC	13[a]		6-20[a]		10.1[a]		2.2-83[a]	10.2		age<46 years, tumor volume < 10.1 cm³,	younger age, small tumor volume
1995	Hall et al.[15]	Retrospective	1991-1994	35	26			48[a]	18-72[a]	LINAC	21[a]	20[a]	7.5-40[a]		28[a]	35[a]	2.4-98[a]	8		younger age, higher KPS	younger age
1996	Larson et al.[17]	Retrospective	1987-1994	189	66			45[a]	2-70[a]	GK	16[a]		5-37.5[a]		6.5[a]		0.3-96[a]	10			younger age, increased KPS, smaller tumor volume, and unifocal tumor
1997	Kondziolka et al.[18]	Retrospective	1987-	107	19		51[b]		3-72[b]	GK(since 1991)		15.5[b]	12-25[b]			6.5[b]	0.88-31.2[b]	30			younger age, smaller tumor volume, and KPS ≥ 70
1999	Cho et al.[19]	Retrospective	1991-1998	71	27			48[a]	16-74[a]	LINAC	17[a]		9-40[a]		10[a]		1-54[a]	7.1			younger age, higher KPS, smaller tumor volume
1999	Sanghavi et al.[60]	Retrospective	1989-1997	30	22			52[a]	13-68[a]	LINAC		12			7.2[a]		0.42-35.1[a]	8[a]	3		
2000	Park et al.[61]	Retrospective	1990-1999	23	22			53[a]	36-80[a]	LINAC (n=13)/GK (n=10)	15[a]		12-20[a]		9.9[a]		0.8-37.9[a]	10.3[a]		NS	
2002	Larson et al.[20]	Prospective phase II	1996-1999	80	14	9:5		53	22-74	GK	15		12-17.5	Marimastat	8		1.6-29.7	8.7	3.8[c]		
2002	Larson et al.[20]	Prospective phase II	1996-1999	80	39	26:13		50	21-77	GK	16		10-20		9.1		0.3-29.1	10.1	3.8[c]		
2005	Mahajan et al.[23]	Retrospective	1998-2003	41	38			54[a]	17-69[a]	LINAC	NR		NR		4.7[a]		0.15-16.3[a]	11[a]			
2005	Hsieh et al.[22]	Retrospective	1998-2003	51	26		58.2	59[b]	17-81[b]	GK	12[b]		15-32[b]		13.6[b]		0.6-64.4[b]	10			age < 50 years, KPS > 90, the use of chemotherapy
2005	Combs et al.[21]	Retrospective	1993-2001	32	32	19:13		56	33-76	LINAC	15		10-20		10		1.2-59.2	10	5	NS	
2008	Schwer et al.[25]	Prospective Phase I	2004-2006	15	11			47[a]	23-65[a]	LINAC			18-36(3 fx)[a]	Gefitinib	41.3[a]		8.4-150.9	10[a]	7[a]		
2008	Kong et al.[24]	Retrospective	2000-2006	114	65			49[a]	5-75[a]	LINAC (n=5)/GK (n=109)	16[a]		12-50[a]		10.6[a]		0.09-79.6[a]	13	4.6	tumor volume < 10cc	NS
2009	Pouratian et al.[29]	Retrospective	1991-2007	48	26			60.7	12.9-76.9	GK	6		3-15		21.3		0.3-110	9.4	7.1	the use of steroid, time to SRS	the use of steroid
2009	Patel et al.[28]	Retrospective	2001-2006	36	26			53	25-70	LINAC	18		12-20		10.4		0.3-60.1	8.4			
2009	Biswas et al.[26]	Retrospective	2000-2007	33	18			57.8[b]	33-81b	LINAC	15		9-20		8.4		0.2-32.2	5.3	3.4	NS	
2009	Kida et al.[27]	Retrospective	-	172	54[b]		52.4		11-80	GK		14.7	8-25			29	7-48.3	14			
2009	Villavicencio et al.[30]	Retrospective	2002-2005	46	26	18:8	56.4		36-82	CK		20	8-25			7	0.4-48.5	7		NS	NS

2011	Elliott et al.[31]	Retrospective	2004-2009	26	16		60	36.5-70.6[a]	GK	15		12-18		1.35		0.27-11.9[a]	12.9		age at diagnosis, age after SRS for recurrence, interval between surgery and recurrence, KPS ≥ 90, RPA class, tumor volume	interval between surgery and recurrence, KPS ≥ 90, tumor volume
2011	Marazano et al.[32]	Retrospective	2001-2008	22	13		55d	27-81[d]	LINAC	17		14-22		5.3		0.6-14	11	4[d]		
2011	Sirin et al.[33]	Retrospective	1998-2010	19	19	13:6	47	23-65	LINAC	16		10-19		13		2-59	9.3	5.7		
2012	Cuneo et al.[35]	Retrospective	2002-2010	63	33		47[a]		LINAC	15[a]		12.5-25[a]	BEV	4.5[a]			11.2[a]	5.2[a]		KPS > 70, age < 50
2012	Cuneo et al.[35]	Retrospective	2002-2010	63	16		48[a]		LINAC	15[a]		12.5-25[a]		5.6[a]			3.9[a]	2.1[a]		KPS > 70, age < 50
2012	Skeie et al.[38]	Retrospective	1996-2007	77	32	12:20	51	27-73[a]	GK	12.2		8-20			12.4		9			tumor volume, RPA class, neurological deficits, time to recurrence, adjuvant therapy, tumor location
2012	Skeie et al.[38]	Retrospective	1996-2007	77	19	7:12	50	27-73[a]	GK+re-operation	12.2		8-20			13.9		15			tumor volume, RPA class, neurological deficits, time to recurrence, adjuvant therapy, tumor location
2012	Park et al.[37]	Retrospective	1987-2010	11	11	8:3	62	46-72	GK	16		13-18	BEV + irinotecan/ TMZ	13.6		1.2-45.1	17.9	14.9		
2012	Koga et al.[36]	Retrospective	1990-2007	9	8	5:3	43[a]	17-64[a]	GK		>20			15[a]		3-47[a]	10.5			
2012	Koga et al.[36]	Retrospective	2007-2010	9	7	4:3	53[a]	27-79[a]	GK		20			13.6[a]		6-19[a]	9			
2012	Conti et al.[34]	Retrospective	2007-2010	23	11		58[c]		CK		20	NR			15.1	NR	7	4		
2012	Conti et al.[34]	Retrospective	2007-2010	23	12		58[c]		CK		20	NR	TMZ		13.8	NR	12	7		
2013	Cabrera et al.[39]	Prospective trial	2010-2011	15	8		53[a]	25-66[a]	LINAC		18	NR	BEV				14.4[a]	3.9[a]		
2014	Clark et al.[40]	Retrospective	2010-2013	21	18		54.1[a]	30-82[a]	LINAC	30 (5-fractions)			BEV	20[a]		3.6-85.6[a]	12.5[a]	11[a]		
2014	Greenspoon et al.[42]	Prospective cohort	2011-2012	31	31		53	36-75	CK	NR		25-35 (5-fractions)	TMZ	12.1		4.9-19.7	9	7	small tumor volume (<3 cm)	
2014	Dodoo et al.[41]	Retrospective	2001-2007	55	35		51.1a	17-81.1a	GK	20		14-22		4.8		0.03-38.1	11.3			
2014	Martinez-Carrillo et al.[43]	Retrospective	1997-2010	87	46	27:19	49.5	26-78	LINAC		18	14-20			4	0.05-34.1	7.5		age, tumor and treatment volume, RPA class, KPS, margin to the planning target volume	KPS > 80, RPA class, margin to the planning target volume
2014	Yazici et al.[44]	Retrospective	2009-2011	37	37	18:19	37	22-69	CK	30		14-32	BEV	24		2-81	10.6	7.9	tumor volume < 24cc	

2015	Bir et al.[45]	Retrospective	2000-2013	36	36[b]	20:16	53	16-82	GK	14	10-20		11.4		7.9		KPS > 70, age ≤ 50, initial post-operative treatment with EBRT, adjuvant SRS for recurrence	
2015	Niranjan et al.[13]	Retrospective	1987-2008	297	153[b]		58	23-89	GK	15	9-25		14	0.26-84.2	10.2	4.3	age < 60 years, KPS ≥ 80, marginal dose ≥ 15Gy, tumor volume ≤ 14cc	age < 60 years, tumor volume ≤ 14cc
2015	Kim et al.[47]	Retrospective	2002-2011	144	29	13:16	61	35-87	GK	15	9-30		11	0.5-40	9.2	3.6		
2015	Kim et al.[47]	Retrospective	2002-2011	144	28	16:12	53	28-73	GK	15	5-20	TMZ	9.8	0.6-49	15.5	6		
2015	Pinzi et al.[48]	Retrospective	2004-2011	128	88		51[a]	18-79[a]	CK	15 (23 for m-SRS group)[a]	6-22 (12-28 for m-SRS group)[a]		2 (10 for m-SRS group)[a]	0.14-83 (0.63-120 for m-SRS group)[a]	10		age<40 years, RPA class 1-2, other therapy after SRS, Radiotherapy=60Gy	other post-SRS therapies (second-line chemotherapy and/or surgery)
2015	Hasan et al.[46]	Retrospective	2007-2014	19	19	13:6	55	28-78	CK	25 (3-5 fractions)	18-35 (3-5 fractions)	BEV/TMZ/ anti-epidermal factor receptor (125)I-mAB 425/combin a-tion	35	0.9-151.7	5.3		frontal lobe tumor, adjuvant therapy with BEV or TMZ, time to first recurrence > 16 months, tumor volume < 36 cc, RPA class < 5, ECOG < 2	
2016	Frischer et al.[50]	Retrospective	NR	42	42	24:18	57.2	15.7-81.9	GK	10	6-16		5.1	0.6-15	9.6	4.4	MGMT methylation	
2016	Holt et al.[51]	Retrospective	2004-2012	34	34	20:14	59.9	29.7-79.4	CK (n=39)/LINAC(n=2)	23.4 (1-3 fractions)	12-30 (1-3 fractions)		9.2	1-100	10.9		tumor volume	prior TMZ therapy
2016	Bokstein et al.[49]	Retrospective	2004-2013	47	33		53.3[a]	24-86[a]	LINAC	18	14-24	BEV/TMZ/ Carboplatin	2.2[a]	0.2-9.5[a]	12.6	4.8	Adjuvant BEV therapy	
2017	Imber et al.[52]	Retrospective	1991-2013	174	174	102:72	54.1	21.8-85.3	GK	16	10-22		7	0.3-39	10.6			younger age at SRS, higher prescription dose, longer interval between original surgery and SRS

2017	Kim et al.[53]	Retrospective	2004-2015	61	61	34:27		58	27-79	GK	16	9-25		7	0.033-35.1	14 (in methylated group)/ 9 (in unmethylated group)	8.5 (in methylated group)/ 4.6 (in unmethylated group)		MGMT methylation
2017	Sutera et al.[54]	Retrospective	2002-2012	65	55			56[a]	30-87[a]	CK (96.1%)/ LINAC(3.9 %)[a]	21[a]	9-30[a]		8.7[a]	0.3-100[a]	10.25[a]	6.6[a]	prior TMZ therapy	prior TMZ therapy
2018	Guseynova et al.[57]	Retrospective	1992-2014	126	126	69:57		56	17-80	GK	12	10-25		3.75	0.04-37.1	7		age < 50 years	
2018	Sharma et al.[58]	Retrospective	1997-2016	53	53	36:17		58	19-82	GK	18	12-24		3.8	0.01-29.7	11	[illegible].4	KPS ≥ 80; tumor volume < 15 cc, homogeneity index > 1.75	KPS ≥ 80; tumor volume < 15cc, homogeneity index > 1.75
2018	Abbassy et al.[55]	Prospective Phase I		9	9	7:2	52.7		28-71	GK	20	18-22	BEV	4.72	2.1-8.8	13	7.5		
2018	Gigliotti et al.[56]	Retrospective	2000-2017	25	20			54[d]	23-74[d]	LINAC	25[d]	27.5[d]		9.83[d]	0.55-92.78[b]	9		Receiving SRS since 2014	
2019	Morris et al.[59]	Retrospective	2009-2015	45	45	21:24		57	20-78	GK	17	13-24	BEV	2.2	0.1-25.2	13.3	5.2		KPS ≤ 70, SRS dose < 18 Gy, use of <2 chemoagents prior to SRS

[a]Including patients with other malignant glioma.

[b]Including patients with upfront adjuvant SRS for residual tumor.

[c]Represented with all study groups.

[d]Including the patients with fractionated stereotactic radiotherapy.

Abbreviations: rGBM, recurrent glioblastoma multiforme; SRS, stereotactic radiosurgery; NR, not reported; NS, not significant; KPS, Karnofsky performance scale; RPA, recursive partitioning analysis; EBRT, external beam radiation therapy; BEV, bevacizumab; TMZ, temozolomide; ECOG, eastern cooperative oncology group performance status; MGMT, O6-methylguanine-DNA-methyltransferase promoter.

Table 1.
Summary of the published literature on stereotactic radiosurgery in patients with recurrent glioblastoma multiforme.

retrospective studies [14–16, 19, 21, 23–26, 28, 32, 33, 35, 39, 40, 43, 49, 51, 54, 56, 60, 61]. The median age ranged from 34 to 54 years. The median prescribed dose ranged from 13 to 30 Gy. The median targeted tumor volume was 4.5 to 41.3 cc. The median overall survival time from the treatment of SRS ranged from 3.9 to 14.4 months, whereas the median progression-free survival time was 2.1 to 11 months.

The first study about LINAC radiosurgery for recurrent GBMs was described by Chamerian et al. [14]. The median prescribed dose was 13.4 Gy, and the median treated tumor volume was 17 cc. The median overall survival time was only 8 months, whereas the median progression-free survival time was 4 months. After that, only one retrospective study of more than 100 patients with recurrent high-grade gliomas treated with LINAC SRS has been reported [16]. Shrieve et al. showed that the median survival time of 72 recurrent GBM patients was 10.2 months [16]. Younger age (less than 46 years) and small tumor volume (less than 10.1 cc) were the significant prognostic factors associated with survival time. There were two studies that enrolled patients with only recurrent GBMs [21, 33]. In 2005, Combs et al. reported 32 patients, including 19 males and 13 females with recurrent GBMs treated with LINAC SRS [21]. The median age was 56 years, ranging from 33 to 76 years. The median prescribed radiation dose was 15 Gy, ranging from 10 to 20 Gy. The median targeted tumor volume was 10 cc with a range of 1.2 to 59.2 cc. The median overall survival time and progression-free survival time were 10 and 5 months, respectively. However, no prognostic factor was significant enough to influence the survival time. In a retrospective study of 19 patients with recurrent GBMs, Sirin et al. also showed that the median overall survival time and progression-free survival time were only 9.3 and 5.7 months, respectively [33]. In the bevacizumab era, three studies reported the combination of LINAC SRS, and bevacizumab improved the overall survival time ranging from 11.2 to 14.4 months [35, 39, 40]. In a retrospective study of 48 patients with recurrent GBMs, Cuneo et al. reported that the median progression-free survival time in recurrent patients who received adjuvant bevacizumab and LINAC SRS was 5.2 months vs. 2.1 months for patients who received LINAC SRS alone. The median overall survival times for patients who received a combination of adjuvant bevacizumab/LINAC SRS and LINAC SRS alone were 11.2 and 3.9 months, respectively. The authors concluded that the combination of salvage radiosurgery and bevacizumab to treat recurrent malignant gliomas seemed to be associated with improved outcomes. Younger age and higher KPS were still significant prognostic factors associated with overall survival time in patients with recurrent GBMs.

3.2 The effect of gamma knife radiosurgery in patients with recurrent GBMs

From 1996 to 2019, a total of 1247 patients with recurrent GBMs in 23 published studies were treated with Gamma Knife SRS [13, 17, 18, 20, 22, 24, 27, 29, 31, 36–38, 41, 45, 47, 50, 52, 53, 55, 57–59, 61]. The median age ranged from 43 to 61 years. The median prescribed marginal dose varied from 6 to 20 Gy. The median targeted tumor volume ranged from 1.35 to 21.4 cc. The median overall survival time ranged from 7 to 30 months, whereas the median progression-free survival time ranged from 3.8 to 14.9 months.

In a retrospective study of 189 patients with recurrent high-grade gliomas treated with Gamma Knife SRS, Larson et al. first reported that the median overall survival time in 66 patients with recurrent GBMs was 10 months [17]. Younger age, smaller tumor volume, higher KPS, and unifocal tumors were significant prognostic factors associated with patients' overall survival times. Several studies reported the impact of a combination of Gamma Knife SRS and adjuvant chemoagents on overall survival times [17, 37, 47, 55, 59]. In 2002, Larson et al. reported a prospective phase II study on patients who received a combination of Gamma Knife SRS, and marimastat had a median overall survival of 8.7 months, whereas the median survival time in patients who received only Gamma Knife SRS alone was 10.1 months. Marimastat did not offer an advantage for patients with recurrent GBMs. However, in a retrospective study of 57 patients with recurrent GBMs, Kim et al. showed that the combination of adjuvant temozolomide and Gamma Knife SRS significantly improved the medium overall survival time from 9.2 to 15.5 months [47]. In the bevacizumab era, two studies reported that the median survival time was approximately 13 months after the combined treatment of Gamma Knife SRS and adjuvant bevacizumab [55, 59].

3.3 The effect of Cyberknife radiosurgery in patients with recurrent GBMs

From 2009 to 2017, a total of 318 patients with recurrent GBMs in eight published studies were treated with Cyberknife SRS [30, 34, 42, 44, 46, 48, 51, 54]. The median age ranged from 37 to 59.9 years. The median prescribed marginal dose ranged from 15 to 30 Gy. The median targeted tumor volume ranged from 2 to 24 cc. The median overall survival time after Cyberknife SRS ranged from 5.3 to 12 months, whereas the median progression-free survival time ranged from 4 to 7.9 months.

The first report on Cyberknife SRS for patients with recurrent GBMs was published by Villavicencio et al. [30]. The median overall survival time in a total of 26 patients with recurrent GBMs was 7 months. No prognostic factor associated with the overall survival time was identified. In 2015, Pinzi et al. reported a retrospective study of more than 100 patients who had recurrent high-grade glioma treated with Cyberknife SRS [48]. Among 88 patients with recurrent GBMs, the median survival time was 10 months after treatment with Cyberknife SRS. Adjuvant second-line chemotherapy and/or surgery were the significant prognostic factors associated with overall survival times. The effect of adjuvant chemoagents, including bevacizumab, temozolomide, and anti-epidermal factor (125)-mAB 425, on the overall survival times was evaluated in four studies [34, 42, 44, 46]. In 2012, Conti et al. compared the effect of a combination of temozolomide and Cyberknife SRS with that of Cyberknife SRS alone on the overall survival times of patients with recurrent GBMs [34]. The progression-free survival time and median survival time in patients who received the adjuvant temozolomide and Cyberknife SRS were 7 and 12 months, respectively. The patients who received Cyberknife SRS alone had a progression-free survival time and median survival time of only 4 and 7 months, respectively. In the bevacizumab era, Yazici et al. revealed that the median survival time in 37 patients with recurrent GBMs was 10.6 months, whereas the median progression-free survival time was 7.9 months [44]. A tumor volume less than 24 cc was the only significant prognostic factor associated with overall survival times.

4. Discussion

4.1 The role of SRS for recurrent GBMs

GBM is an incurable disease with local progression in the majority of patients. The management of recurrent GBMs is a clinically challenging problem, and treatment options are limited [7, 10]. Although reoperation with gross-total removal of the tumor has been shown to improve the overall survival time in patients with recurrent GBMs, surgery may not be preferred for patients with tumors in the eloquent area, older age, or lower performance status [8]. Re-irradiation offers an alternative option for treating recurrent GBMs. In a systematic review and meta-analysis of re-irradiation with external beam radiotherapy for recurrent GBMs, Kazmi et al. showed that the 6- and 12-month overall survival times from the time of re-irradiation were 70 and 34%, respectively, whereas the 6- and 12-month progression-free survival times were 40 and 16%, respectively [11]. The overall toxicity rate was low, ranging from 4 to 10%.

SRS has the ability to combine surgical and radio-oncological treatments to deliver a high dose of focused radiation on the focal tumor lesion and spare the adjacent normal anatomical structures. For recurrent GBMs, the majority of tumors tend to grow within 2 cm of the contrast-enhancing lesion border, and SRS seems to be a reasonable tool to add radiation boost for the focal lesion followed by the standard treatment of initial radiation with 60 Gy in 30 fractions [4, 13]. In our present review, despite the different SRS modalities with the median prescribed dose ranging from 6 to 30 Gy, the overall survival time from the treatment of SRS ranged from 3.9 to 17.9 months, where the progression-free survival time from the treatment of SRS ranged from 2.1 to 14.9 months. Severe prognostic factors, such as small tumor volume, younger age, higher KPS score, and lower RPA class, were mostly suggested to be significantly associated with the overall survival time in patients with recurrent GBMs treated with SRS. These results showed that re-irradiation with the SRS modality are an alternative and feasible method to manage patients with recurrent GBMs.

4.2 The impact of SRS and adjuvant temozolomide for recurrent GBMs

Since 2005, temozolomide, which is an alkylating agent, is the most important FDA-approved chemoagent for the standard treatment of patients with newly diagnosed GBMs [1, 4]. The median overall survival time significantly improved from 12.1 to 14.6 months after the patients with newly diagnosed GBMs received combined treatments with radiotherapy and adjuvant temozolomide. However, the disease frequently progresses within 6–9 months, and the 2-year survival rate is less than 25% [62]. The failure of temozolomide treatment has been found to be associated with the expression of MGMT protein [63–65]. Among the GBM patients with a methylated MGMT promoter, the median overall survival time was 21.7 months after treatment with radiotherapy and temozolomide, whereas the median survival time was 15.3 months in the unmethylated group treated with radiotherapy alone [64].

Due to the blood-brain barrier, temozolomide rechallenge is considered to be a reasonable option in patients with recurrent GBMs. In this review, the combination of SRS and temozolomide was employed in three studies [34, 42, 47]. Cyberknife SRS was performed in two studies, and the other study used the Gamma Knife SRS. The median overall survival time ranged from 9 to 15.5 months, and the median progression-free survival time was approximately 7 months after the time of SRS treatment. In 2012, Conti et al. analyzed the effect of adjuvant temozolomide in recurrent GBM patients treated with Cyberknife SRS [34]. The median overall survival time significantly improved from 7 to 12 months, whereas the median progression-free survival time improved from 4 to 7 months. Based on 57 recurrent GBM patients, Kim et al. also showed that the improved median overall survival time and progression-free survival time were 15.5 and 6 months, respectively [47]. Otherwise, in a retrospective review of 61 patients who received Gamma Knife SRS as a salvage treatment at the time of the first progression, Kim et al. showed that the median overall survival time was 14 months in the methylated MGMT promoter group and 9 months in the unmethylated group [53]. Methylation of the MGMT promoter was significantly corrected with better overall survival times and progression-free survival times. The results mentioned above indicated that the combination of salvage SRS and adjuvant temozolomide may offer an important treatment option to improve the overall survival times in patients with recurrent GBMs.

4.3 The impact of SRS and adjuvant bevacizumab for recurrent GBMs

Bevacizumab is a recombinant human monoclonal antibody that acts against the vascular endothelial growth factor to prevent the growth and maintenance of tumor blood vessels. In 2009, bevacizumab was approved by the USFDA for the treatment of patients with recurrent GBMs [66, 67]. The use of bevacizumab demonstrated a radiological response of up to 40% [68]. However, in a large prospective phase III trial, the use of adjuvant bevacizumab revealed only improvement in the progression-free survival times from 1.5 to 4.2 months but not in the overall survival times [69]. In a systematic review and meta-analysis, Diaz et al. showed that the survival advantage of bevacizumab at recurrence was limited to 4 months [70]. Although bevacizumab may reduce steroid requirements, there was no additional benefit in the health-related quality of life. The role of bevacizumab in combination with other cytotoxic chemoagents remains unclear.

The role of adjuvant bevacizumab in patients with recurrent GBMs treated with SRS has been reported in nine studies, which were included in our review [35, 37, 39, 40, 44, 46, 49, 55, 59]. The median overall survival time ranged from 5.3 to 17.9 months, whereas the median progression-free survival time ranged from 3.9 to 14.9 months. The comparison of SRA with or without adjuvant bevacizumab was investigated in two studies [35, 37]. Among 49 patients with recurrent GBMs, Cuneo et al. showed that the median overall survival time was 11.2 months in patients receiving SRS and adjuvant bevacizumab and 3.9 months in patients receiving SRS therapy alone [35]. The progression-free survival time also improved from 2.1 to 5.2 months. In a case-controlled study of patients with recurrent GBMs treated with SRS and adjuvant bevacizumab plus temozolomide or irinotecan, Park et al. also showed that the median overall survival time and progression-free survival time improved from 12.2 to 17.9 months and 6.7 to 14.9 months, respectively [37]. In a retrospective study and review of the literature, Morris et al. reported that the dual role of bevacizumab and radiosurgery had a benefit in the overall survival times (11.2–17.9 months) and progression-free survival times (3.9–14.9 months). These results showed the potential therapeutic effect of adjuvant bevacizumab in combination with other treatment modalities, such as cytotoxic chemoagents or salvage SRS, in patients with recurrent GBMs.

4.4 The future of SRS for recurrent GBMs

With the advance of molecular diagnostic techniques, newly diagnosed GBMs should be classified based on the mutant status of isocitrate dehydrogenase 1 defined by the updated guidelines of the World Health Organization in 2016 [71]. These molecular profiles influence the overall survival time and the possible therapeutic effects of chemoagents. Similar to the recurrent GBMs, several main molecules, such as MLH1 [72], CASP8 [73], MSH2 [74], and P53 [74], were found to be different from primary GBMs [75]. The molecular features, intra-tumor heterogeneity, immunogenicity, and microenvironment around the tumor contribute to the clinical prognostic outcomes in patients with recurrent GBMs [7, 10]. Reoperation, re-chemotherapy, and re-irradiation currently remain as the standard treatments for most patients with recurrent GBMs [2, 7, 10, 11]. A growing body of literature, including our current review, demonstrates the tolerability and efficacy of salvage SRS for recurrent GBMs, which did not inhibit re-irradiation, followed by a total of

60 Gy typically applied in the first-line treatment [59]. Although younger age is commonly considered as an important independent prognostic factor that is associated with survival, the selected criteria of salvage SRS for better outcomes need to be investigated in further large prospective studies. In the future, individualized precise multi-modality treatment will play an important role in patients with recurrent GBMs, including the combination of cytotoxic chemotherapy, angiogenesis inhibitors, or immunotherapy [76]. Salvage SRS with a combination of other treatment modalities may offer an alternative therapeutic method to manage patients with recurrent GBMs.

5. Conclusion

Our review suggests that salvage SRS is an important treatment protocol for managing patients with recurrent GBMs. The irradiation doses provided by SRS may improve the clinical outcome of patients with recurrent GBMs, which is not hampered by the standard case of 60 Gy prescribed for newly diagnosed GBMs. The dual role of salvage SRS and other cytotoxic chemoagents, such as temozolomide and bevacizumab, also seems to be effective in the management of recurrent GBMs. Further application of salvage SRS combined with other chemoagents or a new treatment modality needs to be investigated.

Conflict of interest

The authors declare no conflict of interest.

Author details

Cheng-Ta Hsieh[1,2,3] and Da-Tong Ju[3*]

1 Division of Neurosurgery, Department of Surgery, Sijhih Cathay General Hospital, New Taipei City, Taiwan

2 Department of Medicine, School of Medicine, Fu Jen Catholic University, New Taipei City, Taiwan

3 Department of Neurological Surgery, Tri-Service General Hospital, National Defense Medical Center, Taipei City, Taiwan

*Address all correspondence to: wxyz670628@yahoo.com.tw

References

[1] Preusser M, de Ribaupierre S, Wöhrer A, Erridge SC, Hegi M, Weller M, et al. Current concepts and management of glioblastoma. Annals of Neurology. 2011;**70**(1):9-21

[2] Weller M, Cloughesy T, Perry JR, Wick W. Standards of care for treatment of recurrent glioblastoma—Are we there yet? Neuro-Oncology. 2013;**15**(1):4-27

[3] Ostrom QT, Cioffi G, Gittleman H, Patil N, Waite K, Kruchko C, et al. CBTRUS statistical report: Primary brain and other central nervous system tumors diagnosed in the United States in 2012–2016. Neuro-Oncology. 2019;**21** (Suppl. 5):v1-v100

[4] Stupp R, Mason WP, van den Bent MJ, Weller M, Fisher B, Taphoorn MJ, et al. Radiotherapy plus concomitant and adjuvant temozolomide for glioblastoma. The New England Journal of Medicine. 2005;**352**(10):987-996

[5] Sanai N, Polley MY, McDermott MW, Parsa AT, Berger MS. An extent of resection threshold for newly diagnosed glioblastomas. Journal of Neurosurgery. 2011;**115**(1):3-8

[6] Hou LC, Veeravagu A, Hsu AR, Tse VC. Recurrent glioblastoma multiforme: A review of natural history and management options. Neurosurgical Focus. 2006;**20**(4):E5

[7] Mallick S, Benson R, Hakim A, Rath GK. Management of glioblastoma after recurrence: A changing paradigm. Journal of the Egyptian National Cancer Institute. 2016;**28**(4):199-210

[8] Bloch O, Han SJ, Cha S, Sun MZ, Aghi MK, McDermott MW, et al. Impact of extent of resection for recurrent glioblastoma on overall survival: Clinical article. Journal of Neurosurgery. 2012;**117**(6):1032-1038

[9] Lu VM, Goyal A, Graffeo CS, Perry A, Burns TC, Parney IF, et al. Survival benefit of maximal resection for glioblastoma reoperation in the temozolomide era: A meta-analysis. World Neurosurgery. 2019;**127**:31-37

[10] Chaul-Barbosa C, Marques DF. How we treat recurrent glioblastoma today and current evidence. Current Oncology Reports. 2019;**21**(10):94

[11] Kazmi F, Soon YY, Leong YH, Koh WY, Vellayappan B. Re-irradiation for recurrent glioblastoma (GBM): A systematic review and meta-analysis. Journal of Neuro-Oncology. 2019; **142**(1):79-90

[12] Jayamanne D, Wheeler H, Brazier D, Newey A, Kastelan M, Guo L, et al. Predicting patterns of failure in temporal lobe GBMs: Possible implications on radiotherapy treatment portals. Radiotherapy and Oncology. 2018;**13**(1):133

[13] Niranjan A, Kano H, Iyer A, Kondziolka D, Flickinger JC, Lunsford LD. Role of adjuvant or salvage radiosurgery in the management of unresected residual or progressive glioblastoma multiforme in the pre-bevacizumab era. Journal of Neurosurgery. 2015;**122**(4):757-765

[14] Chamberlain MC, Barba D, Kormanik P, Shea WM. Stereotactic radiosurgery for recurrent gliomas. Cancer. 1994;**74**(4):1342-1347

[15] Hall WA, Djalilian HR, Sperduto PW, Cho KH, Gerbi BJ, Gibbons JP, et al. Stereotactic radiosurgery for recurrent malignant gliomas. Journal of Clinical Oncology. 1995;**13**(7):1642-1648

[16] Shrieve DC, Alexander E 3rd, Wen PY, Fine HA, Kooy HM, Black PM, et al. Comparison of stereotactic

radiosurgery and brachytherapy in the treatment of recurrent glioblastoma multiforme. Neurosurgery. 1995;**36**(2): 275-282 discussion 82-4

[17] Larson DA, Gutin PH, McDermott M, Lamborn K, Sneed PK, Wara WM, et al. Gamma knife for glioma: Selection factors and survival. International Journal of Radiation Oncology, Biology, Physics. 1996;**36**(5): 1045-1053

[18] Kondziolka D, Flickinger JC, Bissonette DJ, Bozik M, Lunsford LD. Survival benefit of stereotactic radiosurgery for patients with malignant glial neoplasms. Neurosurgery. 1997;**41**(4):776-783 discussion 83-5

[19] Cho KH, Hall WA, Gerbi BJ, Higgins PD, McGuire WA, Clark HB. Single dose versus fractionated stereotactic radiotherapy for recurrent high-grade gliomas. International Journal of Radiation Oncology, Biology, Physics. 1999;**45**(5):1133-1141

[20] Larson DA, Prados M, Lamborn KR, Smith V, Sneed PK, Chang S, et al. Phase II study of high central dose Gamma knife radiosurgery and marimastat in patients with recurrent malignant glioma. International Journal of Radiation Oncology, Biology, Physics. 2002;**54**(5):1397-1404

[21] Combs SE, Widmer V, Thilmann C, Hof H, Debus J, Schulz-Ertner D. Stereotactic radiosurgery (SRS): Treatment option for recurrent glioblastoma multiforme (GBM). Cancer. 2005;**104**(10):2168-2173

[22] Hsieh PC, Chandler JP, Bhangoo S, Panagiotopoulos K, Kalapurakal JA, Marymont MH, et al. Adjuvant gamma knife stereotactic radiosurgery at the time of tumor progression potentially improves survival for patients with glioblastoma multiforme. Neurosurgery. 2005;**57**(4):684-692 discussion 684

[23] Mahajan A, McCutcheon IE, Suki D, Chang EL, Hassenbusch SJ, Weinberg JS, et al. Case-control study of stereotactic radiosurgery for recurrent glioblastoma multiforme. Journal of Neurosurgery. 2005;**103**(2):210-217

[24] Kong DS, Lee JI, Park K, Kim JH, Lim DH, Nam DH. Efficacy of stereotactic radiosurgery as a salvage treatment for recurrent malignant gliomas. Cancer. 2008;**112**(9):2046-2051

[25] Schwer AL, Damek DM, Kavanagh BD, Gaspar LE, Lillehei K, Stuhr K, et al. A phase I dose-escalation study of fractionated stereotactic radiosurgery in combination with gefitinib in patients with recurrent malignant gliomas. International Journal of Radiation Oncology, Biology, Physics. 2008;**70**(4):993-1001

[26] Biswas T, Okunieff P, Schell MC, Smudzin T, Pilcher WH, Bakos RS, et al. Stereotactic radiosurgery for glioblastoma: Retrospective analysis. Radiotherapy and Oncology. 2009;**4**:11

[27] Kida Y, Yoshimoto M, Hasegawa T. Radiosurgery for intracranial gliomas. Progress in Neurological Surgery. 2009; **22**:122-128

[28] Patel M, Siddiqui F, Jin JY, Mikkelsen T, Rosenblum M, Movsas B, et al. Salvage reirradiation for recurrent glioblastoma with radiosurgery: Radiographic response and improved survival. Journal of Neuro-Oncology. 2009;**92**(2):185-191

[29] Pouratian N, Crowley RW, Sherman JH, Jagannathan J, Sheehan JP. Gamma knife radiosurgery after radiation therapy as an adjunctive treatment for glioblastoma. Journal of Neuro-Oncology. 2009;**94**(3):409-418

[30] Villavicencio AT, Burneikiene S, Romanelli P, Fariselli L, McNeely L, Lipani JD, et al. Survival following stereotactic radiosurgery for newly

diagnosed and recurrent glioblastoma multiforme: A multicenter experience. Neurosurgical Review. 2009;**32**(4): 417-424

[31] Elliott RE, Parker EC, Rush SC, Kalhorn SP, Moshel YA, Narayana A, et al. Efficacy of gamma knife radiosurgery for small-volume recurrent malignant gliomas after initial radical resection. World Neurosurgery. 2011;**76** (1–2):128-140 discussion 61-2

[32] Maranzano E, Anselmo P, Casale M, Trippa F, Carletti S, Principi M, et al. Treatment of recurrent glioblastoma with stereotactic radiotherapy: Long-term results of a mono-institutional trial. Tumori. 2011;**97**(1):56-61

[33] Sirin S, Oysul K, Surenkok S, Sager O, Dincoglan F, Dirican B, et al. Linear accelerator-based stereotactic radiosurgery in recurrent glioblastoma: A single center experience. Vojnosanitetski Pregled. 2011;**68**(11): 961-966

[34] Conti A, Pontoriero A, Arpa D, Siragusa C, Tomasello C, Romanelli P, et al. Efficacy and toxicity of Cyberknife re-irradiation and "dose dense" temozolomide for recurrent gliomas. Acta Neurochirurgica. 2012;**154**(2): 203-209

[35] Cuneo KC, Vredenburgh JJ, Sampson JH, Reardon DA, Desjardins A, Peters KB, et al. Safety and efficacy of stereotactic radiosurgery and adjuvant bevacizumab in patients with recurrent malignant gliomas. International Journal of Radiation Oncology, Biology, Physics. 2012;**82**(5):2018-2024

[36] Koga T, Maruyama K, Tanaka M, Ino Y, Saito N, Nakagawa K, et al. Extended field stereotactic radiosurgery for recurrent glioblastoma. Cancer. 2012;**118**(17):4193-4200

[37] Park KJ, Kano H, Iyer A, Liu X, Niranjan A, Flickinger JC, et al. Salvage gamma knife stereotactic radiosurgery followed by bevacizumab for recurrent glioblastoma multiforme: A case-control study. Journal of Neuro-Oncology. 2012; **107**(2):323-333

[38] Skeie BS, Enger PØ, Brøgger J, Ganz JC, Thorsen F, Heggdal JI, et al. Gamma knife surgery versus reoperation for recurrent glioblastoma multiforme. World Neurosurgery. 2012; **78**(6):658-669

[39] Cabrera AR, Cuneo KC, Desjardins A, Sampson JH, McSherry F, Herndon JE 2nd, et al. Concurrent stereotactic radiosurgery and bevacizumab in recurrent malignant gliomas: A prospective trial. International Journal of Radiation Oncology, Biology, Physics. 2013;**86**(5): 873-879

[40] Clark GM, McDonald AM, Nabors LB, Fathalla-Shaykh H, Han X, Willey CD, et al. Hypofractionated stereotactic radiosurgery with concurrent bevacizumab for recurrent malignant gliomas: The University of Alabama at Birmingham experience. Neurooncology Practice. 2014;**1**(4): 172-177

[41] Dodoo E, Huffmann B, Peredo I, Grinaker H, Sinclair G, Machinis T, et al. Increased survival using delayed gamma knife radiosurgery for recurrent high-grade glioma: A feasibility study. World Neurosurgery. 2014;**82**(5):e623-e632

[42] Greenspoon JN, Sharieff W, Hirte H, Overholt A, Devillers R, Gunnarsson T, et al. Fractionated stereotactic radiosurgery with concurrent temozolomide chemotherapy for locally recurrent glioblastoma multiforme: A prospective cohort study. OncoTargets and Therapy. 2014;**7**:485-490

[43] Martínez-Carrillo M, Tovar-Martín I, Zurita-Herrera M, Del Moral-

Ávila R, Guerrero-Tejada R, Saura-Rojas E, et al. Salvage radiosurgery for selected patients with recurrent malignant gliomas. BioMed Research International. 2014;**2014**:657953

[44] Yazici G, Cengiz M, Ozyigit G, Eren G, Yildiz F, Akyol F, et al. Hypofractionated stereotactic reirradiation for recurrent glioblastoma. Journal of Neuro-Oncology. 2014; **120**(1):117-123

[45] Bir SC, Connor DE Jr, Ambekar S, Wilden JA, Nanda A. Factors predictive of improved overall survival following stereotactic radiosurgery for recurrent glioblastoma. Neurosurgical Review. 2015;**38**(4):705-713

[46] Hasan S, Chen E, Lanciano R, Yang J, Hanlon A, Lamond J, et al. Salvage fractionated stereotactic radiotherapy with or without chemotherapy and immunotherapy for recurrent glioblastoma multiforme: A single institution experience. Frontiers in Oncology. 2015;**5**:106

[47] Kim HR, Kim KH, Kong DS, Seol HJ, Nam DH, Lim DH, et al. Outcome of salvage treatment for recurrent glioblastoma. Journal of Clinical Neuroscience. 2015;**22**(3): 468-473

[48] Pinzi V, Orsi C, Marchetti M, Milanesi IM, Bianchi LC, DiMeco F, et al. Radiosurgery reirradiation for high-grade glioma recurrence: A retrospective analysis. Neurological Sciences. 2015;**36**(8):1431-1440

[49] Bokstein F, Blumenthal DT, Corn BW, Gez E, Matceyevsky D, Shtraus N, et al. Stereotactic radiosurgery (SRS) in high-grade glioma: Judicious selection of small target volumes improves results. Journal of Neuro-Oncology. 2016;**126**(3):551-557

[50] Frischer JM, Marosi C, Woehrer A, Hainfellner JA, Dieckmann KU, Eiter H, et al. Gamma knife radiosurgery in recurrent glioblastoma. Stereotactic and Functional Neurosurgery. 2016;**94**(4): 265-272

[51] Holt DE, Bernard ME, Quan K, Clump DA, Engh JA, Burton SA, et al. Salvage stereotactic radiosurgery for recurrent glioblastoma multiforme with prior radiation therapy. Journal of Cancer Research and Therapeutics. 2016;**12**(4):1243-1248

[52] Imber BS, Kanungo I, Braunstein S, Barani IJ, Fogh SE, Nakamura JL, et al. Indications and efficacy of gamma knife stereotactic radiosurgery for recurrent glioblastoma: 2 decades of institutional experience. Neurosurgery. 2017;**80**(1): 129-139

[53] Kim BS, Kong DS, Seol HJ, Nam DH, Lee JI. MGMT promoter methylation status as a prognostic factor for the outcome of gamma knife radiosurgery for recurrent glioblastoma. Journal of Neuro-Oncology. 2017;**133**(3):615-622

[54] Sutera PA, Bernard ME, Gill BS, Quan K, Engh JA, Burton SA, et al. Salvage stereotactic radiosurgery for recurrent gliomas with prior radiation therapy. Future Oncology. 2017;**13**(29): 2681-2690

[55] Abbassy M, Missios S, Barnett GH, Brewer C, Peereboom DM, Ahluwalia M, et al. Phase I trial of radiosurgery dose escalation plus bevacizumab in patients with recurrent/ progressive glioblastoma. Neurosurgery. 2018;**83**(3):385-392

[56] Gigliotti MJ, Hasan S, Karlovits SM, Ranjan T, Wegner RE. Re-irradiation with stereotactic radiosurgery/ radiotherapy for recurrent high-grade gliomas: Improved survival in the modern era. Stereotactic and Functional Neurosurgery. 2018;**96**(5):289-295

[57] Guseynova K, Liscak R, Simonova G, Novotny J Jr. Gamma knife

radiosurgery for local recurrence of glioblastoma. Neuro Endocrinology Letters. 2018;**39**(4):281-287

[58] Sharma M, Schroeder JL, Elson P, Meola A, Barnett GH, Vogelbaum MA, et al. Outcomes and prognostic stratification of patients with recurrent glioblastoma treated with salvage stereotactic radiosurgery. Journal of Neurosurgery. 2018:1-11

[59] Morris SL, Zhu P, Rao M, Martir M, Zhu JJ, Hsu S, et al. Gamma knife stereotactic radiosurgery in combination with bevacizumab for recurrent glioblastoma. World Neurosurgery. 2019;**127**:e523-e533

[60] Sanghavi S, Skrupky R, Badie B, Robins I, Tome W, Mehta MP. Recurrent malignant gliomas treated with radiosurgery. Journal of Radiosurgery. 1999;**2**(3):119-125

[61] Park JL, Suh JH, Barnett GH, Reddy CA, Peereboom DM, Stevens GHJ, et al. Survival after stereotactic radiosurgery for recurrent glioblastoma multiforme. Journal of Radiosurgery. 2000;**3**(4):169-175

[62] Wen PY, Kesari S. Malignant gliomas in adults. The New England Journal of Medicine. 2008;**359**(5): 492-507

[63] Silber JR, Bobola MS, Blank A, Chamberlain MC. O6-methylguanine-DNA methyltransferase in glioma therapy: Promise and problems. Biochimica et Biophysica Acta. 2012; **1826**(1):71-82

[64] Hegi ME, Diserens AC, Gorlia T, Hamou MF, de Tribolet N, Weller M, et al. MGMT gene silencing and benefit from temozolomide in glioblastoma. The New England Journal of Medicine. 2005;**352**(10):997-1003

[65] Hsieh CT, Su IC, Huang CT, Chang CJ, Wang JS. The prognostic value of O6-methylguanine-DNA methyltransferase gene promoter methylation detected by gel-based methylation-specific polymerase chain reaction in patients with glioblastoma multiforme: A systematic review. International Journal of Clinical and Experimental Medicine. 2016;**9**(6): 10899-10906

[66] Kreisl TN, Kim L, Moore K, Duic P, Royce C, Stroud I, et al. Phase II trial of single-agent bevacizumab followed by bevacizumab plus irinotecan at tumor progression in recurrent glioblastoma. Journal of Clinical Oncology. 2009; **27**(5):740-745

[67] Friedman HS, Prados MD, Wen PY, Mikkelsen T, Schiff D, Abrey LE, et al. Bevacizumab alone and in combination with irinotecan in recurrent glioblastoma. Journal of Clinical Oncology. 2009;**27**(28):4733-4740

[68] Chinot OL, Wick W, Mason W, Henriksson R, Saran F, Nishikawa R, et al. Bevacizumab plus radiotherapy-temozolomide for newly diagnosed glioblastoma. The New England Journal of Medicine. 2014;**370**(8):709-722

[69] Wick W, Gorlia T, Bendszus M, Taphoorn M, Sahm F, Harting I, et al. Lomustine and bevacizumab in progressive glioblastoma. The New England Journal of Medicine. 2017; **377**(20):1954-1963

[70] Diaz RJ, Ali S, Qadir MG, De La Fuente MI, Ivan ME, Komotar RJ. The role of bevacizumab in the treatment of glioblastoma. Journal of Neuro-Oncology. 2017;**133**(3):455-467

[71] Louis DN, Perry A, Reifenberger G, von Deimling A, Figarella-Branger D, Cavenee WK, et al. The 2016 World Health Organization classification of tumors of the central nervous system: A summary. Acta Neuropathologica. 2016; **131**(6):803-820

[72] Stark AM, Doukas A, Hugo HH, Mehdorn HM. The expression of mismatch repair proteins MLH1, MSH2 and MSH6 correlates with the Ki67 proliferation index and survival in patients with recurrent glioblastoma. Neurological Research. 2010;**32**(8): 816-820

[73] Martinez R, Setien F, Voelter C, Casado S, Quesada MP, Schackert G, et al. CpG island promoter hypermethylation of the pro-apoptotic gene caspase-8 is a common hallmark of relapsed glioblastoma multiforme. Carcinogenesis. 2007;**28**(6):1264-1268

[74] Stark AM, Witzel P, Strege RJ, Hugo HH, Mehdorn HM. p53, mdm2, EGFR, and msh2 expression in paired initial and recurrent glioblastoma multiforme. Journal of Neurology, Neurosurgery, and Psychiatry. 2003; **74**(6):779-783

[75] Campos B, Olsen LR, Urup T, Poulsen HS. A comprehensive profile of recurrent glioblastoma. Oncogene. 2016; **35**(45):5819-5825

[76] Seystahl K, Gramatzki D, Roth P, Weller M. Pharmacotherapies for the treatment of glioblastoma—Current evidence and perspectives. Expert Opinion on Pharmacotherapy. 2016; **17**(9):1259-1270

Chapter 10

Anticancer Photodynamic Therapy Using Ruthenium(II) and Os(II)-Based Complexes as Photosensitizers

Pavel Kaspler, Arkady Mandel, Roger Dumoulin-White and Mark Roufaiel

Abstract

Photodynamic therapy (PDT) is an approved procedure using a photosensitizer (PS) activated by light to selectively destroy malignant/premalignant cells. Transition metal complexes, such as Ru(II)- and Os(II)-based PSs (Theralase Technologies Inc., Ontario. Canada), are activated in a wide range of wavelengths, are resistant to photobleaching and have a high singlet oxygen quantum yield and ability to produce cytotoxic reactive oxygen species (ROS). Their design allows fine-tuning of the photophysical and photochemical properties. They demonstrate Type I and II photoreactions, and some are activated in hypoxia. High PDT potency and activation under NIR light and even X-ray may provide an advantage over the approved PSs. Their ability to associate with transferrin (Tf) as an endogenous delivery system increases photobleaching resistance, ROS production, selective cellular uptake, and PDT efficacy in combination with a decreased systemic toxicity. This makes these PSs attractive for systemic therapy of recurrent/progressive cancers. Their PDT efficacy has been demonstrated in various in vitro and in vivo clinically relevant models. The unique properties of the mentioned PSs allow bypassing such limitations of PDT as low specific uptake ratio, insufficiently broad absorption band, and low efficacy in hypoxia. One of these PSs (TLD-1433) was successful against non-muscle invasive urinary bladder cancer unresponsive to contemporary anticancer therapies.

Keywords: photodynamic therapy, photosensitizer, transition metal, Ru(II), Os(II), complex, transferrin, selectivity, tumor, cancer, urinary bladder

1. Introduction

Photodynamic therapy (PDT) is an actively developing anticancer modality that offers advantages compared to conventional treatments (ionizing radiation and chemotherapy). PDT utilizes two components, light and a photosensitizing compound (PS) activated by light upon photon absorption and producing in its activated state highly cytotoxic reactive oxygen species (ROS) [1]. The attractiveness of PDT is in the use of safe nonthermal doses of light and nontoxic concentrations of the PS and evoking cytotoxic and immunologic effects upon activation of the PS by light. PDT is supposed to selectively destroy unwanted and/or malignant cells while largely sparing the surrounding healthy tissue. Another desirable property is the ability to induce antigen-specific therapeutic and/or protective immune responses.

Preferential PS uptake by the tumors would make them exclusive targets for cytotoxicity while sparing normal tissues. Light delivery (both source location and emitted energy) can also be controlled more carefully (within the confines of the effective light attenuation in the tissue), which could make PDT a very efficient and safe modality. PDT effects reply upon a variety of photoreactions. The most commonly considered are the two types dependent on oxygen and associated with ROS production: electron transfer from the excited PS generating hydroxyl radical OH among other species (Type I) and energy transfer to a ground-state molecular oxygen 3O2 generating singlet oxygen 1O2 and superoxide radical anions (Type II) [2]. It is proposed that two more types are possible and are oxygen-independent: Type III as the interaction of the activated PS with native free radicals and Type IV as light-induced structural changes in PS allowing it to bind to subcellular targets [3].

PDT has been approved almost 20 years ago as an anticancer treatment. Nevertheless, despite the potential advantages, it is still underutilized clinically. Only a small number of porphyrin- and chlorine-like photosensitizers, as well as one bacteriochlorophyll-based PS, are approved. The number of indications for each photosensitizer is also very limited and includes primarily superficial cancerous/precancerous lesions and other conditions such as actinic keratosis, basal cell carcinoma, high-grade dysplasia in Barrett's esophagus, and age-related macular degeneration. As a palliative measure, PDT is approved for obstructive esophageal or lung cancer and centrally located lung cancer [4, 5]. There are several reasons for this.

One of them is a small depth of penetration of visible light into the tissues restricting PDT to superficial lesions with a thickness not exceeding few millimeters. For deeper organs/tissues, an invasive direct delivery of light is required. Light absorbance of longer wavelengths by the PSs is therefore very advantageous. Light in the range of 650–1350 nm (known as "near-infrared window") [6] has the greatest penetrating ability into biological tissues. This includes parts of red (625–740 nm) and near-infrared (>750 nm) range that can be used for the PS activation.

Another problem is an unsatisfactory selectivity for malignant tissues resulting in PDT-associated damage of normal tissues. For example, Photofrin® is known for this [4]. Prolonged retention of many porphyrin-based PSs in healthy tissues leads to a problem of sensitivity to sunlight and potentially serious damage to the patients' skin and eye [7, 8]. This could be mitigated by delivery systems selectively targeting malignant cells. These systems employ two modes of action [9]. Passive targeting relies upon the morphological and physiological peculiarities of tumor tissue in combination with physicochemical properties of the PS carrier. Active targeting, in contrast, is based on a molecular recognition of the PS carrier by cancer cells such as binding of specific ligands or antibodies to overexpressed cancer cell receptors. Passive PS delivery systems include nanoparticles, fullerenes, and liposomes and have the advantage of protecting the PS from degradation upon injection. Active systems, on the other hand, have the advantage of improved uptake of the PS. The carriers belonging by themselves to passive targeting systems can be nevertheless supplemented with molecular recognition capacity belonging to the features of active systems, such as decoration with Tf to target Tf receptors overexpressed in malignant cells [10–12]. Nevertheless, smaller active targeting systems (such as PS-Tf conjugates discussed further in this chapter) could have an advantage of greater mobility upon intracellular uptake and potentially the advantage of the blood-brain barrier crossing.

Lastly, PDT-induced ROS production strongly relies upon oxygen availability, which is well known for the porphyrin-based PSs [13, 14]. Deep bulky tumors have extensive hypoxic regions, which are also associated with the tumor aggressiveness [15, 16]. Although hypoxic regions still can be treated (at a slower rate) by application of fractionated exposure or inducing reperfusion [17, 18], hypoxia severely decreases PDT efficacy [19]. Together with the limited light penetration, this is another reason why PDT in its current state is usually limited to relatively superficial lesions. This problem could be bypassed by PSs employing photoreactions that have little or no dependency on oxygen.

Considering the said above, an advanced PS should have the ability for targeted delivery; penetration through the blood-brain barrier (BBB) and blood-tumor cell barrier (BTCB); activation by a wide range of wavelengths, including NIR light; and employing of different types of photoreactions enabling induction of immune responses to tumor antigens. Solubility in water and/or saline is a great asset for a successful PS as it makes its delivery both easier and safer, without the use of excipients with potential toxicity/side effects on their own.

Metal-based coordination complexes are among the obvious candidates to satisfy these requirements. Specifically, transition metal complexes possess a wide range of metal oxidation states and the complex geometries [5, 20]. These complexes (e.g., Ru(II) polypyridyl complexes) are of increasing interest as PSs in photodynamic therapy (PDT) and, more recently, for photochemotherapy (PCT) [21]. Importantly, they can have their properties fine-tuned by choosing the central metal and organic ligands (such as bipyridine and 2,2′-biquinoline). These PSs can employ a great variety of excited states associated with the central metal, ligands, or metal-ligand interactions. This is manifested in photoreactions that are ROS-dependent (Type I/II) or ROS-independent (electron transfer to substrates other than molecular oxygen), excitation at different wavelengths, solubility, systemic toxicity, and finally PDT efficacy. Historically, Pt(IV)-, Ru(II)-, and Rh(III)-based complexes were most actively studied as PSs followed by Ir(III) and Os(II) complexes; see the review by Monro et al. [5]. The examples of the most recent studies [22–26] include a summary on the use of ruthenium complexes as PSs in PDT [27].

This chapter reviews the results obtained by our group and collaborators. The properties and PDT efficacy of Theralase Technologies Inc. PSs [28] and Ru(II)- and Os(II)-based complexes are discussed in the perspective of their clinical application.

2. Physical and chemical properties of the transitional metal-based PSs

2.1 Molecular structure

The molecular structure of Ru(II)- and Os(II)-based PSs (later referred to as Ru- and Os-based) is shown in **Tables 1–3**. These are relatively small (approximately 1 kDa) complexes with the ligands involving bipyridine (bip), 2,2′-biquinoline (biq), imidazo[4,5-f][1,10]phenanthroline, and a variable number of thiophene units. A variety of the ligands defines some of the PS properties. For example, the biq ligand is responsible for relatively good absorbance in near-infrared (NIR) light, while the number of thiophene units may be associated with the PS solubility in water [5]. Water solubility, as it was mentioned, represents a serious advantage for this group of PSs as many of the established PSs have poor water solubility [29, 30]. Ru-based PSs are characterized by $^1O_2$ quantum yield that is much higher (up to 99%) than for the established (FDA-approved) porphyrin-based PSs: PPIX, an active metabolite of ALA (0.56) and Photofrin (0.89).

TLD-1011 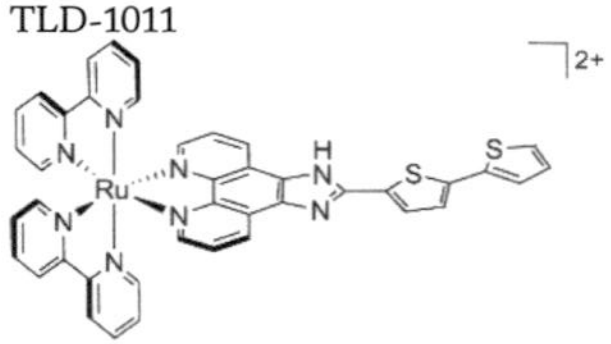 MW = 868.8 $^1O_2$ quantum yield = 0.74 Fluorescent quantum yield = 0.001	TLD-1411 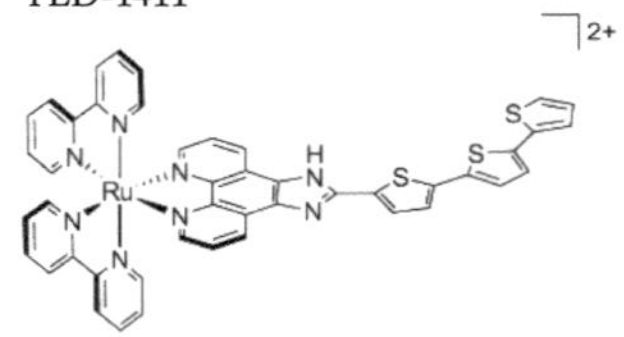 MW = 950.9 $^1O_2$ quantum yield ≈ 0.99 Fluorescent quantum yield < 0.01	TLD-1611 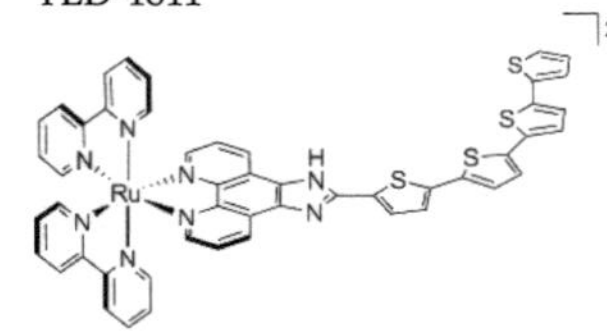 MW = 1033.1 $^1O_2$ quantum yield n/d Fluorescent quantum yield n/d
	TLD-1433 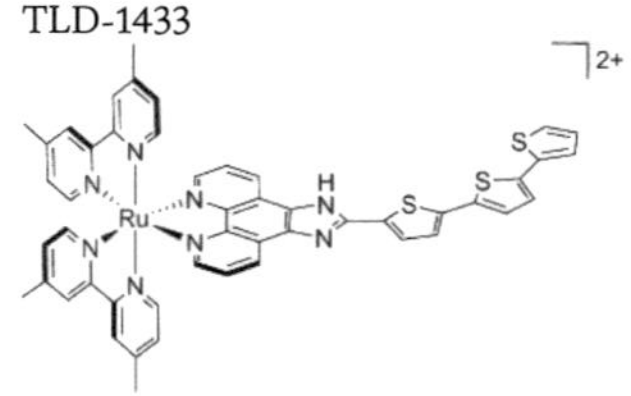 MW = 1007.1 $^1O_2$ quantum yield ≈ 0.99 Fluorescent quantum yield < 0.01	TLD-1633 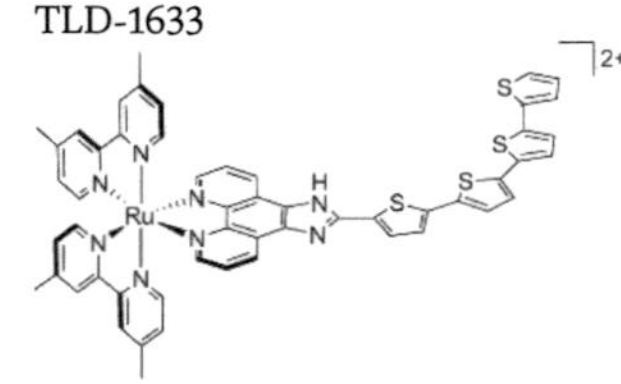 MW = 1089.2 $^1O_2$ quantum yield n/d Fluorescent quantum yield n/d

Table 1.
Ru(II)-based complexes. Quantum yields are measured in solution rather than in cells.

TLD-OsH2B 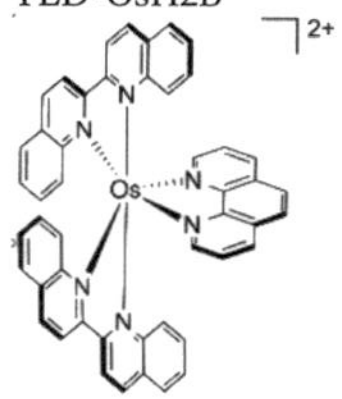 MW = 954.0 $^1O_2$ quantum yield = 0.035 Fluorescent quantum yield = 0.0011	TLD-OsH2IP 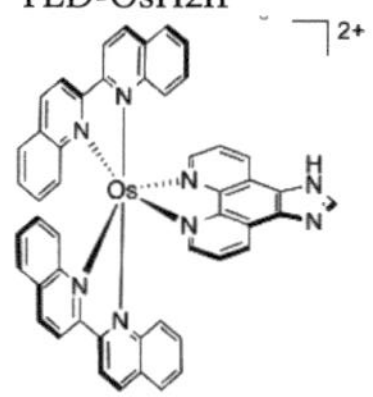 MW = 994.0 $^1O_2$ quantum yield = 0.044 Fluorescent quantum yield =0.0008	TLD-Os10H 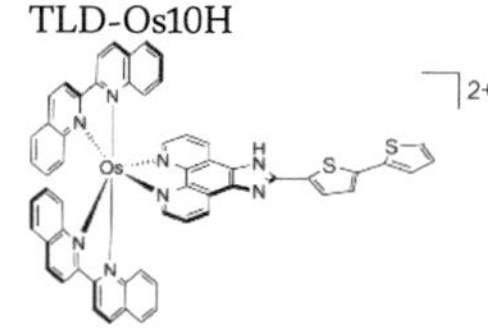 MW = 1158.2 $^1O_2$ quantum yield = 0.035 Fluorescent quantum yield =0.0013	TLD-Os14H 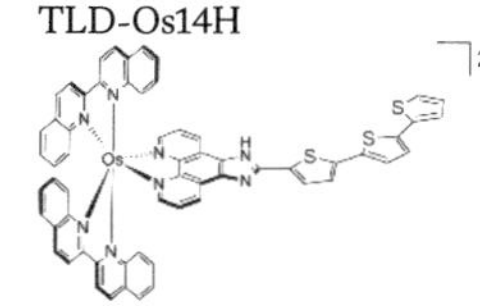 MW = 1240.3 $^1O_2$ quantum yield = 0.03 Fluorescent quantum yield =0.0009
TLD-OsH2dppn 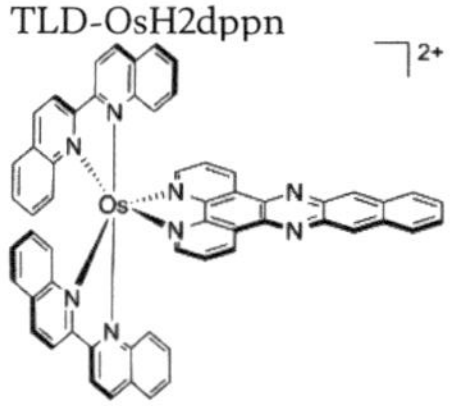 MW = 1106.1 $^1O_2$ quantum yield n/d Fluorescent quantum yield n/d			

Table 2.
Molecular structures of Os(II)-based complexes. Quantum yields are measured in solution rather than in cells.

Bipyridine	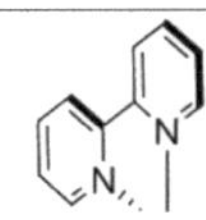
Methylated bipyridine	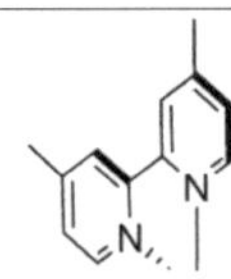
Imidazo[4,5-f][1,10]phenanthroline	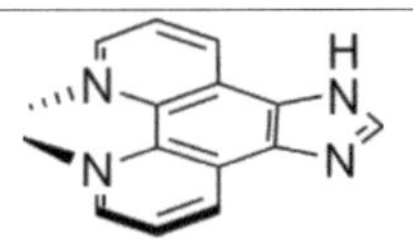
Thiophene	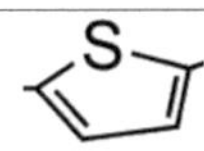
2,2′-biquinoline	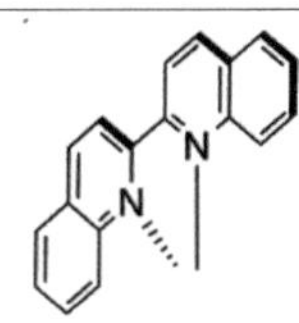
benzo[*i*]dipyrido[3,2-*a*:2′,3′-c]phenazine	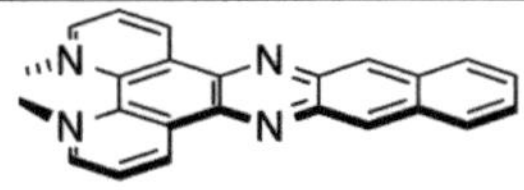

Table 3.
Ligands involved in the PSs' molecular structure.

2.2 Absorbance spectra

The absorbance spectra of the Ru- and Os-based PSs are shown in **Figure 1**. Among the Ru-based PSs, methylation of bidentate ligands (bip) decreases absorbance. An increase in the number of thiophene rings redshifts the main absorbance peak and eventually results in a considerable increase in absorbance at longer wavelengths (see TLD-1633).

Os-based PSs having biq ligands, in contrast to the Ru-based PSs, have similar spectra. They demonstrate rather uniformly located strong main peak at approximately 340 nm attributed to ligand-centered transitions and a characteristic secondary peak at ≈550 nm attributed to metal-to-ligand charge transfer (MLCT) centered on the non-biq ligands. Importantly, these PSs demonstrate consistent

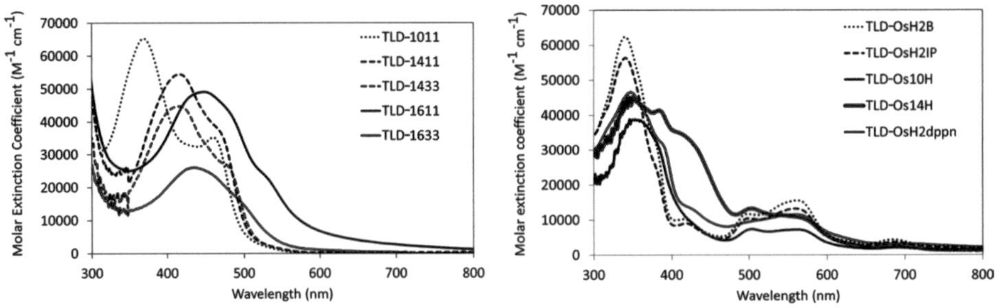

Figure 1.
Absorbance spectra of the Ru(II)- and the Os(II)-based PSs (panels A and B, respectively) in water.

absorbance at longer wavelengths (red to NIR range). The NIR absorbance is attributed to MLCT that involves biq ligands. Altogether, the spectra similarity suggests similar accessible electronic transitions and ground and excited states. Broad absorption band of the Os-based PSs allows for a wider range of photon attenuation coefficients. Considerable absorbance in a clinically important PDT window of 700–900 nm suggests a capacity for one-photon absorption [31]. This asset is emphasized by a good solubility of these PSs in water. Poor solubility in water may hamper PDT potential of PSs even with a good absorbance in this range of the spectrum, as in the case of porphyrin- and phthalocyanine-based PSs [32]. The inclusion of thiophenes and the increase in their number in the ligands (from TLD-OsH2B to TLD-Os14H) not only decreases the main absorbance peak but also markedly redshifts its shape, with a minimal effect on the secondary peak and absorbance in the longer wavelengths (**Figure 1B**).

2.3 Photobleaching resistance

If the PS is resistant to photobleaching, this allows less PS being destroyed by the light exposure. In turn, this makes ROS production and subsequent cytotoxic action more efficient, because the process of conversion of photons to cytotoxicity becomes catalytic without stoichiometric consumption of the PS. This allows making the efficacy of PDT treatment independent on the availability of the PS during the treatment.

The bleaching resistance is hence a very valuable property, especially if the delivered light energy must be increased to achieve the desired PDT efficacy. This could be a drawback though in the case of bleaching-based dosimetry during the treatment [33, 34].

Ru-based PSs show notable bleaching under exposure to green light (525 nm). TLD-1433 is slightly more bleaching resistant than TLD-1411 although they have almost identical absorbance at 525 nm. Nevertheless, more than 50% of each PS remains intact even after 200 Jcm^{-2} of radiant exposure corresponding to $6.6x10^{19}$-absorbed photons per cm^3. Moreover, while bleaching results in the deterioration of the 416–417 nm UV peak, TLD-1433 absorbance in clinically useful range rapidly increases (1.7-fold at 525 nm, 2.0-fold at 625 nm, 1.8-fold at 800 nm) and remains at this level up to the end of light exposure (200 Jcm^{-2}).

Os-based PSs having biq ligands show variable bleaching resistance under green light (525 nm); TLD-OsH2B is the most resistant and TLD-OsH2dppn the most vulnerable. Compared to the Ru-based PS, the bleaching resistance of the Os-based PSs with biq ligands is greater in general, with at least 75% of their initial absorbance retained. The best performers, TLD-OsH2B and TLD-OsH2IP, showed no more than 10% loss of absorbance in the UV peak, with no absorbance loss in green-NIR range. This provides the photobleaching rates in aqueous solution (calculated based on the incident irradiance) equal to $8.7*10^{-28}$ M $h\upsilon^{-1}$ cm^{-2} for TLD-OsH2dppn, $4.1*10^{-27}$ M $h\upsilon^{-1}$ cm^{-2} for TLD-OsH2IP, and $1.5*10^{-2}6$ M $h\upsilon^{-1}$ cm^{-2} for TLD-OsH2B [31]. For comparison, the photobleaching rate for the approved PSs can be much higher (by several orders of magnitude): $5.6*10^{-24}$ M $h\upsilon^{-1}$ cm^{-2} for benzoporphyrin derivative mono acid A (BPD), $7.3*10^{-23}$ M $h\upsilon^{-1}$ cm^{-2} for PPIX, and $4.8*10^{-16}$ M $h\upsilon^{-1}$ cm^{-2} for curcumin [35–37].

2.4 ROS production

Production of ROS represents a final event of the PS activation by light leading to PDT cytotoxicity. Ru-based TLD-1433 is able to generate hydroxyl radical *OH under red light (625 nm, 119 $mWcm^{-2}$), although singlet oxygen $^1O_2$ production is not detected. Importantly, ROS is generated despite very low absorbance of TLD-1433 in red light. This, however, requires certain molecular and ionic environment because ROS is generated only in incomplete DMEM cell culture medium (not complemented with FBS and antibiotics) but not in DI water despite almost identically low absorbance.

Exposure to NIR light (808 nm, 720 $mWcm^{-2}$) produces some amount of ROS (*OH), but it at least an order of magnitude less than under red light. This occurs despite a similar number of absorbed photons and absorbance at 808 nm only 18% less than at 625 nm and greater delivered energy. This may suggest that not only the total delivered energy and number of the absorbed photons but also the photon energy is important for the efficacy in ROS production.

3. Association of the PSs with transferrin

3.1 Delivery platforms

To address the challenge of selective uptake of the PSs by tumors, it would be attractive to utilize serum proteins and natural transmembrane transporters as delivery vehicles. Despite numerous approaches for targeted delivery of the PSs including receptors-assisted uptake (as mentioned in the chapter introduction), neither is related to the use of Tf as a vehicle for transition metal-based complexes. The notable exceptions are the works on the interaction between Tf and Cr(III) complexes [38, 39]. It is also known that Ru(II) complexes can associate with albumin and iron transporter transferrin (Tf) [40, 41]. In addition, overexpression of Tf receptors is a common feature of malignant cells that tend to have an increased Fe^{3+} uptake [42]. The effect of the association of Ru(II)-based PSs with Tf on their photophysical and photobiological properties needs however more elucidation.

3.2 Association signatures and effect of Tf on absorbance spectra

Upon subtraction of the spectra of the complex and Tf from the spectrum of their premix, a characteristic signature of association between the Ru-based complex and Tf can be detected, with two peaks in UV and visible range. The UV peak indicates conformational changes in aromatic rings (the complex itself or transferrin molecule), and the visible range peak is interpreted as an indicator of LMCT (ligand to metal charge transfer) that represents the interaction between the metal of the complex and transferrin [43].

Premixing of Ru-based complexes with apo-Tf (the Tf not saturated with Fe^{3+}) at 4:1 molar ratio demonstrates the signature with UV and visible range peaks (**Figure 2A**). The absorbance increase in UV range could be due to conformation changes either in the Tf molecule or the complex (as both have UV maxima at similar wavelengths). The peak in visible range indicates a new spectral component distinct (redshifted) from the comparable absorbance peak for the PS alone. This indicates the complex-Tf association and is related to the interaction between the metal in the complex and the Tf molecule.

There is also an increase in absorbance between the signature peaks and, importantly, in the long wavelength tail of the spectrum in the visible range and further into the NIR, which is clinically relevant for PDT. Notably, the absorbance of TLD-1433 alone is very low in red to NIR. The increase in absorbance upon the association with Tf is 16.2-fold (MEC = 3125 vs. 193 M^{-1} cm^{-1}) in red (635 nm) and 5.7-fold (MEC = 1676 vs. 294 M^{-1} cm^{-1}) in NIR (800 nm), compared to 5.0-fold (MEC = 8027 vs. 1600 M^{-1} cm^{-1}) increase in the green (535 nm). Notably, the ability of the PS to associate with Tf depends on the number of thiophene rings in the complex. One

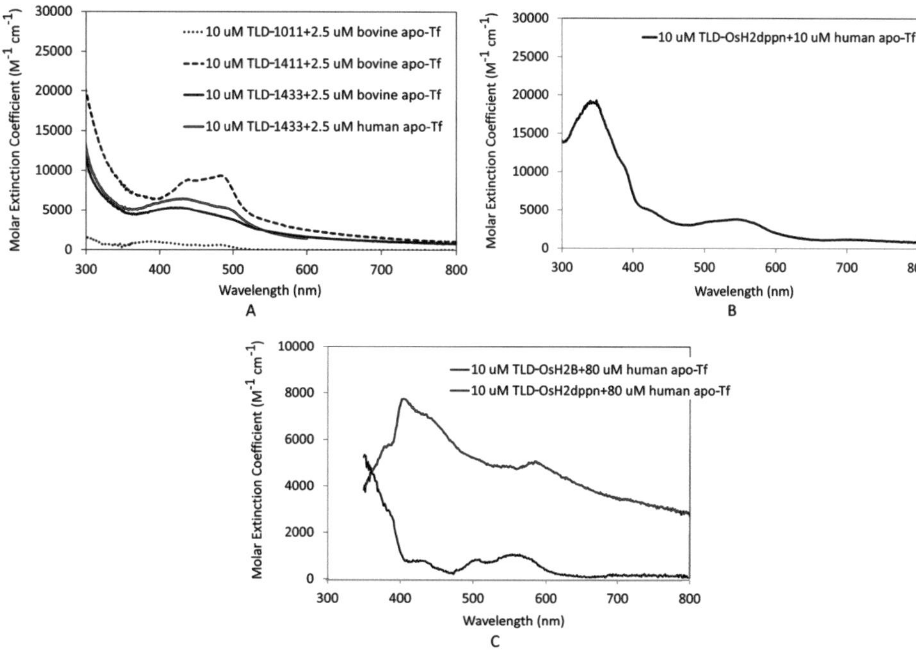

Figure 2.
Spectral signatures of association of the Ru(II)-based (panel A) and Os(II)-based (panels B and C) PSs with apo-Tf. The incubation of Ru-based PSs was performed in 10 mM phosphate buffer +100 mM NaCl (pH = 7.4) and of Os(II)-based PSs in the phosphate buffer (panel B) or incomplete RPMI1640 cell culture media (panel C).

thiophene ring is not enough for this as evident for TLD-1011. Hence, not only metal but also organic ligands play a role in the association of the complex with Tf.

The association signatures seem to be insensitive to the source of apo-Tf and are very similar for bovine and human Tf. The signatures resemble the signature of Fe^{3+}–Tf binding but are not identical to it. Notably, TLD-1433 can also be associated with Fe^{3+} saturated holo-Tf although the magnitude of the association signature is lesser than for apo-Tf [43].

Os-based PSs with biq ligands are also able to associate with apo-Tf, but their signatures (**Figure 2C**) are distinct from those of Ru-based PSs. The visible range peak (observed for TLD-OsH2B and TLD-OsH2dppn but not for TLD-OsH2IP) is however more redshifted (in the range of 500–600 nm), and the signature magnitude is much lesser.

3.3 Stability of the TLD-1433 + Tf association at low pH

Physiologically, when Tf bound with Fe^{3+} is taken up into a cell, it releases iron in endosomes when pH is decreased to ≈5.5 [44]. TLD-1433-Tf conjugate, in contrast, remains stable during the gradual acidification emulating this process [43]. This is evident by the stability of absorbance at the two peaks of the signature across different pH values.

Notably, an association of TLD-1433 with holo-Tf also survives the acid environment. The magnitude of the signature peaks is 31–33% lower than for TLD-1433 & apo-Tf at pH = 7.4, but by pH = 5 it increases so the UV peak magnitude catches up with that of TLD-1433 & apo-Tf, and the visible peak magnitude even becomes about 20% greater. Hence, TLD-1433 may remain associated with Tf in the acidic endosome environment. Acidification resistance does not hold however for the increased absorbance in green to NIR range. The increase in red-NIR range due to the association of TLD-1433 with Tf deteriorates completely at low pH, and only in the green range, it shows some resistance: 16% remaining for TLD-1433 & apo-Tf and 66% for TLD-1433 & holo-Tf.

3.4 Effect of Tf on photobleaching

Association with Tf markedly decreases the extent and rate of photobleaching of TLD-1433 under green light (525 nm, 130 $mWcm^{-2}$). At $0.93*10^{20}$ absorbed photons per cm^3, more than 59% of TLD-1433 remains intact in 1:1 TLD-1433 & Tf premix. At the comparable absorbed light ($0.23*10^{20}$ absorbed photons per cm^3), 74% of TLD-1433 in the premix persists compared to 45% of TLD-1433 alone [43]. As mentioned above, a decreased bleaching allows for more efficient ROS production with less PS expended, so the advantage of TLD-1433 & Tf conjugate is evident.

3.5 Effect of Tf on ROS production

Association of TLD-1433 with Tf dramatically increases ROS production upon irradiation with red light (625 nm, 119 $mWcm^{-2}$). In this case, $^1O_2$ is generated, which does not happen with TLD-1433 alone. The production of *OH is increased twofold at $1.9*10^{22}$ absorbed photons per cm^3 [43]. The association with Tf is therefore advantageous for ROS production considering that *OH is not only an extremely cytotoxic ROS but can also be produced from $^1O_2$ [45]. The association with Tf is, however, unable to improve ROS production by TLD-1433 under NIR (808 nm, 720 $mWcm^{-2}$) despite the increase in absorbance in this range.

4. In vitro PDT

Transition metal-based PSs hence are able to absorb light at clinically relevant wavelengths and produce cytotoxic ROS, and the association with Tf is beneficial in that. This warrants assessment of this capacity in biological systems. In vitro, the PDT effects are tested using clinically relevant human cancer cell lines (human glioblastoma U87 cells, human bladder cancer HT1376 cells) or nonhuman cells relevant for preclinical models (rat bladder cancer AY27 cells).

4.1 Ru-based PSs

The comparative efficacy of the Ru-based PSs on U87 cells is shown in **Table 4**. PDT efficacy of the Ru-based PSs can be very efficient in green light (LD50 in sub-nanomolar range) and moderately efficient in red light (LD50 in micromolar range in red light), but they are not active in NIR light. Notably, the efficacy of the PSs in red light is observed despite negligible absorbance (measured in water). In complete cell culture medium (and potentially intracellularly), absorbance in red is increased due to associaiton of the PSs with proteins but is still low compared to that at the shorter wavelengths.

Depending on the PS, the maximal PDT effect did not reach 100% cell kill. The data at 45 Jcm^{-2} PDT are not shown, but the increase in the light radiant exposure from 45 to 90 Jcm^{-2} significantly ($P < 0.05$) decreased LD50 for the PDT effect in green light. In red light, the PDT efficacy also could be increased with the increase in the radiant exposure from 45 to 90 and then to 180 Jcm^{-2}. This can be explained by the insufficient number of incident photons per a given concentration of the PS at lower radiant exposure but not by a difference in quantum efficacy of the PDT that

U87 cells	Dark	Green	Red	NIR
		530 nm	625 nm	808 nm
		90 Jcm^{-2}	90 Jcm^{-2}	400-600 Jcm^{-2}
		108 $mWcm^{-2}$	125 $mWcm^{-2}$	150 $mWcm^{-2}$
TLD-1411	LD50 (μM): 101.5 (CI95 = 87.8–117.4)	LD50 (μM):0.00595 (CI95 = 0.0050–0.0074)	LD50 (μM): 0.909 (CI95 = n/d-12.36)	Insufficient cell kill
		Maximal kill (%): 49.41 (CI95 = 46.9–52.0)	Maximal kill (%): 71.17 (CI95 = 33.7–124.1)	
	N = 28	N = 9	N = 5	
MEC (water)		2520	151	86
TLD-1433	LD50 (μM): 192.9 (CI95 = 146.8–253.3)	LD50 (μM): 0.00702 (CI95 = 0.00261–0.01891)	LD50 (μM):3.57 (CI95 = 2.99–4.40)	Inconsistent and low cell kill
		Maximal kill (%): 65.9 (CI95 = 59.1–72.8)	Maximal kill (%): 76.2(CI95 = 66.7–85.8)	
	N = 118	N = 32	N = 32	
MEC (water)		3094	158	294
TLD-1611	LD50 (μM): 62.9 (CI95 = 44.9–92.5)	LD50 (μM): 0.002 (CI95 = 0.00117–0.0040)	Inconsistent and low cell kill	No cell kill
		Maximal kill (%):74.8 (CI95 = 65.7–83.9)		
	N = 31	N = 9		
MEC		24,263	4635	1167
TLD-1633	LD50 (μM): 31.13 (CI95 = 14.85 to 63.68)	LD50 (μM): 0.000574 (CI95 = 2.403e-006–0.005691)	Inconsistent and low cell kill	No cell kill
		Maximal kill (%): 100.8 (52.2–171.0)		
	N = 14	N = 6		
MEC (water)		7468	741	0
Photofrin®	LD50 (μM): 2974 (CI95 = 245.5–36,027)	LD50 (μM): 0.20 (CI95 = 0.16–0.25)	LD50 (μM): 0.23 (CI95 = 0.17–0.31)	No cell kill
		Maximal kill (%): 79.7 (CI95 = 72.5–87.0)	Maximal kill (%): 91.8 (CI95 = 83.2–100.4)	
	N = 45	N = 18	N = 26	
MEC (water)		6947	3046	209

The cells were incubated with the PS for 4 h, and the PS was removed before PDT. The dose–response provides LD50 (μM) and maximal cell kill (%) for a green and red light and a cell kill for a fixed PS concentration for NIR light. The data are presented as means and their 95% confidence intervals (SEM for NIR PDT).

Table 4.
In vitro PDT efficacy of Ru(II)-based PSs on U87 cells, in comparison to the FDA-approved Photofrin®.

depends only on the photon energy but not on the radiant exposure. The increase in the number of thiophenes in the PS complexes decreases LD50 for the green light and hence increases PDT efficacy. The dark toxicity is however also increasing. In HT1376 cells, LD50 in red light (90 Jcm^{-2}) is 15.0 μM (CI95 = 9.1–24.9 μM, N = 30).

This is a greater value than for U87 cells and suggests lesser PDT sensitivity. The total PDT cell kill is however high, 98.5% (CI95 = 85.6–111.4%). Dark toxicity is, in contrast, low, with LD50 exceeding 200 μM. Importantly, the efficacy of the Ru-based PSs exceeds the efficacy of FDA-approved Photofrin® in green light, although not in red light (**Table 4**). Judging by LD50, the Ru-based PSs have higher dark toxicity than Photofrin®, but this is of less importance because, in addition to their solubility in water, they are effective at much lesser, nontoxic concentrations.

Pure PDT effect elucidates the PS efficacy for PDT neglecting its dark toxicity, which is justifiable scientifically to reveal mechanisms of the PS action. Clinically, however, in the case of selective uptake of the PS into cancer cells vs. normal cells, cancer cell kill can be achieved both by PDT-mediated and cytotoxic mechanisms, and the total PDT-induced cell kill becomes relevant. Considering this, total cell kill close to 100% can be achieved in green light in sub-micromolar (20 nM for TLD-1633, 30 nM for TLD-1433, and 200 nM for TLD-1411) or even sub-nanomolar range (0.5 nM for TLD-1611). For comparison, Photofrin® achieved 100% total cell kill in U87 cells only at concentrations above 300 nM.

Clinically, the balance between the efficacy and safety of the PS is characterized by the therapeutic ratio that indicates how far a dose for a desired therapeutic effect is from the dose that causes undesired toxicity. Dividing PDT effect LD50 to dark toxicity LD50 provides small numbers that are not convenient to operate with. It is easier therefore to use inverted therapeutic ratio, ITR = Dark LD50/PDT effect LD50. In U87 cells, ITR = 17,061 for TLD-1411, 27,486 for TLD-1433, 31,460 for TLD-1611, and 54,252 for TLD-1633 under green light PDT. This exceeds the ITR = 14,870 for Photofrin® and shows thus a clear clinical advantage of Ru-based PSs over an established porphyrin-based PS.

4.2 Os-based PSs

The comparative efficacy of the Os-based PSs on U87 cells is shown in **Table 5**.

Additionally, in HT1376 cells, TLD-OsH2IP has a dark LD50 > 200 μM, N = 43, red light PDT LD50 = 15.0 μM (CI95 = 9.1–24.9, N = 30), and a NIR light PDT LD50 = 39.0 μM (CI95 = 30.6–49.6, N = 5). TLD-OsH2dppn has dark LD50 = 203.2 μM (CI95 = 190.2–217.1, N = 61), red light PDT LD50 = 4.1 μM (CI95 = 2.9–5.7, N = 26) and NIR light PDT LD50 = 27.4 μM (CI95 = 7.2–100.4, N = 9).

The presence of imidazo[4,5-f][1,10]phenanthroline and adding dppn to the complex increase PDT efficacy of the Os-based PSs, although it does not exceed the efficacy of Ru-based PSs. Similarly to the PDT LD50, ITR of the Os-based PSs in red light is also not better than that of Photofrin®; in U87 cells, ITR = 4.9 for TLD-OsH2B, 24.8 for OsH2IP, and 14.7 for TLD-OsH2dppn. In HT1376 cells, ITR > 13.3 for TLD-OsH2IP and equals to 49.6 for TLD-OsH2dppn. The advantage of the Os-based PSs, however, is their PDT activity in NIR light, which both Ru-based PSs and Photofrin® are lacking. ITR for NIR PDT is greater than 5.1 for TLD-OsH2IP and equal to 7.4 for TLD-OsH2dppn.

Another set of experiments focused at three Os-based PSs with bis ligands [31] supplements the data on red light PDT (625 nm, 90Jcm^{-2}, 450 mWcm^{-2}). In U87 cells, TLD-OsH2IP is the most efficient PS (LD50 = 57 ± 4 μM) exceeding both TLD-OsH2dppn (LD50 = 87 ± 12 μM) and TLD-OsH2B (125 ± 12 μM). In HT1376 cells, TLD-OsH2dppn is the most efficient (LD50 = 83 ± 4 μM); the remaining two PSs have similar LD50 (121 ± 10 μM for TLD-OsH2B and 141 ± 14 μM for TLD-OsH2IP). The inferiority of TLD-OsH2B in red light over the two other PSs is best reproduced across the presented datasets although comparative efficacy of TLD-OsH2IP and TLD-OsH2dppn is less consistent.

U87 cells	Dark	Green	Red	NIR
		530 nm	625 nm	808 nm
		90 Jcm^{-2}	90 Jcm^{-2}	400-600 Jcm^{-2}
		108 $mWcm^{-2}$	125 $mWcm^{-2}$	150 $mWcm^{-2}$
TLD-OsH2B	LD50 (μM):395.7 (CI95 = 323.4–484.1)	LD50 (μM):36.0(CI95 = 19.4–365.4)	LD50 (μM):81.5(CI95 = 16.9–393.3)	Kill (%):32.1 (SEM = 14.3)
		Maximal kill (%): 70.7 (CI95 = 19.9–121.6)	Maximal kill (%): 114.3 (CI95 = 7.6–220.9)	
	N = 43	N = 7	N = 12	N = 4
MEC (water)		12,328	3632	2269
TLD-OsH2IP	LD50 (μM):145.8 (CI95 = 67.6–314.6)	LD50 (μM): 3.1 (CI95 = 2.1–13.2)	LD50 (μM): 12.2 (CI95 = 9.2–15.8)	Kill (%): 63.8 (SEM = 13.5)
		Maximal kill (%): (CI95 = 30.67–107.9)	Maximal kill (%): 54.0 (CI95 = 51.5–56.6)	
	N = 20	N = 10	N = 4	N = 4
MEC (water)		10,761	3119	1957
TLD-OsH2dppn	LD50 (μM): 179.1 (CI95 = 112.6–284.8)	LD50 (μM): 0.16 (CI95 = 0.08–0.34)	LD50 (μM): 12.2 (CI95 = 0.7–577.6)	Inconsistent and low cell kill
		Maximal kill (%): 84.2 (CI95 = 70.5–97.8)	Maximal kill (%): 79.1 (CI95 = -2.0–160.3)	
	N = 20	N = 10	N = 4	
MEC (water)		10,486	4828	2273
TLD-Os14H	LD50 (μM): 141.2 (CI95 = 107.8–185.0)	LD50 (μM): 2.1 (CI95 = 1.6–3.4)	LD50 (μM): 2.4 (CI95 = 1.8–3.3)	Kill (%): 24.2 (SEM = 4.7)
		Maximal kill (%): 59.4 (CI95 = 46.6–72.3)	Maximal kill (%): 78.2 (CI95 = 69.0–87.5)	
	N = 54	N = 33	N = 53	N = 10
MEC (water)		11,716	2914	1376

The cells were incubated with the PS for 4 h, and the PS was removed before PDT. The dose–response provides LD50 (μM) and maximal cell kill (%) for a green and red light and a cell kill for a fixed PS concentration for NIR light. The data are presented as means and their 95% confidence intervals (SEM for NIR PDT).

Table 5.
In vitro PDT efficacy of Os(II)-based PSs on U87 cells (90 Jcm^{-2}).

Importantly, the dataset presented in [31] provides LD50 for NIR PDT (808 nm, 600 Jcm^{-2}, 900 $mWcm^{-2}$), in contrast to the cell kill at a single concentration presented in **Table 5**. TLD-OsH2IP proves to be most effective among the three in U87 cells (LD50 = 45 ± 5 μM), whereas TLD-OsH2B was the most effective PS for HT1376 cells (LD50 = 121 ± 8 μM). For this wavelength, therefore, the efficacy of TLD-OsH2dppn was the lowest, in contrast to the red light PDT.

Concentration-wise, the PDT efficiency is almost always similar in red and NIR light. The exception is greater efficacy of TLD-OsH2dppn in red vs. NIR in HT1376 cells ($P < 0.001$). In U87 cells, ITR is 3.3–9.6 for red PDT and 4.2–12.0 for NIR

PDT. In HT1376 cells, it is, respectively, 4.6–6.1 and 2.6–6.1. As in the dataset shown in **Table 5**, this is far behind the ITR value for Photofrin®, but considerable PDT activity in NIR is a decisive asset. This advantage is reinforced by the similar LD50 for red and NIR PDT, which means that (at certain light exposure conditions) NIR PDT can be at least not worse than red PDT.

One should remember however that NIR PDT needs much more energy to be delivered, NIR range photons carry less energy, and absorbance is lesser than for the red range. Red light PDT is still more efficient per absorbed photon than NIR PDT because similar LD50 in μM is achieved at a much lesser number of absorbed photons ($P < 0.001$). Hence, the NIR PDT advantage of the Os-based PSs must be realized by increasing the delivered energy of light. This does not pose a problem because no thermal effects are observed for 808 nm at 600 Jcm^{-2}.

4.3 Effect of Tf on in vitro PDT efficacy

Additional apo-Tf increases red light PDT efficacy of the Ru-based TLD-1433 in AY27 cells, together with a decrease in dark toxicity [43]. The PDT improvement effect is however significant (PDT effect LD50 = 11.6–11.9 μM vs. 17.0 μM with no additional Tf, $P < 0.05$) only after a relatively short (30 minutes) TLD-1433 incubation before PDT. If the incubation time is increased to 90 minutes, the beneficial effect of the additional Tf is not anymore evident, masked by the increased TLD-1433 PDT efficacy.

4.4 PDT efficacy in hypoxia

Hypoxia in tumors is one of the major challenges for anticancer therapy because both conventional radiotherapy and PDT rely upon oxygen, a mediator of damage to cancer cells. It is known at the same time that the tumors with hypoxic cores are clinically more aggressive [15].

This means that any modality effective under hypoxic conditions is extremely valuable. Among the four Ru-based and six Os-based PSs, Ru-based TLD-1633 and Os-based TLD-OsH2B proved to be active in hypoxic conditions (at 0.1–0.5% O_2) after red light PDT (625 nm, 90 Jcm^{-2}, 125 $mWcm^{-2}$). Incubation with ALA (having its metabolite PPIX as photosensitizer) is used as a negative control (an oxygen-dependent PS). For TLD-1633, hypoxia resistance is observed at a concentration as low as 4 μM, with significantly non-zero PDT effect = 67.3% cell kill in normoxia ($P = 0.022$) and 46.2% in hypoxia ($P = 0.036$), at moderate (25% cell kill) dark toxicity. For TLD-OsH2B, PDT effect is evident only at 320 μM. PDT effect reaches significantly non-zero effect: 59.8% in hypoxia ($P = 0.006$) vs. 42.2% in normoxia ($P = 0.0006$), and at considerable (53% kill) dark toxicity. For both PSs, hypoxia resistance occurs at concentrations above the PDT LD50.

It is noteworthy that TLD-1633 is active at low oxygen concentration corresponding to $pO_2 = 0.76$ mmHg. It is very encouraging because it is known that anticancer efficacy of conventional treatment progressively decreases at pO_2 below a critical threshold of 15–35 mmHg [46, 47].

High dark toxicity of the OsH2B hypoxia-effective concentration is a clear limitation, but this demonstrates anyways a possibility of hypoxia-effective Os-based PSs that, as it was shown, have also PDT activity in NIR. NIR light has greater penetration depth into tissues than visible light, and this, together with the PS activity under hypoxia, will pose a double benefit for PDT of bulk tumors.

5. In vivo PDT

5.1 Selective uptake by tumors

Intracellular accumulation of TLD-1433 was detected earlier, and association with Tf facilitated this process [43]. Hence, one needs to explore whether this translates to the selectivity of TLD-1433 uptake into tumors in vivo.

TLD-1433 is able to accumulate selectively in tumor tissue vs. normal ones even without premixing with Tf. In AY27 rat urinary bladder tumors, characteristic staining can be seen co-localized with tumors (**Figure 3**) 1 h after instillation of 50 μg/mL TLD-1433.

TLD-1433 accumulation in the tumors is at least one order of magnitude greater than in the adjacent apparently normal tissue: 77 ± 18 mg/kg, N = 6 vs. 0.4 ± 0.09, N = 6, P = 0.007.

The concentration in a tumor, therefore, reaches estimated 76 μM, which is far exceeding in vitro PDT effect LD_{50} for U87 cells in green light (**Table 4**). Moreover, the foci of coloration are visible outside of a major tumor. This suggests a possibility of detection of very small malignant lesions not readily visible macroscopically without staining by the PS.

Association of TLD-1433 with apo-Tf is able to increase selectiveness of the PS accumulation in subcutaneous CT26.WT (murine colon adenocarcinoma) tumors in BalbC mice (**Figure 4**). Four hours after systemic injection of 10 mg/kg TLD-1433 premixed with apo-Tf (molar ratio = 1:1), significantly more TLD-1433 is found in a tumor vs. adjacent muscle tissue (P = 0.038); the selectivity ratio is about 1.8. With TLD-1433 injected, the uptake into a tumor is not significantly different from the adjacent muscle tissue.

Averaging of the individual tumor/muscle uptake ratios for each animal confirms the results shown above. The ratio is significantly above 1 upon injection of the TLD-1433-Tf premix (1.81 ± 0.14, N = 5, P = 0.005) indicating the uptake selectivity. With TLD-1433 alone injected, the uptake into the tumors is not selective (0.74 ± 0.18, N = 4, P = 0.247). This firmly suggests that the association of TLD-1433 with apo-Tf increases selectivity of TLD-1433 uptake by a tumor. Apo-Tf per se cannot be taken up because it has to bind Fe^{3+} to be recognized by the cell surface TfR. Since selective improvement of the uptake of TLD-1433 & apo-Tf premix by the tumors is

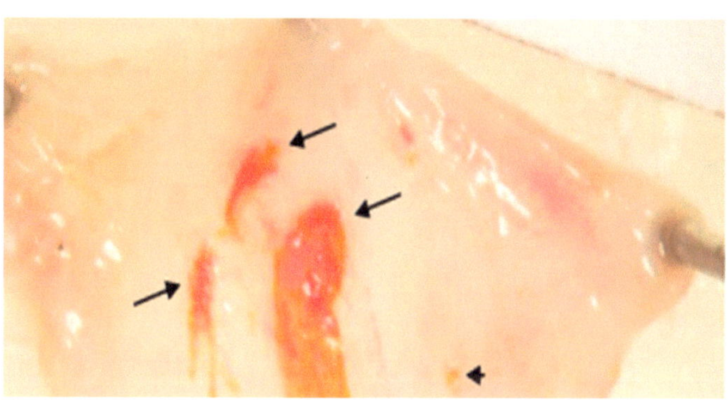

Figure 3.
Accumulation of TLD-1433 in AY27 orthotopic urinary bladder tumors in fisher rats. The bladder was examined 1 h after instillation of 50 μg/mL TLD-1433. The arrows denote the areas of coloration by TLD-1433 implying its accumulation in the lesions.

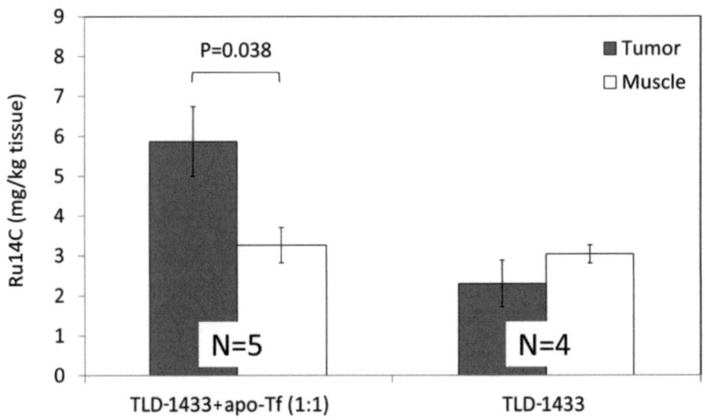

Figure 4.
Accumulation of TLD-1433 without or with apo-Tf at different molar ratios in CT26.WT tumors in BalbC mice 4 h after systemic (IV) injection (10 mg/kg). N = 5 for TLD-1433 & apo-Tf group; N = 4 for TLD-1433 group.

demonstrated, one can anticipate two possible scenarios: (1) TLD-1433 & apo-Tf still manages to bind Fe^{3+}, and (2) TLD-1433 & apo-Tf conjugate can be recognized by TfR and taken up by the cell without the need to bind Fe^{3+}.

5.2 In vivo PDT efficacy

5.2.1 Light penetration

Assessing PDT efficacy in vivo is a necessary step on the way to potential clinical applications. It has however its own challenges to be addressed. Light exposure regime is one of them.

The penetration depth of light at different PDT conditions is crucial for the PDT success. For example, a small penetration depth of green light is because of a strong attenuation by intrinsic chromophores, such as hemoglobins and cytochromes. The calculations estimate the energy attenuation up to 1/8 cm^{-1} in

TLD-OsH2B	MEC (in water)	No PS	4.5 mg/kg	9 mg/kg	
Green	12,328	0.10–15	0.10	0.01↓	
Red	3632	0.60	0.30↓	0.08↓	
NIR	2269	0.55	0.22↓	0.15↓	
TLD-OsH2IP	**MEC (in water)**	**No PS**	**2.25 mg/kg**	**3 mg/kg**	**9 mg/kg**
Green	10,761	0.10–15	0.07↓	0.005↓	0.06↓
Red	3119	0.60	0.70	0.29↓	0.05↓
NIR	1957	0.55	0.79	0.37↓	0.08↓
TLD-Os14H	**MEC (in water)**	**No PS**	**0.9 mg/kg**	**1.8 mg/kg**	**9 mg/kg**
Green	11,716	0.10–15	0.04↓	0.06↓	0.06↓
Red	2914	0.60	0.22↓	0.07↓	0.05↓
NIR	1376	0.55	0.11↓	0.08↓	0.08↓

Table 6.
Light attenuation in a phantom tumor (proportion of energy penetrating to the bottom of 1-cm-thick phantom vs. surface) in green (525 nm), red (635 nm), and NIR (808 nm) light.

skin and 1/20 cm^{-1} in a tumor that has a higher density of vasculature and hence more absorbing chromophores [48]. High absorbance of light by the PS is a very desirable property contributing to its efficacy. This could be a double-edged sword however because high absorbance of the PS close to the tumor surface can shield the deeper tissue from the light exposure and hence result in undertreatment of a tumor. The measurements using a tissue-emulating phantom (a piece of meat having a size of an experimental tumor with an overlaying piece of shaved mouse skin) show indeed that the Os-based PSs (TLD-OsH2B, TLD-Os2IP, and TLD-Os14H) affect the penetration of light into a tumor at different wavelengths. Without PSs, 85–90% of energy is lost across the tumor thickness (about 1 cm) for green (525 nm, 40 $mWcm^{-2}$), 40% for red (635 nm, 150 $mWcm^{-2}$) and 45% for NIR (808 nm, 300 $mWcm^{-2}$) photons. The PSs injected into a tumor further diminishes the light penetration (**Table 6**).

It is noteworthy that the increase in light attenuation across the wavelengths is PS-specific. At the minimal used dose for each PS, TLD-OsH2B does not attenuate green light penetration, TLD-OsH2IP does not attenuate in red and NIR, while TLD-Os14H does this at all three wavelengths. Also, the increase in the PS concentration results in a progressive and disproportional increase in light attenuation. Notably, the absorbance of the PS measured in water (see **Figure 1**) is not translated directly into the PS-dependent light attenuation in the tumor phantom.

The limitations of light penetration can be also illustrated by the distribution of PDT-induced damage in tumors. The damage inflicted by red light (660 nm, 90 J/cm^{-2}, 125 $mWcm^{-2}$) PDT to CT26.WT subcutaneous tumors in BalbC mice after systemic administration of 10 mg/kg of the 1:1 TLD-1433 & apo-Tf premix clearly diminishes as it goes deeper into a tumor (**Figure 5C,D**). The damage area is not necessarily decreased, but the magnitude of the damage has a definite gradient with coagulative necrosis near the surface and the "general damage" that cannot be defined as coagulative necrosis. The damage is incomplete even when TLD-1433 is associated with apo-Tf (which is expected to facilitate PDT effect as evident from in vitro experiments). Notably, the skin on the way of the light beam is not damaged, which can suggest selectivity of the PS uptake into a tumor. Considering that red light is still delivering 60% of the incident energy at 10 mm depth (**Table 6**), much more shallow damage (up to about 3 mm) suggests a steep gradient of PDT efficacy as the delivered energy falls below a certain threshold.

The observed damage should be clearly attributed to PDT but not dark toxicity of the PS in a tumor because, without light, there is no visible damage (**Figure 5B**).

Figure 6 shows representative examples of coagulative necrosis as a result of damage and a pattern of gradual transition of the damaged zone from an intact tumor to the necrotic area.

5.2.2 Thermal effect

Thermal effect is another consideration because it can potentially occur in a tumor upon light irradiation. For green light, this is possible due to absorption by intrinsic hemoglobin. Hyperthermia is known and used as an anti-tumor modality [49], but in PDT studies, the thermal effect may mask PDT-specific mechanisms of tumor damage.

In the subcutaneous tumor model (CT26.WT tumor in BalbC mice), continuous-wave irradiation with red (635 nm, 150 $mWcm^{-2}$) or green (525 nm, 40 $mWcm^{-2}$) light does not show any signs of overheating at the tumor surface. The temperature does not exceed 31–35°C at the end of irradiation even with TLD-Os14H injected intratumorally.

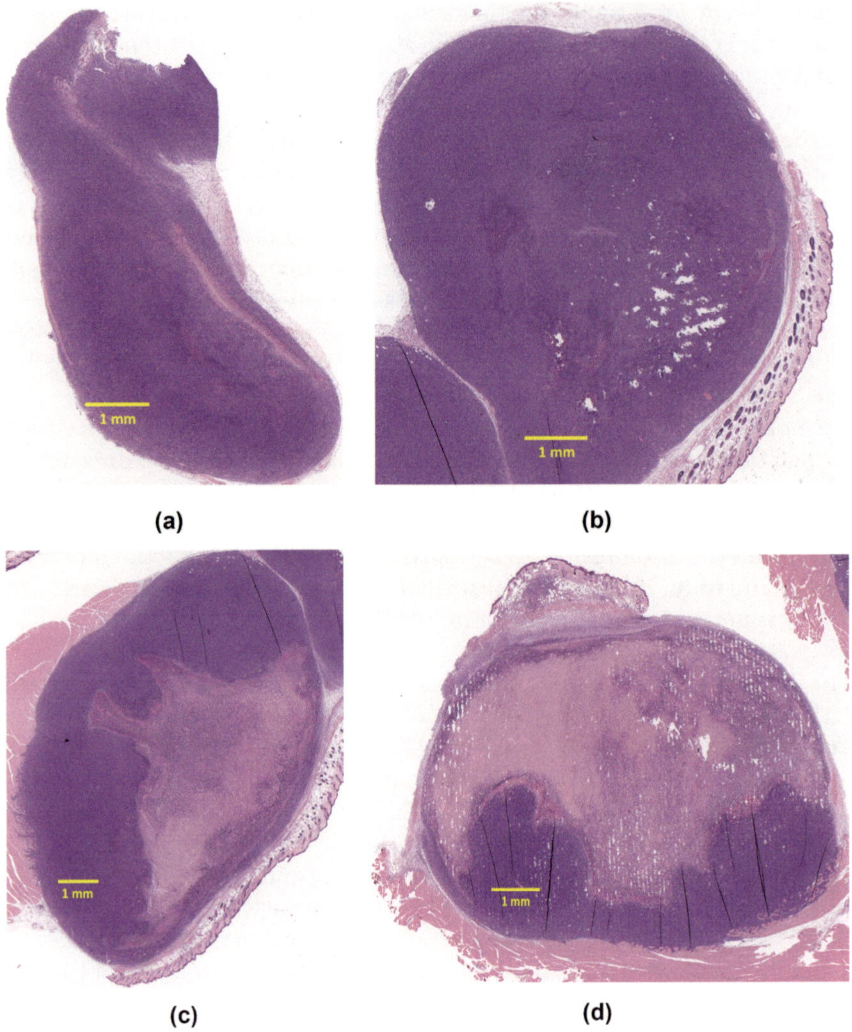

Figure 5.
Tumor damage (H&E staining) after red light (660 nm, 90Jcm^{-2}, 125 mWcm^{-2}) PDT to CT26.WT subcutaneous tumors in BalbC mice after systemic administration of 10 mg/kg TLD-1433 as 1:1 TLD-1433 & apo-Tf premix. The PDT was performed 4 h after the administration, and the tumors harvested 2 days post-PDT. The Panel a shows untreated tumor, the Panel b shows PS-injected tumor with no irradiation, and the Panels c-d show PDT-treated tumors.

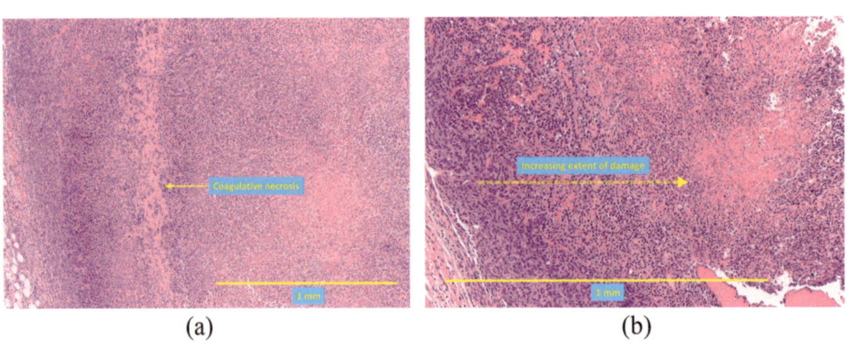

Figure 6.
Coagulative necrosis and "general damage" in a PDT-treated tumor. The Panel a shows an example of coagulative necrosis area; the Panel b shows a gradient transition from non-damaged tumor area to the necrotic one through the area of "general damage".

Within a tumor, a combination of deeper-penetrating light and less absorbance by the PS also does not result in considerable thermal effect. Under NIR light alone (808 nm, 600 Jcm^{-2}, 300 $mWcm^{-2}$), the temperature increases only by 4.8°C (from 26.9 to 31.7°C) during 30 minutes of irradiation. In the presence of Ru-based TLD-1433 (50 mg/kg intratumorally in 100 μL per 20 g BW), the temperature rapidly increases from 28.4°C to 33.6°C (by 5.2°C) at 50 Jcm^{-2} delivered to a tumor and only by 8.1°C at the end (600 Jcm^{-2}). The temperature reaches no more than 36.5°C showing no PDT-dependent thermal effect. TLD-1433 is responsible only for 3.3°C (41%) of the total PDT-induced increase. Notably, in euthanized animals, the total increase in temperature is similar to that in live animals (although with more linear increase dynamics). This may mean that the active removal of heat by circulating blood is not critical in maintaining the temperature within the safe range during PDT.

5.2.3 PDT effect

In CT26.CL25 subcutaneous tumor model in BalbC mice, intratumoral injection of TLD-1411 or TLD-1433 at 1/20 MTD (1.8 and 5.2 mg/kg, respectively) green (525 nm, 192 Jcm^{-2}, 200 $mWcm^{-2}$) light PDT resulted in a fast reduction or complete regression of the tumors and a temporary (8–9 days) delay in their growth [50]. This effect was statistically significant ($P < 0.05$) only for TLD-1433 translating to an increased survival (about 15% of the animals surviving beyond the 90 days follow-up period).

The dose of both PSs has to be increased to 1/2 MTD (18 and 52 mg/kg, respectively) to obtain significant ($P < 0.01–0.05$) PDT effect of greater magnitude, with only continuous-wave PDT effective. About 50% of the animals survived beyond 60 days for TLD-1411 and about 75% beyond 90 days for TLD-1433. **Figure 7** shows an example of the PDT-induced tumor damage and subsequent regression.

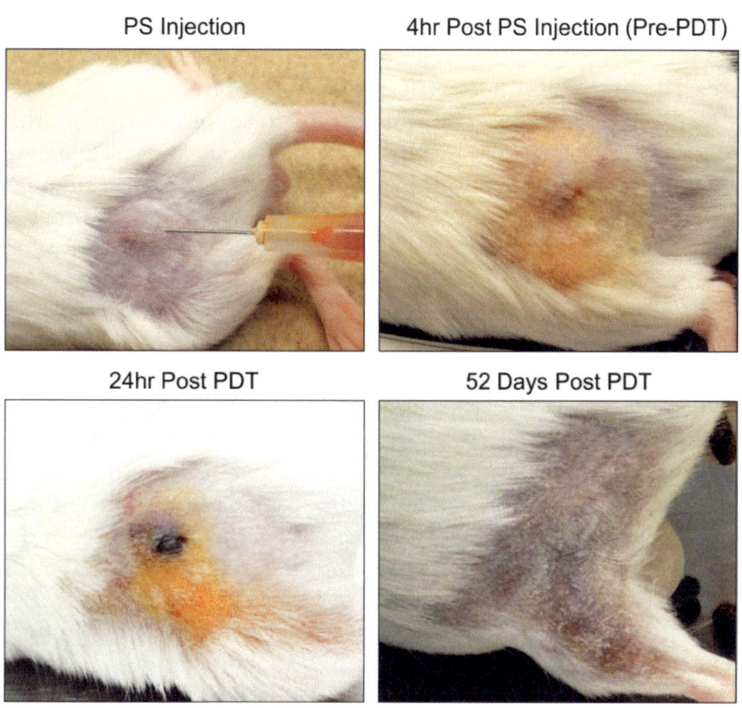

Figure 7.
An example of successful tumor destruction by 53 mg/kg TD1433-mediated PDT under continuous-wave green light (525 nm, 192 Jcm^{-2}, 200 $mWcm^{-2}$).

These results are obtained with a green light that has only a superficial light penetration. TLD-1433-mediated (50 mg/kg =47% MTD) PDT using deeper-penetrating NIR light (808 nm, 600 Jcm^{-2}, 400 $mWcm^{-2}$) does not reach however the efficacy of green light PDT despite 6.7 times greater radiant exposure [43]. Only a trend to improvement in survival (P = 0.164–0.179 vs. dark toxicity and light only) could be observed. This is not surprising by itself considering that TLD-1433 has extremely low absorbance in NIR. Nevertheless, the P values allow hypothesizing that a significant effect could be achieved with more powerful experimental design or greater delivered light energy.

More encouraging is a beneficial effect of combining TLD-1433 with Tf. A highly significant PDT effect in the animals survival can be observed when 4:1 TLD-1433 & apo-Tf premix (50 mg/kg TLD-1433) is injected instead of TLD-1433 only (P = 0.0182–0.0032 vs. dark toxicity and light only). No dark toxicity for tumors (effect of the premix with no light on tumor growth) is detected. Although the difference vs. TLD-1433-induced PDT (P = 0.0633) still does not reach statistical significance threshold, the P value, again, is small enough to talk about a trend toward the improvement. The result reinforces the valuable finding of the benefit of TLD-1433-Tf premix in PDT efficacy improvement under NIR light. This is especially noteworthy because the absorbance of TLD-1433-Tf in NIR range is still very low compared to the absorbance in green light despite the facilitating effect of Tf.

Anyways, 600 Jcm^{-2} NIR PDT is able to maintain about 70% of the animals surviving beyond 90 days follow-up (vs. only about 30% after PDT mediated by TLD-1433 that was not mixed with Tf), which is not less than survival after 192 Jcm^{-2} green light PDT. This is especially encouraging considering that NIR PDT is not effective in vitro, either with or without Tf. The failure to detect in vitro PDT effect in NIR is possibly because the short-term viability assay (reflecting metabolic suppression rather than actual cell death) could be not sufficient to detect the effect of NIR that has less energy per photon. The effect *in vivo*, in contrast, is assessed by the long-term follow-up of tumor growth. The activity of the Ru-based complexes under NIR is known from literature [51] but involves multiphoton excitation. In contrast, the results presented above demonstrate the ability of the PSs to be activated by NIR in a continuous-wave regime via single-photon excitation. Moreover, TLD-14333-Tf premix has an additional benefit of decreased systemic toxicity, with MTD more than twofold greater than that for injection of TLD-1433 only [50].

This double benefit of using apo-Tf as a delivery vehicle for TLD-1433 resembles the already mentioned effect in vitro for red light PDT using AY27 cells where TLD-1433-Tf decreased dark toxicity and increased PDT efficacy. Note however that in vitro experiments using cancer cell line determined dark toxicity in cancer cells and hence can be rather an estimate for dark toxicity of the PS in tumors. In contrast, in vivo model considered the benefit for systemic toxicity.

NIR PDT efficacy in vivo can be also demonstrated by direct quantitation of the tumor damage. Even suboptimal PDT (200 instead of 600 Jcm^{-2}) shows a trend (P = 0.104, df = 8, one-tailed) to an increase in the relative area of damage in a tumor as compared to the tumors not subjected to PDT (dark and tumor alone data pooled). The damage area is increased to 33.4 ± 10.2% (N = 4) vs. 17.1 ± 2.5% (N = 6). The effect is only moderate and does not reach statistical significance, but this could be because of suboptimal (200 Jcm^{-2}) radiant exposure.

Among the Os-based PSs (TLD-OsH2B, TLD-OsH2IP, TLD-OsH2dppn), the MTD values vary. TLD-OsH2B is the most toxic (MTD = 1.25 mg/kg) and TLD-OsH2dppn the least toxic (MTD = 47 mg/kg), which is more than one magnitude of difference [31]. For comparison, in vitro dark LD50 for three PSs were much closer to one another (416–617 μM for U87 cells and 476–744 μM for HT1376 cells). As it was mentioned already, however, in vitro dark toxicity for cancer cells and in vivo MTD as systemic toxicity is not directly comparable.

TLD-OsH2IP-mediated (3 mg/kg = 1/2 MTD) continuous-wave red light PDT (635 nm, 192 or 266 Jcm^{-2}) significantly slows down the tumor growth and increases survival vs. light only group ($P < 0.01$). The effect is however temporary (like TLD-1433, as discussed above). Increasing the radiant exposure to 266 Jcm^{-2} allows for a better result, with the cases of tumor regression and survival significantly increased vs. both dark and light only groups ($P < 0.01$) and about 80% of the animals surviving beyond the 50 days follow-up. Considering high photostability of TLD-OsH2IP, further increase in power and energy density for red light PDT is possible. This could potentially allow achieving complete tumor-suppressing success, at least in the framework of this in vivo model.

We have discussed previously that NIR effect is potentially possible even at suboptimal settings with Ru-based TLD-1433-Tf formulation. This formulation has an absorbance in NIR higher than TLD-1433 but still lower than Os-based TLD-OsH2dppn (MEC = 777–1459 vs. 2273 $M^{-1}\,cm^{-1}$, respectively). Hence, we could expect NIR PDT effect for TLD-OsH2dppn because this PS absorbs much better in NIR than TLD-1433. The PDT effect is indeed observed at 3 mg/kg of the PS and 800 nm and 600 Jcm^{-2}, with about 60% of the animals surviving beyond 50-day follow-up vs. dark and light only groups ($P < 0.01$ and 0.0001, respectively). This result further demonstrates the potential of NIR PDT application using transition metal-based PSs. The NIR PDT still requires delivery of at least 3 times more

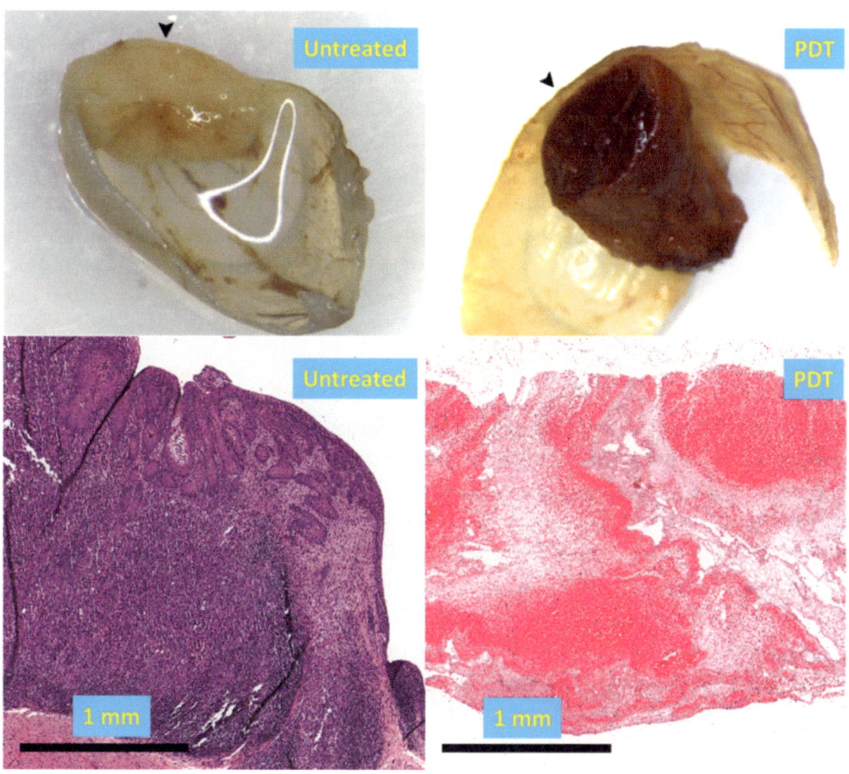

Figure 8.
Damage to muscle noninvasive AY27 tumor induced orthotopically in fisher rats' urinary bladder 2 days after TLD-1433-mediated green light (535 nm, 90 Jcm^{-2}) PDT. TLD-1433 at 6 mg/mL was instilled into bladders, and PDT performed after 1 h of incubation and TLD-1433 washing out of the bladder cavity. The macroscopic image and H&E images are shown.

photons than for red light PDT to match it in efficacy (considering the difference in absorbance and quantum energy), but this does not pose a serious problem because of thermal safety of the light exposure as it was discussed above.

Another anticancer application of PDT using transition metal-based PSs is urothelial non-muscle invasive bladder cancer [52]. As it was mentioned above, Ru-based TLD-1433 accumulated selectively in the orthotopic urinary bladder tumors (instillation with 0.05 mg/mL). At higher concentration of TLD-1433 (6 mg/mL) that is more relevant for the future clinical applications, green light (535 nm, 90 Jcm^{-2}) PDT causes full depth (2–3 mm) necrosis in a tumor that showed a deep red coloration (**Figure 8**). Importantly, PDT spared the muscle and urothelial tissue adjacent to the tumors, with only a transient local inflammation of the adjacent urothelium. This is a decisive advantage because the collateral muscle damage impairing the bladder function was a reason for the failure of the prior clinical trials on bladder cancer PDT.

6. Clinical PDT efficacy

The results of the preclinical research allowed planning and initiation of a clinical trial for non-muscle invasive bladder cancer (NMIBC) at the Princess Margaret Cancer Center in Toronto, Canada. It is noteworthy that although several other Ru-based complexes (NAMI-A, KP1019, and KP1339) have currently entered clinical trials as antineoplastic drugs, TLD-1433 is meanwhile the only transition metal complex tested in a trial as a PS for PDT [5, 53].

TLD-1433-mediated PDT (525 nm, 3 W, target dose = 90 Jcm^{-2}) with intravesical irradiation demonstrated safety and efficacy of the PS in patients with non-muscle invasive urinary bladder cancer (NMIBC) who were previously unresponsive to contemporary anticancer therapy, including the intravesical therapy with Bacillus Calmette-Guérin (BCG) [54]. At therapeutic dose (0.70 mg per cm^2 of bladder surface), 2 of 3 patients were tumor-free at the 180-day posttreatment, with no essential adverse effects and minimal systemic absorption of the PS (complete clearance from the plasma within 72 hrs) and no photosensitivity reactions. This outcome is successful enough to warrant further advance to a phase II trial.

7. PS activation by ionizing radiation

It is worth noting that at least one of the PSs under discussion, TLD-1433, can be activated not only by nonionizing electromagnetic radiation but also by ionizing one (X-ray). Transition metal complexes are theoretically prone to this because the atoms of transitional metals can attenuate X-rays. For example, Ru attenuates X-ray photons at 75 keV to an extent comparable to iodine, an established X-ray imaging agent [55]. Activation of the PS by X-ray is very advantageous because it allows treatment of the tumors located considerably deeper than reachable by NIR. TLD-1433 retains its functionality after 75 keV irradiation at doses up to 20Gy and retains its ability to generate postirradiation *OH signal under subsequent red light exposure. In cultured human glioblastoma U87 cells, 20 μM TLD-1433 exerted non-zero radio-enhancement effect after 75 keV X-ray exposure (5 Gy) at the magnitude of 37% cell kill ($P = 0.020$, $df = 3$), at dark toxicity of 20% cell kill ($P = 0.009$, $df = 3$). Moreover, the effect can be detected in vivo in CT26.WT tumors induced in BalbC mice. At 1 Gy, X-ray resulted in a 2.9-fold increase in coagulative necrosis area in the tumors on day 2 postexposure vs. TL1433 alone and X-ray alone groups pooled

($P = 0.007$, df = 15) [56]. It is noteworthy that thermal effects at these conditions are highly unlikely because 1 Gy deposits only 0.001 J per gr tissue, which, at the estimated average specific heat capacity $C \approx 3.7\ J\ g^{-1}\ K^{-1}$ [57], provides a very small (0.0003°C) increase in temperature.

8. Conclusions

In vitro and in vivo data suggest that transition metal-based complexes are versatile as PSs with diverse photophysical, photochemical, and biological properties. This includes activation over a wide range of wavelengths and high singlet oxygen yield and photobleaching resistance. The Ru(II)-based PSs may have very high cytotoxic efficacy far exceeding the established porphyrin-based PSs. The Os(II)-based PSs are notable in their PDT activity at deeper-penetrating NIR light PDT. Moreover, even Ru(II)-based PSs could be effective in vivo under NIR light. Transition metal-based PSs demonstrate both Type I and Type II photoreactions and can be active in hypoxic conditions, presenting the potential for the treatment of bulky hypoxic tumors. These properties are further facilitated by their ability to associate with endogenous metal transporter molecules, like human apo-Tf, which enables their targeted endocytosis. Furthermore, the association with Tf increases absorptivity at longer wavelengths (far red to NIR range), ROS generation, and finally tumor destroying potential. The observed capacities of the PSs may allow overcoming notorious challenges of PDT: the necessity for deeper light penetration, the selectivity of accumulation in tumors, and activity under hypoxic conditions. Finally, the research has led to the first clinical trial for this class of PSs, with a successful outcome and potential to further clinical advance. This raises justified hopes that with the ongoing technological improvements, such as the development of transition metal complexes (including the advanced Theralase PSs discussed above), and personalized dosimetry with a treatment planning approach, PDT has the potential to become integrated into the mainstream of cancer treatment.

Acknowledgements

The authors are grateful to the employees of Theralase Inc. for ensuring a very helpful and benevolent working atmosphere and particularly appreciate the contribution of the members of its research team, both past (Jamie Fong, Kamola Kasimova, Yaxal Arenas, and Savo Lazic) and present (Manjunatha Ankathatti Munegowda) for their experimental work and publications used in this chapter. The next acknowledgement is of the invaluable help and crucial support by Prof. Lothar Lilge at Princess Margaret Cancer Centre, Toronto, Ontario, Canada, and his group (including Sarah Forward and Carl Fisher) and of the staff of the other departments, facilities, and services at the center for doing their best to make our work going smoothly and effectively. We greatly appreciate the collaboration with Prof. Sherri McFarland at Acadia University, Wolfville, Nova Scotia, Canada, and her group.

Conflict of interest

No conflict of interest has been declared.

Author details

Pavel Kaspler*, Arkady Mandel, Roger Dumoulin-White and Mark Roufaiel
Theralase Inc., Toronto, Canada

*Address all correspondence to: pkaspler@theralase.com

References

[1] Henderson BW, Dougherty TJ, editors. Photodynamic Therapy: Basic Principles and Clinical Applications. 1st. ed. London: CRC Press; 1992. 480 p

[2] Dolmans DEJGJ, Fukumura D, Jain RK. Photodynamic therapy for cancer. Nature Reviews. Cancer. 2003;**3**:380-387. DOI: 10.1038/nrc1071

[3] Scherer KM, Bisby RH, Botchway SW, Parker AW. New approaches to photodynamic therapy from Type I, II and III to Type IV using one or more photons. Anti-Cancer Agents in Medicinal Chemistry. 2017;**17**:171-189. DOI: 10.2174/18715206 16666160513131723

[4] Van Straten D, Mashayekhi V, de Bruijn H, Oliveira S, Robinson D. Oncologic photodynamic therapy: Basic principles, current clinical status and future directions. Cancers. 2017;**9**:1, E19-54. DOI: 10.3390/cancers9020019

[5] Monro S, Colón KL, Yin H, Roque J 3rd, Konda P, Gujar S, et al. Transition metal complexes and photodynamic therapy from a tumor-centered approach: Challenges, opportunities, and highlights from the development of TLD-1433. Chemical Reviews. 2018. DOI: 10.1021/acs.chemrev.8b00211 [Epub ahead of print]

[6] Smith AW, Mancini MC, Nie S. Bioimaging: Second window for in vivo imaging. Nature Nanotechnology. 2009;**4**:710-711. DOI: 10.1038/nnano.2009.326

[7] Matsuoka M, editor. Infrared Absorbing Dyes. New York: Springer Science+Business Media; 1990. 220 p

[8] Dougherty TJ, Gomer CJ, Henderson BW, Jori G, Kessel D, Korbelik M, et al. Photodynamic therapy. Journal of the National Cancer Institute. 1998;**90**:889-905

[9] Hodgkinson N, Kruger CA, Abrahamse H. Targeted photodynamic therapy as potential treatment modality for the eradication of colon cancer and colon cancer stem cells. Tumour Biology. 2017;**39**:1-17. DOI: 10.1177/1010428317734691

[10] Zhang H, Hou L, Jiao X, Ji Y, Zhu X, Zhang Z. Transferrin-mediated fullerenes nanoparticles as Fe^{2+}-dependent drug vehicles for synergistic anti-tumor efficacy. Biomaterials. 2015;**37**:353-366. DOI: 10.1016/j.biomaterials.2014.10.031

[11] Gijsens A, Derycke A, Missiaen L, De Vos D, Huwyler J, Eberle A, et al. Targeting of the photocytotoxic compound AlPcS4 to Hela cells by transferrin conjugated PEG-liposomes. International Journal of Cancer. 2002;**101**:78-85. DOI: 10.1002/ijc.10548

[12] Paszko E, Vaz GM, Ehrhardt C, Senge MO. Transferrin conjugation does not increase the efficiency of liposomal Foscan during in vitro photodynamic therapy of oesophageal cancer. European Journal of Pharmaceutical Sciences. 2013;**48**:202-210. DOI: 10.1016/j.ejps.2012.10.018

[13] Bonnett R. Chemical Aspects of Photodynamic Therapy. 1st ed. London: CRC Press; 2000. 324 p

[14] Ethirajan M, Chen Y, Joshi P, Pandey RK. The role of porphyrin chemistry in tumor imaging and photodynamic therapy. Chemical Society Reviews. 2011;**40**:340-362. DOI: 10.1039/b915149b

[15] Pouysségur J, Dayan F, Mazure NM. Hypoxia signalling in cancer and approaches to enforce tumour regression. Nature. 2006;**441**:437-443. DOI: 10.1038/nature04871

[16] Noman MZ, Messai Y, Carré T, Akalay I, Méron M, Janji B, et al. Microenvironmental hypoxia orchestrating the cell stroma cross talk, tumor progression and antitumor response. Critical Reviews in Immunology. 2011;**31**:357-377. DOI: 10.1615/CritRevImmunol.v31.i5.10

[17] Freitas I. Role of hypoxia in photodynamic therapy of tumors. Tumori. 1985;**71**:251-259. DOI: 10.1177/030089168507100306

[18] Dang J, He H, Chen D, Yin L. Manipulating tumor hypoxia toward enhanced photodynamic therapy (PDT). Biomaterials Science. 2017;**5**:1500-1511. DOI: 10.1039/c7bm00392g

[19] Feng L, Cheng L, Dong Z, Tao D, Barnhart TE, Cai W, et al. Theranostic liposomes with hypoxia-activated prodrug to effectively destruct hypoxic tumors post photodynamic therapy. ACS Nano. 2017;**11**:927-937. DOI: 10.1021/acsnano.6b07525

[20] Ashfaq M, Najam T, Shah SS, Ahmad MM, Shaheen S, Tabassum R, et al. DNA binding mode of transition metal complexes, a relationship to tumor cell toxicity. Current Medicinal Chemistry. 2014;**2**:3081-3094. DOI: 10.2174/0929867321666140601201803

[21] Rohrabaugh TN, Collins KA, Xue C, White JK, Kodanko JJ, Turro C. New Ru(ii) complex for dual photochemotherapy: Release of cathepsin K inhibitor and 1O2 production. Dalton Transactions. 2018;**47**:11851-11858. DOI: 10.1039/c8dt00876k

[22] Ellahioui Y, Patra M, Mari C, Kaabi R, Karges J, Gasser G, Gómez-Ruiz S. Mesoporous silica nanoparticles functionalised with a photoactive ruthenium(ii) complex: Exploring the formulation of a metal-based photodynamic therapy photosensitiser. Dalton Transactions 2018. DOI: 10.1039/c8dt02392a [Epub ahead of print]

[23] Le Gall T, Lemercier G, Chevreux S, Tücking KS, Ravel J, Thétiot F, et al. Ruthenium (II) polypyridyl complexes as photosensitizers for antibacterial photodynamic therapy: A structure-activity study on clinical bacterial strains. ChemMedChem. 2018;**13**: 2229-2239. DOI: 10.1002/cmdec.201800392

[24] Lin K, Zhao ZZ, Bo HB, Hao XJ, Wang JQ. Applications of ruthenium complex in tumor diagnosis and therapy. Frontiers in Pharmacology. 2018;**9**:1323. DOI: 10.3389/fphar.2018.01323. eCollection 2018.

[25] Pickens RN, Neyhouse BJ, Reed DT, Ashton ST, White JK. Visible light-activated co release and $^1o_2$ photosensitizer formation with Ru(II),Mn(I) complexes. Inorganic Chemistry. 2018;**57**:11616-11625. DOI: 10.1021/acs.inorgchem.8b01759

[26] Zhang P, Huang H. Future potential of osmium complexes as anticancer drug candidates, photosensitizers and organelle-targeted probes. Dalton Transactions. 2018;**47**:14841-14854. DOI: 10.1039/c8dt03432j

[27] Lilge L. Use of ruthenium complexes as photosensitizers in photodynamic therapy. In: Holder AA, Lilge L, Browne WR, Lawrence MAW, Bullock JL Jr, editors. Ruthenium Complexes. Photochemical and Biomedical Applications. Weinheim, Germany: Wiley-VCH Verlag GmbH & Co. KGaA; 2017. pp. 117-137. DOI: 10.1002/9783527695225

[28] Metal-Based Coordination Complexes as Photodynamic Compounds and Their Use. US Provisional Patent #61801674. Filed Mar 15 2013; US nonprovisional/PCT

application filed Mar. 17, 2014, PCT/US14/30194

[29] Li Y, Wang J, Zhang X, Guo W, Li F, Yu M, et al. Highly water-soluble and tumor-targeted photosensitizers for photodynamic therapy. Organic & Biomolecular Chemistry. 2015;**13**:7681-7694. DOI: 10.1039/c5ob01035g

[30] Uruma Y, Nonomura T, Yen PY, Edatani M, Yamamoto R, Onuma K, et al. Design, synthesis, and biological evaluation of a highly water-soluble psoralen-based photosensitizer. Bioorganic & Medicinal Chemistry. 2017;**25**:2372-2377. DOI: 10.1016/j.bmc.2017.02.050

[31] Lazic S, Kaspler P, Shi G, Monro S, Sainuddin T, Forward S, et al. Novel osmium-based coordination complexes as photosensitizers for panchromatic photodynamic therapy. Photochemistry and Photobiology. 2017;**93**:1248-1258. DOI: 10.1111/php.12767

[32] Chin Y, Lim SH, Zorlu Y, Ahsen V, Kiew LV, Kiew LV, et al. Improved photodynamic efficacy of Zn(II) phthalocyanines via glycerol substitution. PLoS One. 2014;**9**:e97894. DOI: 10.1371/journal.pone.0097894

[33] Wilson BC, Patterson MS, Lilge L. Implicit and explicit dosimetry in photodynamic therapy: A new paradigm. Lasers in Medical Science. 1997;**12**:182-199. DOI: 10.1007/BF02765099

[34] Pogue BW, Elliott JT, Kanick SC, Davis SC, Samkoe KS, Maytin EV, et al. Revisiting photodynamic therapy dosimetry: Reductionist & surrogate approaches to facilitate clinical success. Physics in Medicine and Biology. 2016;**61**:R57-R89. DOI: 10.1088/0031-9155/61/7/R57

[35] Aveline B, Hasan T, Redmond RW. Photophysical and photosensitizing properties of benzoporphyrin derivative monoacid ring a (BPD-MA). Photochemistry and Photobiology. 1994;**59**:328-335. DOI: 10.1111/j.1751-1097.1994.tb05042.x

[36] Dovigo LN, Pavarina AC, Ribeiro APD, Brunetti IL, Costa CA de S, Jacomassi DP, et al. Investigation of the photodynamic effects of curcumin against *Candida albicans*. Photochemistry and Photobiology. 2011;**87**:895-903. DOI: 10.1111/j.1751-1097.2011.00937.x

[37] Valentine RM, Brown CTA, Moseley H, Ibbotson S, Wood KJ. Monte Carlo modeling of in vivo protoporphyrin IX fluorescence and singlet oxygen production during photodynamic therapy for patients presenting with superficial basal cell carcinomas. Journal of Biomedical Optics. 2011;**16**:048002. DOI: 10.1117/1.3562540

[38] Toneatto J, Garcia PF, Argüello GA. Advances on the interaction of polypyridyl Cr(III) complexes with transporting proteins and its potential relevance in photodynamic therapy. Journal of Inorganic Biochemistry. 2011;**105**:1299-1305. DOI: 10.1016/j.jinorgbio.2011.07.013

[39] Garcia PF, Toneatto J, Silvero MJ, Argüello GA. Binding of [Cr(phen)3](3+) to transferrin at extracellular and endosomal pHs: Potential application in photodynamic therapy. Biochimica et Biophysica Acta. 2014;**1840**:2695-2701. DOI: 10.1016/j.bbagen.2014.06.010

[40] Dömötör O, Hartinger CG, Bytzek AK, Kiss T, Keppler BK, Enyedy EA. Characterization of the binding sites of the anticancer ruthenium(III) complexes KP1019 and KP1339 on human serum albumin via competition studies. Journal of Biological Inorganic

Chemistry. 2013;**18**:9-17. DOI: 10.1007/s00775-012-0944-6

[41] Śpiewak K, Brindell M. Impact of low- and high-molecular-mass components of human serum on NAMI-A binding to transferrin. JBIC, Journal of Biological Inorganic Chemistry. 2015;**20**:695-703. DOI: 10.1007/s00775-015-1255-5

[42] Shen Y, Li X, Dong D, Zhang B, Xue Y, Shang P. Transferrin receptor 1 in cancer: A new sight for cancer therapy. American Journal of Cancer Research. 2018;**8**(6):916-931 eCollection 2018

[43] Kaspler P, Lazic S, Forward S, Arenas Y, Mandel A, Lilge L. A ruthenium(II) based photosensitizer and transferrin complexes enhance photo-physical properties, cell uptake, and photodynamic therapy safety and efficacy. Photochemical & Photobiological Sciences. 2016. [Epub ahead of print]. DOI: 10.1039/c5pp00450k

[44] Quarles CD Jr, Randunu KM, Brumaghim JL, Marcus RK. Metal retention in human transferrin: Consequences of solvent composition in analytical sample preparation methods. Metallomics. 2011;**3**:1027-1034. DOI: 10.1039/c1mt00094b

[45] Ueda J, Takeshita K, Matsumoto S, Yazaki K, Kawaguchi M, Ozawa T. Singlet oxygen-mediated hydroxyl radical production in the presence of phenols: Whether DMPO-*OH formation really indicates production of *OH? Photochemistry and Photobiology. 2007;**77**:165-170. DOI: 10.1562/0031-8655(2003)0770165SOM HRP2.0.CO2

[46] Höckel M, Vaupel P. Tumour hypoxia: Definitions and current clinical, biologic, and molecular aspects. Journal of the National Cancer Institute. 2001;**93**:266-276. DOI: 10.1093/jnci/93.4.266

[47] Hu YL, DeLay M, Jahangiri A, Molinaro AM, Rose SD, Carbonell WS, et al. Hypoxia-induced autophagy promotes tumour cell survival and adaptation to antiangiogenic treatment in glioblastoma. Cancer Research. 2012;**72**:1773-1783. DOI: 10.1158/0008-5472.CAN-11-3831

[48] Shi G, Monro S, Hennigar R, Colpitts J, Fong J, Kasimova K, et al. Ru(II) dyads derived from α-oligothiophenes: A new class of potent and versatile photosensitizers for PDT. Coordination Chemistry Reviews. 2015;**282**:127-138. DOI: 10.1016/j.ccr.2014.04.012

[49] Raaphorst GP, Heller DP, Bussey A, Ng CE. Thermal radiosensitization by 41″C hyperthermia during low dose-rate irradiation in human normal and tumour cell lines. International Journal of Hyperthermia. 1994;**10**:263-270. DOI: 10.3109/02656739409009347

[50] Fong J, Kasimova K, Arenas Y, Kaspler P, Lazic S, Mandel A, et al. A novel class of ruthenium-based photosensitizers effectively kills in vitro cancer cells and in vivo tumors. Photochemical & Photobiological Sciences. 2015;**14**:2014-2023. DOI: 10.1039/c4pp00438h

[51] Yu B, Ouyang C, Qiu K, Zhao J, Ji L, Chao H. Lipophilic tetranuclear ruthenium(II) complexes as two-photon luminescent tracking non-viral gene vectors. Chemistry - A European Journal. 2015;**21**:3691-3700. DOI: 10.1002/chem.201405151

[52] Lazic S, Kaspler P, Mandel A, Jewett MAS, Kulkarni G, Lilge L. MP61-06. Photodynamic therapy for non-muscle invasive bladder cancer mediated by instilled photosensitizer TLD-1433 and green light activation. The Journal of Urology. 2016;**195**:E805. DOI: 10.1016/j.juro.2016.02.880

[53] Thota S, Rodrigues DA, Crans DC, Barreiro EJ. Ru(II) compounds: Next-generation anticancer metallotherapeutics? Journal of Medicinal Chemistry. 2018;**61**:5805-5821. DOI: 10.1021/acs.jmedchem.7b01689

[54] Kulkarni GS, Lilge L, Mandel A, Perlis N, Nesbitt M, Dumoulin-White R, et al. TLD-1433 photodynamic therapy for BCG-unresponsive NMIBC - a phase IB clinical study. In: 19th Annual Meeting of the Society of Urologic Oncology (SUO). Phoenix, AZ, USA; 2018

[55] NIST: X-Ray Mass Attenuation Coefficients – Ruthenium. 2018. Available from https://physics.nist.gov/PhysRefData/XrayMassCoef/ElemTab/z44.html [Accessed: 26 December 2018]

[56] Mandel A, Kaspler P, Roufaiel M, Munegowda MA, Lilge L. X-ray and photon mediated in vitro and in vivo activity of ruthenium(II) compounds. In: 16th International Photodynamic Association (IPA) World Congress. Coimbra, Portugal; 2017

[57] Giering K, Lamprecht I, Minet O, Handke A. Determination of the specific heat capacity of healthy and tumorous human tissue. Thermochimica Acta. 1995;**251**:199-205. DOI: 10.1016/0040-6031(94)02047-R

Chapter 11

Theranostics Application of Graphene-Based Materials in Cancer Imaging, Targeting and Treatment

Neha Karki, Anita Rana, Himani Tiwari, Pushpa Negi and Nanda Gopal Sahoo

Abstract

Recent advancements in graphene-based nanomaterials provide the opportunity that compliments the limitations of conventional drug delivery systems (DDSs) through simultaneous targeting of the anticancer drug to the cancer cell by reducing the side effects of other administration routes. Graphene with its extraordinary electronic properties like larger surface area, possibilities of surface modification, can efficiently target the tumor cell. At the same time, nanocarriers have the advantages of immune clearance adulteration of physicochemical properties of anticancer drug. The DDSs can be made by biodegradable nanocarriers such as proteins, peptides, biocompatible polymers, antibodies, polymer-drug conjugates, etc. Graphene-supported DDSs in cancer therapy also supports the co-delivery of therapeutic agents, antioxidants, SiRNA, shRNA, etc. as the co-delivery approach, which provide additive or synergistic therapeutic efficacy and can reduce toxic effects.

Keywords: graphene, nanocarrier, cancer imaging, drug delivery, DDSs

1. Introduction

As a promising interdisciplinary field, nanotechnology acts as a bridge for various disciplines, such as material sciences, engineering, physics and chemistry, and is dedicated to the production of different materials in the nanometer scale (<100 nm), with assorted physical, chemical and mechanical properties. Although nanoscience and nanotechnology are new research interests, the application of nanomaterials for humankind was well-known since ancient times. Among the periodic elements, carbon has the intense ability of catenation and great tendency to form various hybrid orbitals (e.g., sp, sp^2, and sp^3) which results in the formation of various smart compounds having different physical and chemical properties according to their structure [1, 2]. Due to the properties mentioned above, carbon have tendency of forming different allotropes of different dimensions, like quantum dots (0D), carbon nanotubes (1D), fullerenes (0D), graphene (2D), graphite (3D), among which, graphene got lot of attention in the past decade. Graphene has hexagonally packed honeycomb like geometry in which a unit layer of carbon atoms are arranged in two-dimensional (2D) lattice [3–6]. The hybrid orbital of carbon-carbon atoms are in sp^2 hybridized form, in which the in-plane σ (C–C) bonds are much stronger than the out-of-plane π (C–C) bonds, which is highly accountable for the delocalized array of electrons and come up with the weak polar interaction between graphitic layers of the graphene sheets as well as with graphene and other molecules.

In scheming a potent drug delivery carrier, besides its physicochemical constancy in the biological surroundings, reactivity and toxic issues, diffusivity, immunogenicity, interactions with biological systems, drug loading and release characteristics, blood circulation half-life, drug transportation ability of the biological medium to aim the cells within tissues, etc. are the significant issues (**Figure 1**). Due to the electrostatic interaction and presence of different alkali and alkaline earth metal ions *viz.* Na, Mg, etc. in the physiological medium, the graphene sheets tends to agglomerate which results in reduction of their surface area, decreasing their solubility and increasing their toxicity. Therefore, surface modification of graphene nanosheets is required to overcome such physical and biological effects. Covalent functionalization and noncovalent physisorption are the two well-known strategies universally applied for surface modification to construct desired modified graphene nanosheets [7–9].

Number of research groups have been investigating the surface modification of GO with different kinds of biocompatible polymers as a nanodrug carrier for development of targeted drug delivery systems. The polymers are selectively preferred according to their functional groups, bioavailability and compatibility in the cell medium [10]. Therefore responding to specific stimulus, surface fabrication of GO with various polymers for this particular drug delivery application is limited [11]. For well-organized diagnosis, expressive intracellular drug release is elected over the contemporary arrival of the drug in the system.

With the innovation of the smart material graphene, the curiosity of researchers remarkably moved toward graphene and its oxygenated derivatives from the previously invented other nanomaterials of carbon family, and various scientists are working to organize the surface modification of graphene through the spacious understanding of different functionalization methods [12–14]. From the chemical

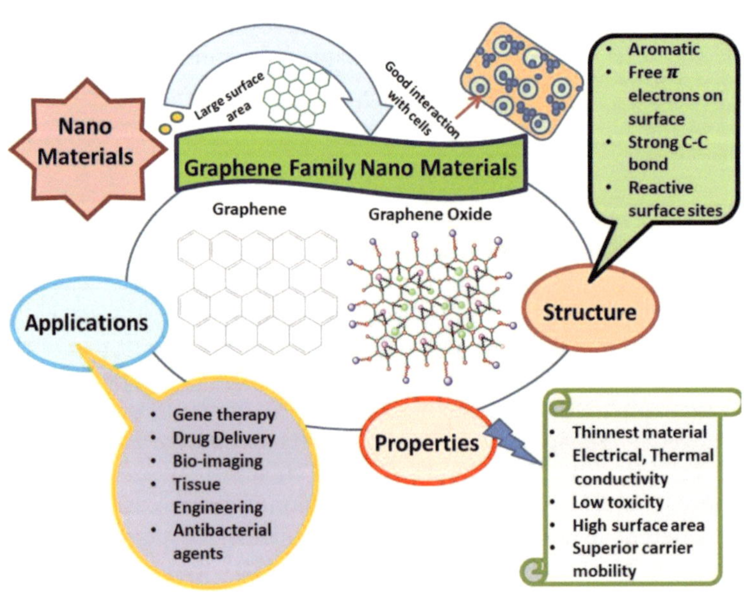

Figure 1.
Properties and applications of graphene oxide.

point of view, production of graphene oxide that possesses many reactive oxygen-containing groups is appropriate for advance modification and relative aspects of GO sheets, or we can say that the reactivity of GO is highly desirable.

Beside this, graphene is sparingly soluble in the water, polar solvents and in the cell environment due to aromatic character [15]. Graphene oxide on the other hand has water contact angle of 30.7° [16] and proficient of composing weak hydrogen bonds and metal incorporated complex ion due to the polar oxygenated groups present on the basal plane and negatively charged carboxylic groups present on the edge site [17–20]. The distinctive arrangement of graphene oxide and its strong carbon-carbon covalent bonding provides outstanding thermal and electrical conductivity with very low thermal expansion quotient. These properties of graphene are also significantly affected by alteration such as edge scattering defect [21] and isotopic doping [22] due to diffusion or localization of phonons at the defect sites. Light absorption and optical imaging are highly dependent on the total number of layers present in GO sheets, as they increase accordingly with the number of layers present in GO [23]. Optoelectronic devices based on GO derivatives are developed as tunable IR detectors, modulators and emitters by electrophysiology and charge multiplexers [24]. This capability to organize the rearrangement and partition of surface electrons can be oppressed in emergent bio-imaging applications [25, 26].

The GO sheets are highly influenced by the divalent ions and some specific polymers which play a crucial role in mechanical properties of GO sheets by inter connecting both the molecules [27, 28]. Due to the superior mechanical properties of GO, it has been reported that by incorporating the different polymers with it, the tensile strength of the respective polymer increases. Graphene supported polymethyl methacrylate (PMMA) and poly-L-lactic acid (PLLA) drastically amplifies the young's modulus and hardness of these polymer nanocomposites for mechanical applications [29].

With reference to different physicochemical properties of nanomaterials of graphene family, it can be projected that they will demonstrate numerous mutual connections with biological moieties such as cells and tissues depending on chemical modification, thickness and dimensions of graphene sheets, etc. [30, 31]. With more supplementary data of graphene application in biomedical field, research on its cellular activity and other intracellular processes is rising. Introduction of polar and reactive oxygenated functionalities give rise to oxidative force in objective cells is supposed to be the effective mechanism for potency of graphene oxide [32, 33]. Due to their dose dependent cytotoxicity and bactericidal activity, graphene-based materials are being explored for applications in antimicrobial products. A number of studies have been performed reporting the antibacterial activities of CNTs, graphene, GO and rGO against *Escherichia coli* and *Staphylococcus aureus* bacteria with rGO having the strongest antibacterial effectiveness [34–38]. With reference to the various studies discussed above, it is apparent that shape and size, of graphene-based materials importantly take part in determining their interactions with cell membrane and intracellular uptake. Moreover *in vitro* studies in various cell lines along with broad perspective of various mechanisms dependent on graphene-based materials are being increasingly explored for various applications in antimicrobial products. In the end, we will briefly discuss the prospects and future challenges regarding graphene-based materials as cancer imaging, targeting and treatment applications.

2. Synthesis of graphene oxide and its surface modification

Different methods are used to set up the preparation of graphene sheets according to its structural and chemical behavior with various biocompatible molecules.

The methods are widely categorized as colloidal suspension (size specific), arc discharge (electric charge specific), and chemical or mechanical exfoliation. For the broad and extensive production of graphene sheets, mechanical exfoliation method were not used as it is expensive but for the fabrication of electronic devices it is widely applied. Graphene oxide (GO) the oxygenated derivative and replacement of graphene is synthesized by the chemical exfoliation method, in which the sp2-hybridized C–C hybrid orbitals breaks and the different oxygenated groups such as hydroxyl, carboxyl and epoxy are introduced [39]. The surface modifications of the graphene sheets are site specific as the bulky group carboxyl attached toward the edges of the sheets while on the other hand hydroxyl and epoxy groups tends to form bond with the basal plane of the graphene sheets [40, 41]. These oxygenated and highly reactive functional groups offers reactive handles for a range of surface-functionalization reactions covalently and non-covalently, which can be used to build up surface modified GO, its biocompatible composites. For the large-scale synthesis of graphene, the most common methods required exfoliation of graphene. The only variances among graphene made by different methodologies are the defect content and yield of their products [42]. Various methods are available for graphene synthesis, but for the large production of graphene oxide (GO) oxidative-exfoliation methods give excellent results. There are some additional treatments required to reduce typically defective graphene-like nanosheet into reduced graphene oxide (RGO) [43]. During the oxidation process of graphene, functional groups containing oxygen attached to the surface increase the distance among graphitic layers and responsible for enhancing the exfoliation by weakening the van der Waals forces [44]. After the oxidation process, several washing steps are required so that oxidizing agents and some other impurities removed from graphite oxide to enhance the exfoliation. For large-scale washing of graphite oxide, different conventional approaches such as filtration process [45], centrifugation process [46], and dialysis process [47] are mostly used. Among all these processes infiltration processes, after some time, particles of graphite oxide choke the filter pores and make it time-consuming process.

2.1 Synthesis of graphene oxide (GO)

For the synthesis of graphene oxide, the most used source of graphite is flake graphite, which occurs as a natural mineral which further use to purify to remove heteroatomic contamination [48]. GO prepared by the use of flake graphite have the property to easily dispersed in water hence used on a large scale [49]. This expanded form of graphite powder has been used for the synthesis of GO sheets by the following method.

2.1.1 Modified Hummer's method

Graphene oxide is synthesized by modified Hummer's method using graphite powder [50]. In this method, in a round bottom flask, a mixture of 1 g of $NaNO_3$ and calculated graphite powder are mixed. In this mixture drop by drop, 46 mL of H_2SO_4 was added in an ice water bath with continuous stirring. After 4 h stirring without any pause at 32°C temperature, 6 g of $KMnO_4$ was poured into a slurry mixture of $NaNO_3$ and graphite. Later 2 h continuous stirring 92 mL of DD water was combined in it at 95°C. Again after 2 h, 200 mL of DD water was poured in it and leave for 1 h for constant stirring. Lastly, at room temperature, 20 ml of H_2O_2 was mixed and mixed it repeatedly for 1 h. The obtained supreme oxidized product washes by 10% HCl solution for purification by abundant quantity by ion free water. Finally, it is filtered by 0.2 μm Nylon membranes until neutralizing the final product.

2.2 Surface functionalization of GO

From the last decades, the interest has increased in the scientific community for the use of graphene oxide (GO) in biological and biomedical field applications [51]. GO is a two dimensional material with a large surface area containing single-layer sheets of carbon atoms with sp^2 hybridization and carbon sites with sp^3 hybridization in which hydrophilic functional groups with oxygen are present [52]. Thus, GO has many possibilities for surface functionalization due to outstanding solubility in water [53]. There are different methods for the functionalization of the surface of graphene oxide; some of them are discussed below (**Figure 2**).

The nanocarrier thus synthesized was characterized by some advanced spectroscopic techniques, like RAMAN (**Figure 3**), Fourier Transform infrared (FT-IR) (**Figure 4**), Transmittance Electron Microscope (TEM) (**Figure 5**). Thermal stability and quantitative analysis were characterized by Thermo gravimetric Analyzer TGA under a nitrogen atmosphere at a heating rate of 10°C/min from 30 to 600°C (**Figure 6**).

2.2.1 Covalent functionalization of GO

During the processes of oxidation and exfoliation of graphite, there is a large extent of carboxylic group forms on the graphene surface. These groups better modified by different methods; one of them is covalent functionalization. In covalent functionalization, graphene is coupled with reagents, such as 1-ethyl-3-(3-dimethyllaminopropyl) carbodiimide (EDC) and N-hydroxysuccinimide (NHS) [54], or can also be converted to acyl chlorides using thionyl chloride (SOCl) [55]. Covalent functionalization is a multipurpose methodology for modification

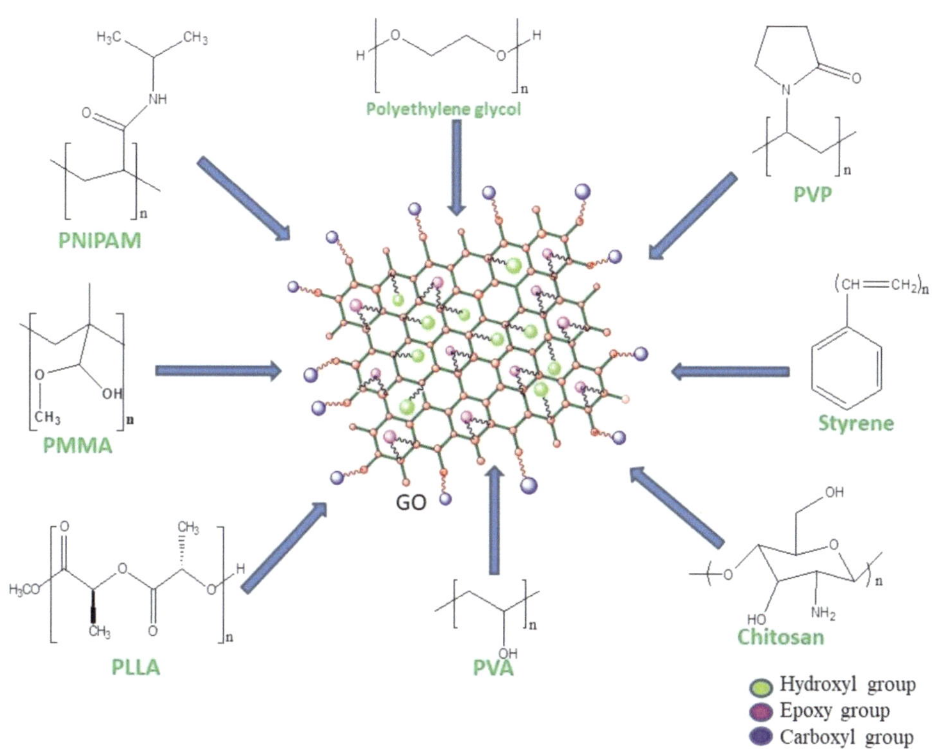

Figure 2.
Surface modification of graphene oxide.

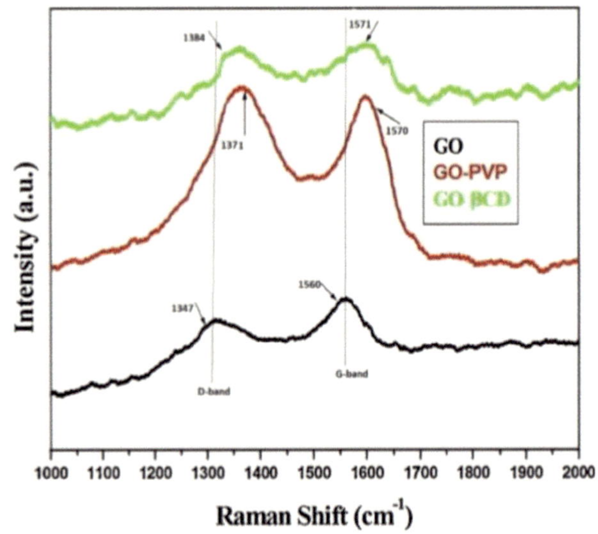

Figure 3.
Raman spectra for GO, GO-PVP, and GO-β-CD.

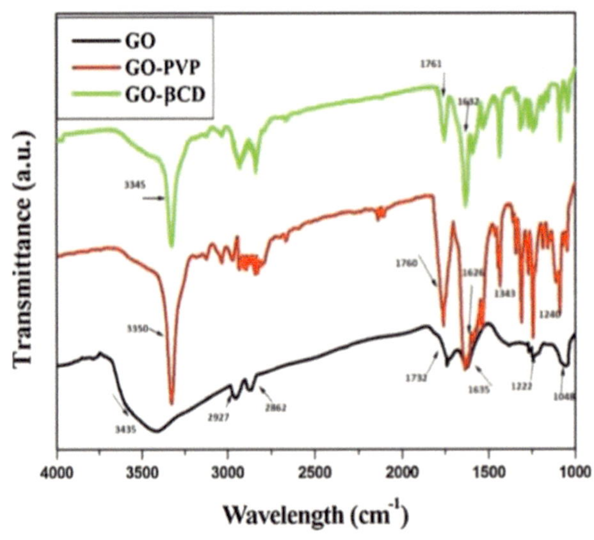

Figure 4.
Fourier transform infrared (FT-IR) spectra of GO, GO-PVP and GO-βCD.

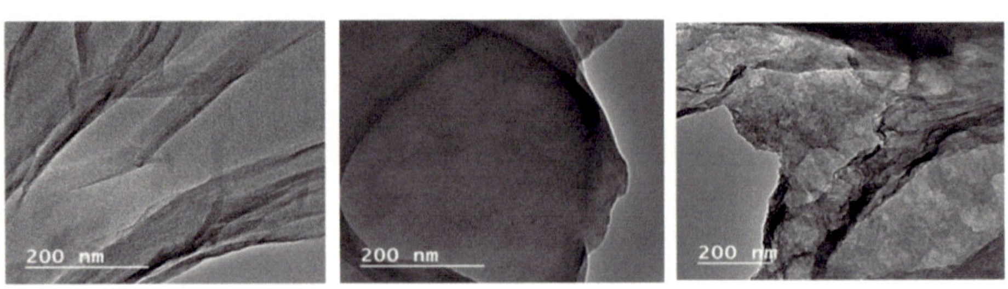

(a) (b) (c)

Figure 5.
TEM images of (a) GO (b) GO-PVP, and (c) GO-β-CD.

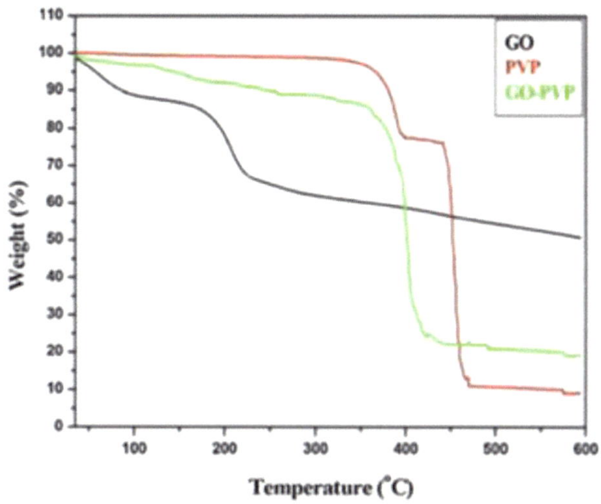

Figure 6.
TGA analysis of GO, PVP, and GO-PVP.

of graphene surface which tailoring the chemical properties as well as electronic properties of graphene [56]. The methodology of GO functionalization by covalent functionalization depends on the environments of the reaction, nature of solvent, temperature condition, different functional groups of the incoming molecules, and other factors like reaction time. When polymer attach to the GO nanosheets it creates stress on GO surface, the covalent mode of functionalization is helpful in controlling the chemical properties of GO and reduces the stress caused by polymer [57]. GO surfaces have the ability for excellent covalent functionalization which makes it a unique nanomaterial which is helpful in developing studies of biological system. According to previous studies functionalization of GO shows excellent results when perform its use in targeted drug delivery applications [58]. There are chances of this because GO surface has the affinity for the adsorption of huge amount of hydrophobic drugs easily and due to specificity of covalent functionalization it releases the drug to particular regions of organisms. This functionalization of GO is also applicable in other biological activities like anti-bacterial activity, bioimaging [59], and photo-dynamic therapy [60]. Even though some procedures of graphene surface modification by covalent functionalization have validated efficient results but some methods generate some supplemental defects on the surface of graphene which are responsible for the changes in graphene structure.

2.2.2 Non-covalent functionalization of GO

Non-covalent functionalization is a more effective method in order to make maximum use of the inherent structure and mechanical properties of graphene oxide or graphene. Non-covalent functionalization is largely preferred in place of covalent functionalization as it does not alter the structure and electronic properties of graphene and it simultaneously introduces new chemical groups on the surface. The most common examples of non-covalent functionalization on graphene surface include polymer wrapping, π-π interactions, electron donor-acceptor complexes, hydrogen bonding, and van der Waals forces. Non-covalent functionalization of graphene results in the enhancement of dispersibility, biocompatibility, and reactivity, binding capacity, or sensing properties. Non-covalent interactions also known as supramolecular interactions are found in all types of materials that experience attractive as well as repulsive forces between them. These type of interactions are found in many natural and synthetic systems [61, 62]. In comparison to covalent bonds the energies of individual non-covalent interactions are normally lower [63]. In graphene, two types of π-π interactions occur between the electron-rich and electron-poor regions, which influence its interaction with other molecules or nanomaterials. This is commonly seen in the face-to-face and edge-to-face arrangement [64]. Graphene materials, with the π-π interactions have dissociation energies less than 50 kJ mol^{-1}. The weakest forces, that is, London-dispersion forces or van der Waals interactions are responsible for the non-covalent interaction affect all atoms in close proximity. The hydrophobic effects caused by different types of interactions are influence not only dispersibility of GO but recognition interactions [65, 66].

3. Challenges in nanotheranostics designing

In forthcoming nanotheranostics will be accepted as an efficient nanomedicine due to their unique properties like imaging, target selectivity and ability to load the drug in nanocarrier. In the process of nanotheranostics evolution as a potential nanoplatform various challenges encountered for detection of clinical complications. An appropriate technology is required for the treatment and selection of effective therapeutic agents for respective diseases like metallic nanocrystals, image-contrasting agents and choosing an efficient therapeutic agents for corresponding diseases like metallic nanocrystal and concatinate them as nanomaterial. The advanced nanomaterial high selectivity to the target site is required for advance nanotheranostic for excellent delivery of drug targeted nanotheranostic should contain delivery and loading capacity. The biocompatible material should be used in the preparation of nanotheranostics the normal tissue should not damage and easily excreted by human system. Whole designing of nanotheranostics will cheap with no side effects to body.

3.1 Pharmacokinetic and toxicological aspects

The introduction of a new drug to the site is not only expensive, but also time consuming. It includes discovery, clinical testing, development, and approval. Improving safety/efficacy ratio of marketed drugs is more cost-effective. All this can be done by controlling the time, rate, and place of drug release in the body through a drug-delivery system. Hence, a drug-delivery system could be seen as an interface between the patient and the drug [67]. Since past decades, a growing number of drugs were discovered and were optimized for an enhanced efficiency. However, about 40% of the new drugs, especially those based on biomolecules, like peptides, nucleotides, or proteins, often present a low bioavailability and are rejected by the pharmaceutical industry [68]. For controlled release the ideal materials must control certain important issues like easy reach to the target site in the body, ability to transport the necessary volume of active compounds, and a certain level of release with a certain speed, apart from the properties needed to ensure a better and safe interaction with the human body [69].

4. Graphene-based composites in various biomedical application

Graphene is considered as the finest and most durable monolayer capable of free existence. The specific 2D geometry and presence of pi electrons in graphene basal plane further applied for valuable drug loading via hydrophobic interactions and π-π stacking. Furthermore, large surface area of graphene allows for high density surface fabrication via different surface modification. A number of research on the in vivo behavior and bioactivity of graphene (**Figure** 7) has been investigated previously.

4.1 Drug delivery

Graphene is the finest and most durable monolayer material which is capable of free existence. In graphene, its 2D structure and presence of delocalized π electrons on its surface can be used for effective drug loading via hydrophobic interactions and π-π stacking. In addition to this, large surface area of graphene allows it for high density bio-functionalization via both covalent and non-covalent surface modification methods. Various studies based on the in vivo behaviour and bioactivity of graphene shows that the nanocarriers interact with the cell membranes and enter into the cells by endocytosis. For targeted drug delivery to the cell nucleus, it is essential that the drug carrier escapes endosomal compartment and release loaded drug into the cytosolic compartments [70, 71]. This process proposed a strategy to reverse cancer drug resistance in DOX resistant MCF-7/ADR cells by loading DOX on graphene oxide surface via physical mixing [72]. High pH dependent release for drug loading with of DOX was observed *in vitro*. GO enhanced accumulations of DOX in MCF-7/ADR cells causing higher cytotoxicity in comparison to free DOX. It is well known that pH is acidic in the cancer micro environment, intracellular lysosomes and endosomes. This fact has been exploited to achieve active drug release in the tumor tissue/cells using chemical modification of graphene [73–76]. For chemotherapeutic efficacy use of graphene-based materials has also been explored for co-delivery of multiple drugs. Zang et al. [77] Loading of DOX and CPT in controlled way inside the same drug delivery system resulted in remarkably higher toxicity in MCF-7 cells compared with GO-loaded only with DOX or CPT. Thus, graphene and GO-modified magnetic nanoparticles results in various biomedical applications in the field of drug delivery, MRI and bioimaging.

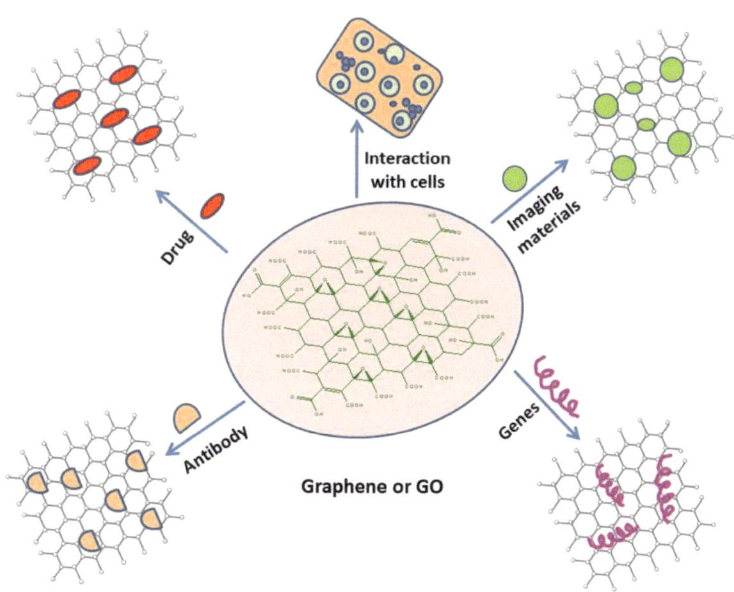

Figure 7.
Graphene-based composites for various biomedical applications.

Attachment of nanoparticles such as iron oxide with graphene-based nanomaterial makes them super paramagnetic in property and can be useful in drug delivery applications [78]. The resulting magnetic hybrids dispersed uniformly in aqueous solution before and after loading of DOX. Magnetic hybrids show agglomeration behavior in acidic medium and redispersion behavior observed in basic medium. This pH triggered magnetic behavior of GO-Fe_3O_4 nanoparticle hybrids can be help in controlled drug delivery. Similar pH-dependent drug release system was reported for 5-FU-loaded nanohybrid system composed of graphene nanosheets (GN), carbon nanotube (CNT) and Fe_3O_4 [79].

4.2 Gene delivery

Gene therapy is used in many expanding area to treat genetic disorders like Parkinson's disease, cystic fibrosis and cancer. An effective gene therapy needs efficient and safe gene vectors that also protect DNA from nuclease degradation as well as facilitate DNA uptake with high transfection efficiency [80, 81]. According to review of literature, graphene has been reported for wide applications in the field of gene delivery, gene-drug co-delivery and protein delivery with. PEI has been extensively investigated as nonviral gene vector having strong electrostatic interactions with negatively charged phosphates of RNA and DNA. Chemical modification is very easy in PEI which offers increased transfection efficiency, cell selectivity and reduced cytotoxicity however low biocompatibility and high toxicity of (Polyethyleneimine) PEI limit its use for biomedical applications [82]. Chitosan-GO complex are also used for simultaneous drug and gene delivery [83]. Chitosan-GO converts pDNA into stable nano-sized complexes. Amine-terminated PEGylated GO was effectively used to deliver high protein payloads due to non-covalent interactions with surface of PEG-GO [84]. Bone morphogenic protein-2 (BMP-2) was loaded onto Ti substrate coated with alternate layers of positively (GO-NH_3+) and negatively (GO-COO-) charged GO nanosheets with high loading efficacy and conserved bioactivity. Osteogenic differentiation of MSCs was enriched on Ti coated GO surfaces carrying BMP-2 than only Ti surface with BMP-2. In vivo studies in mouse also exhibited vigorous new bone formation with Ti-GO-BMP2 implants compared to Ti or Ti-GO or Ti-BMP2 implants and making the new composite a very effective carrier for therapeutic drug delivery [85]. All above studies have highlighted potential of graphene-based materials as drug and gene delivery vehicles *in vitro* studies though there is a necessity to validate their potential in vivo with particular focus on safety, biodistribution and efficacy.

4.3 Tissue engineering

Tissue engineering is an interdisciplinary field that endeavors to develop biological substitutes to resolve, retain or enhance functionality of a tissue or whole organ [86]. Recently, graphene-based materials have been used to treat wound healing, stem cell engineering, regenerative medicine and tissue engineering. Hydrogels have viscoelastic and transport properties to mimicking natural tissues [87], but their weak mechanical properties can limit their use in many tissue engineering applications. Graphene has a platform for tailoring various functionalities on flat surfaces with outstanding mechanical properties like high elasticity, strength, flexibility. Potentially, graphene has a wide range of applications in the field of hydrogels, biodegradable films, electrospun fibers and other tissue engineering scaffolds. When GO incorporated into PVA-based hydrogels it potentially increases tensile stability (132%) and compressive strength (36%) of composite hydrogel without altering their cytoaffinity [88]. According to Lu et al. graphene-based composite materials are applicable for wound healing by formulating graphene containing chitosan-PVA nanofibrous scaffolds. These three groups, chitosan-PVA-graphene electrospun fibers, chitosan-PVA fibers were also studied without graphene and control (no scaffold), to check wound healing affinity in mice and rabbit [89]. Graphene containing samples healed the wound completely in faster rate in comparison to without graphene-based samples in both mice and rabbit. Graphene-based materials also have applications in the area of musculoskeletal tissue engineering using mouse myoblast C2C12 cell lines [90]. Cellular behavior on graphene derivatives are enhanced by the Surface roughness and surface oxygen content and adsorption of serum proteins. Thus, graphene materials can be useful in reinforcing tissue engineering scaffolds due to its mechanical and electrical properties. Graphene materials have properties like large surface area which adsorb proteins/DNA and can be useful in many therapeutic applications. For instance, Mahmoudi et al. [91] recently reported protective role of GO and protein-coated GO surfaces in amyloid beta fibrillation process, which is implicated in various neurodegenerative disorders. However, along with detailed *in vitro* characterization of scaffolds, more emphasis should be placed on their evaluation in vivo with respect to inflammatory responses, biocompatibility and regenerative potential.

5. Application of graphene in bioimaging

Graphene-based nanomaterials have been widely explored in biomedical fields such as bioimaging, drug delivery, theranostics, and so on. The recent advances in bioimaging of graphene-based nanomaterials, including graphene, graphene oxide, reduced graphene oxide, graphene quantum dots, and their derivatives, the synthetic methods of graphene-based nanomaterials are included in situ synthesis and binding method. The bioimaging modalities, including optical imaging (fluorescence [FL], two-photon FL), positron emission tomography/single-photon emission computed tomography, magnetic resonance imaging, photoacoustic imaging, Raman imaging, and multimodal imaging are highlighted (**Figure 8**).

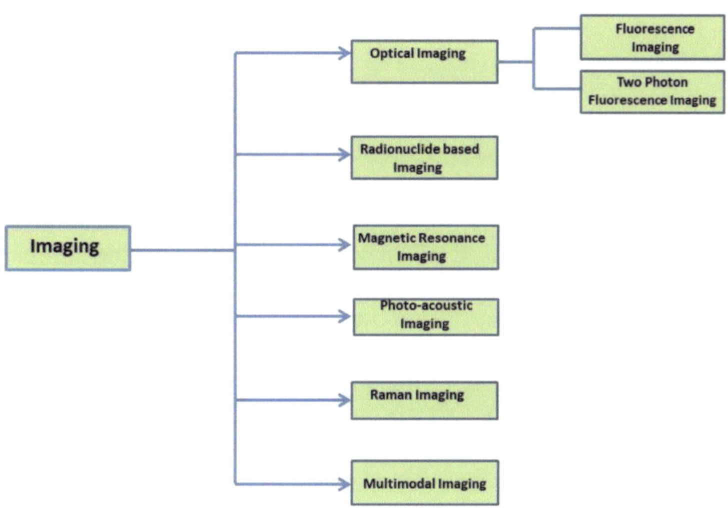

Figure 8.
Different types of bioimaging graphene-based bioimaging.

5.1 Optical imaging

GO- and rGO-based composites are extensively used in the bioimaging field as the arrangement of tissues were comprehend with the help of optical imaging and with the application of unique characteristics of photon-based visible light [92]. As compared to the other progression GO derivatives has immense superiority including high-sensitivity non-ionizing energy, relative and economical advantage, real-time imaging, multiplexing capability, short range free space optical communication [93]. Although, this advancement is affected by low tissue penetration (0–2 cm), high tissue spreading of photons in the visible spectra region and considerable conditions because of tissue auto fluorescence and light absorption by macronutrients, oxygen binding groups and even by water molecules [94]. GO-based composites were dynamically developed for future aspects of different optical imaging techniques, such as (Fluorescence Imaging) FL imaging and (Two-Photon Fluorescence Imaging) TPFI.

5.1.1 Fluorescence imaging

Fluorescence imaging is a nonpersistent technique depends on the intensity of photons emitted from the probe used for fluorescent imaging [95]. A number of research groups focused on organic fluorescent dyes to fabricate GO and rGO *in vitro* and in vivo FL optical imaging. Liu and coworkers subjugated firstly a visible near infrared fluorescent dye, Cyanin 7 (Cy7), complexed with nGO-PEG and form a imaging system (nGO-PEG-Cy7) for in vivo FL imaging of tumor xenografted mice. The nGO-PEG-Cy7 supposed to be enriched in the tumor over time after intravenous vaccination. Prominent uptake of nGO was observed in the infected area compared with other healthy parts of the mouse after 24 h postinjection for different types of tumor modalities. The result shows high tumor accumulation of nGO-PEG-Cy7 based on the improved permeability and retention effect of malignant tumors [96]. Apart from compiling with organic fluorescent dyes, the other non-fluorescence dyes or porphyrin rings are also directly coated on the graphene surface for this particular imaging. Chen and coworkers reported GO conjugated multifunctional system composed of VEGF-loaded (vascular endothelial growth factor) IR-Dye-800 (e.g., GO-IR-Dye-800-VEGF) for fluorescence imaging of ischemic limb cells in the aquatic posterior limb ischemia mold [97]. Further IR-800 dye was firstly compile with the six headed amino groups of poly ethylene glycol (PEG), then later VEGF was loaded onto the two available basal planes of GO via physisorption. The IR-800 shows the same account of FL emission spectra variation even after combing it with various other components at the particular specific maximum wavelength of 800 nm. This specific imaging property of the fluorescence active compounds is used extensively in the imaging application of the GO-based compounds. When we compared the ischemic limbs with the nonischemic limbs the fluorescence intensity ischemic limbs are stronger than that of nonischemic limbs at after intravenous vaccination, explains that GO-IR800-VEGF could exclusively be used to target ischemic limb sowing the enlarged permeability of blood cells. At 24 h time point p.i., the mice were sacrificed and organs of GO-IR800 and GO-IR800-VEGF-injected mice were harvested for *ex vivo* imaging. Interestingly, both of GO-IR800 and GO-IR800-VEGF were mainly distributed throughout the entire ischemic tissue below the ligation site. When we functionalized a biocompatible polymer on the GO surface it acts as a linkage between the GO and these fluorescence active dye [98]. Recently graphene quantum dots are also came into the scenario as they show some photoluminescent properties when incorporated with GO. The lattices inside the GQDs play an important role in functionalization process as well as show some extraordinary characteristics such as zig zag geometry, electron hole mobile electron carriers, high photostability and lower toxic index [99]. Nahain and its research group demonstrate the particular sized GQDs with the fluid known as hyaluronic acid for proficient CD44-targeted delivery to tumor-effective BALB/c mice, representing the intense fluorescence image of the tumor cell line [100]. However, the QY of GQDs still needs to be improved for further bioimaging applications. Meanwhile, further surface modification is also necessary to improve the optical belongings of GQDs and improve the tumor accrual rate.

5.1.2 Two-photon fluorescence imaging

Due to some background noise disturb the fluorescence imaging due to single photon fluorescence imaging Two-Photon Fluorescence Imaging came into the picture. Two-Photon Fluorescence Imaging has fascinated much concentration because of its potential applications in fundamental study and medical diagnostics [101]. With the help of TPFI more detailed examination of various in vivo activities of deep located tumorous cells. Compared with one photon excitation using simple continuous-wave lasers, two-photon nonlinear excitation usually uses a nonlinear femtosecond laser to obtain a high reflux of excitation photons. Recently, graphene-based nanomaterials aroused considerable interest in the field of TPFI. Wang and Gu et al. first reported transferrin functionalized GO-PEG with strong two-photon luminescence as a nonbleaching optical probe for three-dimensional TPFI and laser-based cancer microsurgery, using an ultrafast pulsed laser as the excitation source [102]. Gong group employed nitrogen doping GQDs (N-GQDs) with an average size of ~3 nm as efficient two photon fluorescent probes for cellular and deep-tissue imaging [103]. Taking dimethylformamide as solvent and nitrogen sources, the nitrogen was successfully doping to GQDs by a facile one-pot solvothermal method. Obviously, the TPFI using N-GQDs as fluorescent probe is particularly suitable for in vivo investigation of biostructures in the 800–1500 μm region.

5.2 Radionuclide-based imaging

Optical imaging cannot provide quantitative results and sometimes may be interfered by FL quenching of fluorescent dyes, light absorption and scattering of tissues, and autofluorescence background. Radiolabeling method would be able to accurately track the labeled substances in vivo in a quantitative manner with excellent sensitivity (~10–11–10–12 mol/L) and nearly no penetration depth limit. The radionuclide-based imaging mainly contains PET and SPECT. PET and SPECT images are acquired over a nominally low background signal and require little signal amplification [104]. Graphene-based nanomaterials as promising nanoplatforms are playing an important role in PET/SPECT imaging. In 2011, Liu et al. reported a method to label nGO-PEG with 125I by anchoring iodine atoms on the defects and edges of GO [105]. After that a number of studies have been developed based on this method. Cai group explored in vivo active tumor targeting using 64Cu-labeled nGO-PEG [106]. In comparison to PET, SPECT is ~10 times less sensitive (~10–10–10–11 mol/L); however, SPECT enables concurrent imaging of multiple radionuclides of different energies [107]. Cornelissen et al. explored the use of anti-HER2 antibody (trastuzumab)-conjugated nGO, radiolabeled with 111In-benzyl-diethylenetriaminepentaacetic acid (BnDTPA) via π-π stacking, for in vivo targeting and SPECT imaging. The radiolabeled nGO-trastuzumab conjugates demonstrated better pharmacokinetics compared with radiolabeled trastuzumab without NGO, with more rapid clearance from the circulation [108].

5.3 Magnetic resonance imaging

Noninvasive technique MRI have been extensive used for the detection of morphological feature of tissue related bioscience in comparison to other optical imaging. But somehow the lower sensitivity for the detection of different concentration and inappropriate signaling time has been assigned as the huge drawbacks of MRI [109]. While the biomolecules and ions with paramagnetic nature of metal ions having manganese (Mn) and gadolinium (Gd) as major contributions are reported as the toxic in most of the cases [110]. Whereas such metallic ions can be incorporated with GO utilizing chelation procedure in between metals and different graphene layers [111]. The Gd (gadolinium) incorporated graphene oxide and amidoamine polymer dendrimer-based composite for the delivery of anti-cancerous drugs on the targeting sites have been reported by Wei et al. [112]. The composite of nitrogen doped graphene oxide have been studied for the detection of tumor containing sites on the defective cells. Starting from GO andiron hydrate the reduced graphene oxide-based composites were synthesized by Liu et al. following autoclave-based thermal treatment methodology. The hydrophobic interaction-based functionalization of polyetheneglycol and maleic anhydride-alt-1-octadecene molecule with iron-based nanoparticles were reported by the same to restore the magnetic properties along with the enhancement of thermal stability of developed solutions [113]. Graphene oxide/iron oxide nanoparticle-based system was fabricated to study and diagnosis of pancreatic cancer by Fu et al. [114]. The graphene and iron nanoparticle-based composite was reported as the magnificent composite to help the surgeons into the preparations of cancer cells. The dual mapping is main device that can easily radiate the difference in between normal and RLN tissues, thus further the lymph nodes can be treated with laser. The penetration effects of lower energy waves are much larger and deeper, while the radio waves worked as the low scatter for biomedical systems, i.e., tissues, cells or organs, etc. the PAI cells photographic technique, which take advantage of the absorption of longer wavelength containing waves into thermal energy for thermal expansion [115].

5.4 Photoacoustic imaging

The reduced graphene nanomaterials are irreplaceable candidates to absorb near infra-red light in comparison to graphene oxide that reflects sp^2 hybridization of carbon [116]. The reduced nature of reduced GO reflects hydrophobic nature of the graphene oxide thus finally result its poor water solubility. In order to find out a unique solution, the microwave heating-based-reduced graphene sheets having lower oxygen containing functional groups were synthesized by Patel et al. [117]. The Hummers method has been utilized to reduce the major oxygen content present in the graphitic powder, the methodology of Hummers method includes the acidic oxidations. The GO sheets can also be reduced to rGO by single step thermal reduction methodology and reported rGO possess excellent stability and lesser cell toxicity [118].

5.5 Raman imaging

The advanced characterizations technique, i.e., the RAMAN technique is excellently advanced tool for the analytical and experimental extension for the detection of related various biochemical problems. The RAMAN spectrum including D and G bands exactly mentions and elaborates the enhancements of combinations of various nanoparticles [119]. The folic acid hybrid incorporated Ag/GO composite have been developed for specifically targeting of defective cancerous cells [120].

The in situ synthesis of gold- and GO-based composites have been incorporated in HeLa 229 cells which have been found to display excellent peaks and shifts in Raman spectra. The gold nanoparticle incorporated with nitrogen doped graphene oxide was reported by Ma and coworkers. The in situ synthesis of gold nanocomposites were also assumed to have physical forces of attraction between NOPs and gold particles. The further modifications of GO and reduced graphene sheets with 2-mercaptopyridine were reported by the non-covalent linkage [121]. Gold-based GO composites were reported for the development of good substrate than the Au NPs. Similarly, polyethylene glycol functionalized gold/copper nanoparticles along with graphene were incorporated through CVD method by the group of Tan et al. [122]. The unique Raman signals of graphite-based nanoparticles were reported along with further cell labeling and SERS detection. Recently, bio-imaging applications with more modalities have gained excellent popularity in recent decade [123].

5.6 Multimodal imaging

The multimodality of such imaging applications has been referred as the better technique over the individual imaging technique for the higher accuracy and for the better diagnosis [124, 125]. While the multiphase analysis of single agent lack the potential problem on the probe, i.e., tissues blood for the further removal of impurities along with several doses [126]. Liu et al. have developed rGO-IONP for triple modulation, i.e., FL, PA along with MR [127]. The rGO-based composites of iron and GO have been synthesized via hydrothermal methodology where the polyethylene glycol was incorporated with poly(maleicanhydride-alt-1-octadecene) (C18PMH-PEG), further NIR was performed for the detection of magnetic absorbance. Similarly, Chen et al. reported the graphene oxide-based composite of PEG having non-covalent interactions, i.e., π-π stacking for the detection of tumorous cells. The recent reports of Wu et al. have synthesized the BaGdF5 nanoparticles which were reported to formulate on the graphene oxide sheets in moderate presence of polyethylene glycol. In the transmission electron microscopy (TEM), the exact morphology of GO/BaGdF5-based PEG composite was shown. This showed excellent separation of layers, along with the accuracy in size of sheets, where the size was reported to exist as smaller than corresponding pure GO sheets. While the SAED (selected area electron diffraction) spectra showed the excellently good crystal nature of BaGdF nanoparticles having cubic shape [128].

6. Conclusion and future prospects

The unique ability of catenation of carbon and tendency to form various hybrid orbitals results in the formation of various smart compounds with different physical and chemical properties. Its 2D hexagonally packed unique structure of in-plane sigma C—C bonds accounts for certain physical and chemical properties in biological media has led to its varied applications in the field of drug delivery, gene delivery, tissue engineering and various imaging techniques, etc. The electrostatic interaction and presence of metallic ions in biological media tends to agglomerate and reduces the surface area of graphene sheets. Therefore, covalent and non-covalent methods of surface modifications are used to increase the efficacy of graphene sheets. Further surface fabrication of GO with various polymers allows its use in the fields of drug delivery, tissue engineering and different imaging techniques. Surface modification by way of exfoliation is used for large scale synthesis of graphene. Modified Hummer's method is a common procedure of synthesizing GO from the natural mineral source, i.e., flake graphite. The carboxylic group is found on the surface of graphite during the process of oxidation and exfoliation is modified by covalent functionalization making its use possible in the studies of biological systems and also found applications in biological activities like anti-bacterial activity, bioimaging and photodynamic therapy. Non-covalent functionalization has added advantage of not altering the structure or electronic properties of graphene while introducing new chemical groups on its surface. This results in enhancement of its dispersibility, biocompatibility, reactivity, binding capacity and sensing properties. Graphene has the properties of high surface region, distinctive geometry and structure, flexibility, extra ordinary physico-chemical properties, counting the high fracture strength, high Young's modulus, great thermal and electrical conductivity, highly mobile charge carriers and biocompatibility. All mentioned properties makes graphene a valuable and important material for applications in biological systems and other biomedical processes.

In contrast to pristine graphene synthesized GO has high dispersibility in physiological media leading to better contact with biologically important organic molecules. Outstanding thermal and electrical conductivity and very low thermal expansion quotient of GO allows its use in energy conversion storage devices and bio sensors. GO derivative-based optoelectronic devices have been developed as IR detectors and electrophysiological modulators and emitters. The optical properties like intense light transmittance, fluorescence, photoluminescence and high mobility of charge make graphene an important material for application in MRI and biomedical imaging. Superior mechanical properties of GO like high tensile strength and extensive stiffness has enabled its use in the field of biomedical implant and tissue engineering. Cell-graphene and biomolecule-graphene studies have opened a vast area of GOs exploration in the fields of cellular biology, genomics and development of antibiotics, etc. Despite its varied uses certain challenges still remain in the field of nanotheranostic designing in terms of bioavailability, selectivity, biocompatibility and safety. In the field of pharmacology, better targeted and relatively lower dose drug delivery with graphene complex has proved cheaper and efficient than the discovery of newer drug. Graphene-based materials as drug and gene delivery vehicles have used successfully in *in vitro* studies, however much research in in vivo studies is still in early stages. Many researchers have focused on developing graphene-based materials for wound healing, stem cell imaging, regenerative medicine and tissue engineering. Graphene finds its application in bio imaging by way of optical imaging, fluorescence Imaging (FL) and two photon fluorescence imaging (TPFI), etc. High sensitivity non-ionizing energy, real time imaging, multiplexing capability, short range free space optical communication and economic advantages makes GO derivative superior for use in optical imaging. However, low tissue penetration, high tissue spreading of photons in the visible spectra, tissue auto fluorescence and light absorption by oxygen binding groups and water limits the use of GO derivatives in optical imaging. Labeling of fluorescent dyes on GO surface and their detection by photons emission from probe has been enabled the development of fluorescent imaging technique for the study of biological systems. Recently certain desirable properties of GQDs like luminescence, zig zag geometry, electron hole mobile electron carriers, high photostability and lower toxic index have enabled development of better FL imaging system. The limitations of FL imaging leads to development of TPFI using non-linear femto second laser to obtain a high reflux of excitation photons, thereby enabling the development of better and deeper fluorescent imaging probes. Radio labeling of graphene-based nanomaterials has increased the sensitivity of qualitative imaging studies like PET/SPECT further doped GO has found its application in MRI for detailed study of different tissues in humans. Past few years have witnessed the development of graphene from a little known nanoparticle to wide spread interest in the field of development of graphene-based nanomaterial for applications in biochemical and biophysical systems and processes. However, much research work is still desired to enable commercial scale applications of GO-based nanomaterials.

Acknowledgements

Authors acknowledge the financial assistance from NMHS research grant KU/NMHS/MG/2016/002/8603/007, GBPIHED, Kosi-Katarmal, Almora, India.

Author details

Neha Karki[1], Anita Rana[1], Himani Tiwari[1], Pushpa Negi[2] and Nanda Gopal Sahoo[1*]

1 Department of Chemistry, Prof. Rajendra Singh Nanoscience and Nanotechnology Centre, Kumaun University, Nainital, Uttarakhand, India

2 Department of Chemistry, Graphic Era Hill University, Uttarakhand, India

*Address all correspondence to: ngsahoo@yahoo.co.in

References

[1] Hoboken NJ, Depan D, Shah J, Misra RDK. Controlled release of drug from folate-decorated and graphene mediated drug delivery system: Synthesis, loading efficiency, and drug release response. Materials Science and Engineering C. 2011;**31**(7):1305-1312

[2] Allen MJ, Tung VC, Kaner RB. Honeycomb carbon: A review of graphene. Chemical Reviews. 2010;**110**(1):132-145

[3] Geim AK, Novoselov KS. The rise of graphene. Nature Materials. 2007;**6**:183-191

[4] Novoselov KS, Falko VI, Colombo L, Gellert PR, Schwab MG, Kim K. A roadmap for graphene. Nature. 2012;**490**:192-200

[5] Karki N, Tiwari H, Pal M, Chaurasia A, Bal R, Joshi P, et al. Functionalized graphene oxides for drug loading, release and delivery of poorly water soluble anticancer drug: A comparative study. Colloids and Surfaces, B: Biointerfaces. 2018;**169**:265-272

[6] Romberg B, Hennink WE, Storm G. Sheddable coatings for long-circulating nanoparticles. Pharmaceutical Research. 2008;**2**(1):55-71

[7] Yang K, Hu L, Ma X, Ye S, Cheng L, Shi X, et al. Multimodal imaging guided photothermal therapy using functionalized graphene nanosheets anchored with magnetic nanoparticles. Advanced Materials. 2012;**24**(14):1868-1872

[8] Pal K, Maiti UN, Majumder TP, Debnath SC, Ghosh S, Roy SK, et al. Switching of ferroelectric liquid crystal doped with cetyltrimethylammonium bromide-assisted Cds nanostructures. Nanotechnology. 2013;**24**:125702

[9] Lin J, Chen X, Huang P, Hu SH, Chen YW, Hung WT, et al. Quantum-dot-tagged reduced graphene oxide nanocomposites for bright fluorescence bioimaging and photothermal therapy monitored in situ graphene-based nanomaterials for bioimaging. Advanced Drug Delivery Reviews. 2016;**105**:242-254

[10] Sagadevan S, Pal K. Chowdhury ZZ, Scalable synthesis of CdS–graphene nanocomposite spectroscopic characterizations. Materials in Electronics. 2017;**28**(22):17193-17201

[11] Wong CW, Chan YS, Jeevanandam J, Pal K, Bechelany M, Elkodous MA, et al. Response surface methodology optimization of mono-dispersed MgO nanoparticles fabricated by ultrasonic-assisted sol–gel method for outstanding antimicrobial and antibiofilm activities. Journal of Cluster Science. 2020;**31**:367-389

[12] Yang M, Yao J, Duan Y. Graphene and its derivatives for cell biotechnology. The Analyst. 2013;**138**(1):72-86

[13] Liu K, Zhang JJ, Cheng FF, Zheng TT, Wang C, Zhu JJ. Green and facile synthesis of highly biocompatible graphene nanosheets and its application for cellular imaging and drug delivery. Journal of Materials Chemistry. 2011;**21**(32):12034e40

[14] Feng L, Zhang S, Liu Z. Graphene based gene transfection. Nanoscale. 2011;**3**(3):1252-1257

[15] Taherian F, Marcon V, Van der Vegt NFA, Leroy F. What is the contact angle of water on graphene? Langmuir. 2013;**29**(5):1457-1465

[16] Xue Y, Liu Y, Lu F, Qu J, Chen H, Dai L. Functionalization of graphene oxide with polyhedral oligomeric silsesquioxane (POSS) for multifunctional applications. Journal of Physical Chemistry Letters. 2012;**3**(12):1607-1612

[17] Hsieh CT, Chen WY. Water/oil repellency and work of adhesion of liquid droplets on graphene oxide and graphene surfaces. Surface and Coating Technology. 2011;**205**(19):4554-4561

[18] Hasan SA, Rigueur JL, Harl RR, Krejci AJ, Gonzalo-Juan I, Rogers BR, et al. Transferable graphene oxide films with tunable microstructures. ACS Nano. 2010;**4**(12):7367-7372

[19] Yang ST, Chang Y, Wang H, Liu G, Chen S, Wang Y, et al. Folding/aggregation of graphene oxide and its application in Cu^{2+} removal. Journal of Colloid and Interface Science. 2010;**351**(1):122-127

[20] Cote LJ, Kim F, Huang J. Langmuir-Blodgett assembly of graphite oxide single layers. Journal of the American Chemical Society. 2008;**131**(3):1043-1049

[21] Nika DL, Pokatilov EP, Askerov AS, Balandin AA. Phonon thermal conduction in graphene: Role of Umklapp and edge roughness scattering. Physical Review B. 2009;**79**(15):155413

[22] Jiang JW, Lan J, Wang JS, Li B. Isotopic effects on the thermal conductivity of graphene nanoribbons: Localization mechanism. Journal of Applied Physics. 2010;**107**(5):054314

[23] Kravets VG, Grigorenko AN, Nair RR, Blake P, Anissimova S, Novoselov KS, et al. Spectroscopic ellipsometry of graphene and an exciton-shifted Van Hove peak in absorption. Physical Review B. 2010;**81**(15):55413

[24] Wang F, Hamdi M. Strictly non-blocking conditions for the central-stage buffered clos-network. IEEE Communications Letters. 2008;**12**(3):206-208

[25] Ma X, Tao H, Yang K, Feng L, Cheng L, Shi X, et al. A functionalized graphene oxide–iron oxide nanocomposite for magnetically targeted drug delivery, photothermal therapy, and magnetic resonance imaging. Nano Research. 2012;**5**:199-212

[26] ShenAJ LDL, Cai XJ, Dong CY, Dong HQ, Wen HY, Dai GH, et al. Multifunctional nanocomposite based on graphene oxide for *in vitro* hepatocarcinoma diagnosis and treatment. Journal of Biomedical Materials Research Part A. 2012;**100**(9):2499-2506

[27] Park S, Lee KS, Bozoklu G, Cai W, Nguyen ST, Ruoff RS. Graphene oxide papers modified by divalent ions—Enhancing mechanical properties via chemical cross-linking. ACS Nano. 2008;**2**(3):572-578

[28] Park S, Dikin DA, Nguyen ST, Ruoff RS. Graphene oxide sheets chemically cross-linked by polyallylamine. Journal of Physical Chemistry C. 2009;**113**(36):15801-15804

[29] Barun D, Prasad KE, Ramamurty U, Rao CNR. Nano-indentation studies on polymer matrix composites reinforced by few-layer graphene. Nanotechnology. 2009;**20**(12):125705

[30] Sanchez VC, Jachak A, Hurt RH, Kane AB. Biological interactions of graphene-family nanomaterials: An interdisciplinary review. Chemical Research in Toxicology. 2011;**25**(1):15-34

[31] Bianco A. Graphene: Safe or toxic? The two faces of the medal. Angewandte Chemie, International Edition. 2013;**52**(19):4986-4997

[32] Stone V, Johnston H, Schins RPF. Development of in vitro systems for nanotoxicology: Methodological considerations. Critical Reviews in Toxicology. 2009;**39**(7):613-626

[33] Oberdörster G, Oberdörster E, Oberdörster J. Nanotoxicology: An

emerging discipline evolving from studies of ultrafine particles. Environmental Health Perspectives. 2005;**113**(7):823-839

[34] Kang S, Herzberg M, Rodrigues DF, Elimelech M. Antibacterial effects of carbon nanotubes: Size does matter! Langmuir. 2008;**24**(13):6409-6413

[35] Kang S, Pinault M, Pfefferle LD, Elimelech M. Single-walled carbon nanotubes exhibit strong antimicrobial activity. Langmuir. 2007;**23**(17):8670-8673

[36] Akhavan O, Ghaderi E. Toxicity of graphene and graphene oxide nanowalls against bacteria. ACS Nano. 2010;**4**(10):5731-5736

[37] Hu W, Peng C, Luo W, Lv M, Li X, Li D, et al. Graphene-based antibacterial paper. ACS Nano. 2010;**4**(7):4317-4323

[38] Tazawa H, Tatemichi M, Sawa T, Gilibert I, Ma N, Hiraku Y, et al. Oxidative and nitrative stress caused by subcutaneous implantation of a foreign body accelerates sarcoma development in Trp53+/− mice. Carcinogenesis. 2006;**28**(1):191-198

[39] Bourlinos AB, Gournis D, Petridis D, Szabo T, Szeri A, Dekany I. Graphite oxide: Chemical reduction to graphite and surface modification with primary aliphatic amines and amino acids. Langmuir. 2003;**19**(15):6050-6055

[40] He HY, Klinowski J, Forster M, Lerf A. A new structural model for graphite oxide. Chemical Physics Letters. 1998;**287**(1):53-56

[41] Lerf A, He H, Forster M, Klinowski J. Structure of graphite oxide revisited. The Journal of Physical Chemistry. B. 1998;**102**(23):4477-4482

[42] Banhart F, Kotakoski J, Krasheninnikov AV. Structural defects in graphene. ACS Nano. 2010;**5**(1):26-41

[43] Paton KR. Scalable production of large quantities of defect-free few-layer graphene by shear exfoliation in liquids. Nature Materials. 2014;**13**(6):624-630

[44] Marcano DC. Improved synthesis of graphene oxide. ACS Nano. 2010;**4**(8):4806-4814

[45] Becerril HA. Evaluation of solution-processed reduced graphene oxide films as transparent conductors. ACS Nano. 2008;**2**(3):463-470

[46] Li D, Muller MB, Gilje S, Kaner RB, Wallace GG. Processable aqueous dispersions of graphene nanosheets. Nature Nanotechnology. 2008;**3**(2):101-105

[47] Shih CJ, Lin S, Sharma R, Strano MS, Blankschtein D. Understanding the Ph-dependent behavior of graphene oxide aqueous solutions: A comparative experimental and molecular dynamics simulation study. Langmuir. 2011;**28**(1):235-241

[48] Wissler M. Graphite and carbon powders for electrochemical applications. Journal of Power Sources. 2006;**156**(2):142-150

[49] Ishikawa T, Nagaoki T. Shin tansokogyo (New Carbon Industry). 2nd ed. Tokyo: Kindaihensyusya; 1986. pp. 125-136

[50] Hummers WS, Offeman RE. Preparation of graphitic oxide. Journal of the American Chemical Society. 1958;**80**(6):1339

[51] Xie C, Lu X, Han L, Xu J, Wang Z, Jiang L, et al. Biomimetic mineralized hierarchical graphene oxide/chitosan scaffolds with adsorbability for immobilization of nanoparticles for biomedical applications. ACS Applied Materials & Interfaces. 2016;**8**(3):1707-1717

[52] Loh KP, Bao Q, Eda G, Chowalla M. Graphene oxide as a chemically tunable

platform for optical applications. Nature Chemistry. 2010;**2**(12):1015-1024

[53] Mahmoudi N, Simchi A. On the biological performance of graphene oxide-modified chitosan/polyvinyl pyrrolidone nanocomposite membranes: *In vitro* and *in vivo* effects of graphene oxide. Materials Science and Engineering: C. 2017;**70**(1):121-131

[54] Song MM, Xu HL, Liang JX, Xiang HH, Liu R, Shen YX. Facile fabrication of water-dispersible nanocomposites based on hexa-*peri*-hexabenzocoronene and Fe_3O_4 for dual mode imaging (fluorescent/MR) and drug delivery. Materials Science and Engineering C. 2017;**77**(71):904-911

[55] Panahi F, Fareghi-Alamdari R, Dangolani SK, Nezhad AK, Golestanzadeh M. Graphene grafted N-methyl-4-pyridinamine (G-NMPA): An efficient heterogeneous organocatalyst for acetylation of alcohols. Chemistry Select. 2017;**2**(1):474-479

[56] Paulus GLC, Wang QH, Strano MS. Covalent electron transfer chemistry of graphene with diazonium salts. Accounts of Chemical Research. 2013;**46**:160-170

[57] Lin Y, Ehlert GJ. Superhydrophobic functionalized graphene aerogels. ACS Applied Materials & Interfaces. 2011;**3**(7):2200-2203

[58] Yin T, Liu J, Zhao Z, Zhao Y, Dong L, Yang M, Zou J. Redox sensitive hyaluronic acid decorated graphene oxide for photothermally controlled tumor cytoplasm selective rapid drug delivery. Advanced Functional Materials. 2017;**27**:1604620-1604631

[59] Li A, Ma H, Liu J. Graphene oxide coated Fe_3O_4@$MSiO_2$ Nps for magnetic controlled bioimaging. RSC Advances. 2016;**6**(68):63704-63710

[60] Wei Y, Zhou F, Zhang D, Chen Q, Xing D. Graphene oxide based smart drug delivery system for tumor mitochondria-targeting photodynamic therapy. Nanoscale. 2016;**8**(6):3530-3538

[61] Atabia F, Gargarib SLM, Hashemic M, Yaghmaeia P. Doxorubicin loaded DNA aptamer linked myristilated chitosan nanogel for targeted delivery to prostate cancer. Iran Journal of Pharmacy Research. 2017;**16**(1):35-49

[62] Lehn JM. Supramolecular Chemistry: Concepts and Perspectives. Vol. 99. New York: Wiley; 1995. pp. 4763-4768

[63] Atkins P, de Paula J. Physical Chemistry. New York: W. H. Freeman; 2002

[64] Smithrud DB, Sanford EM, Chao I, Ferguson SB, Carcanague DR, Evanseck JD, et al. Solvent effects in molecular recognition. Pure and Applied Chemistry. 1990;**62**(12):2227-2236

[65] Southall NT, Dill KA, Haymet ADJ. A view of the hydrophobic effect. The Journal of Physical Chemistry. B. 2002;**106**(3):521-533

[66] Zhang ZX, Huang HL, Yang XM, Zang L. Tailoring electronic properties of graphene by pi-pi stacking with aromatic molecules. Journal of Physical Chemistry Letters. 2011;**2**(15):2897-2905

[67] Butte K, Momin M, Kurhade S, Kar S. Intravesical drug delivery system for bladder: An overview. International Journal of Pharmaceutical, Chemical and Biological Sciences. 2013;**3**(3):680-681

[68] Li N, Zhao P, Astruc D. Anisotropic gold nanoparticles: Synthesis, properties, applications, and toxicity. Angewandte Chemie International Edition. 2014;**53**(7):1756-1789

[69] Argyo C, Weiss V, Bräuchle C, Bein T. Multifunctional Mesoporous

silica nanoparticles as a universal platform for drug delivery. Chemistry of Materials. 2013;**26**(1):430-434

[70] Liu Z, Robinson JT, Sun X, Dai H. PEGylatednanographene oxide for delivery of water-insoluble cancer drugs. Journal of the American Chemical Society. 2008;**130**(33):10876-10877

[71] Yang K, Wan J, Zhang S, Zhang Y, Lee ST, Liu Z. In vivo pharmacokinetics, long-term biodistribution, and toxicology of PEGylated Graphene In mice. ACS Nano. 2010;5(1):516-522

[72] Jing W, Yin-song W, Xiao-ying Y, Yuan-yuan L, Jin-rong Y, Rui Y, et al. Graphene oxide used as a carrier for adriamycin can reverse drug resistance in breast cancer cells. Nanotechnology. 2012;**23**(35):355101

[73] Depan D, Shah J, Misra RDK. Controlled release of drug from folate-decorated and graphene mediated drug delivery system: Synthesis, loading efficiency, and drug release response. Materials Science and Engineering C. 2011;**31**(7):1305-1312

[74] Zhang L, Xia J, Zhao Q, Liu L, Zhang Z. Functional graphene oxide as a nanocarrier for controlled loading and targeted delivery of mixed anticancer drugs. Small. 2010;**6**(4):537-544

[75] Bai H, Li C, Wang X, Shi G. A Ph-sensitive graphene oxide composite hydrogel. Chemical Communications. 2010;**46**(14):2376-2378

[76] Yang X, Zhang X, Liu Z, Ma Y, Huang Y, Chen Y. High-efficiency loading and controlled release of doxorubicin hydrochloride on graphene oxide. Journal of Physical Chemistry C. 2008;**112**(45):17554-17558

[77] Zhang L, Xia J, Zhao Q, Liu L, Zhang Z. Functional graphene oxide as a nanocarrier for controlled loading and targeted delivery of mixed anticancer drugs. Small. 2010;**6**(4):537-544

[78] Yang X, Zhang X, Ma Y, Huang Y, Wang Y, Chen Y. Superparamagnetic graphene oxide–Fe_3O_4 nanoparticles hybrid for controlled targeted drug carriers. Journal of Materials Chemistry. 2009;**19**(18):2710-2714

[79] Fan X, Jiao G, Gao L, Jin P, Li X. The preparation and drug delivery of graphene-carbon nanotube–Fe_3O_4 nanoparticle hybrid. Journal of Materials Chemistry B. 2013;**1**(20):2658-2664

[80] Shen H, Zhang L, Liu M, Zhang Z. Biomedical applications of graphene. Theranostics. 2012;**2**(3):283-294

[81] Yang ZR, Wang HF, Zhao J, Peng YY, Wang J, Guinn BA, et al. Recent developments in the use of adenoviruses and immunotoxins in cancer gene therapy. Cancer Gene Therapy. 2007;**14**(7):599-615

[82] Jager M, Schubert S, Ochrimenko S, Fischer D, Schubert US. Branched and linear poly(ethylene imine)-based conjugates: Synthetic modification, characterization, and application. Chemical Society Reviews. 2012;**41**(13):4755-4767

[83] Bao H, Pan Y, Ping Y, Sahoo NG, Wu T, Li L, et al. Chitosan-functionalized graphene oxide as a nanocarrier for drug and gene delivery. Small. 2011;7(11):1569-1578

[84] Shen H, Liu M, He H, Zhang L, Huang J, Chong Y, et al. PEGylated graphene oxide-mediated protein delivery for cell function regulation. ACS Applied Materials & Interfaces. 2012;**4**(11):6317-6323

[85] La WG, Park S, Yoon HH, Jeong GJ, Lee TJ, Bhang SH, et al. Delivery of a therapeutic protein for

bone regeneration from a substrate coated with graphene oxide. Small. 2013;**9**(23):4051-4060

[86] Langer R, Vacanti JP. Biodegradable polymer scaffolds for tissue engineering. Tissue Engineering. Science. 1993;**260**(14):920-926

[87] Sant S, Hancock MJ, Donnelly JP, Iyer D, Khademhosseini A. Biomimetic gradient hydrogels for tissue engineering. Canadian Journal of Chemical Engineering. 2010;**88**(6):899-911

[88] Zhang L, Wang Z, Xu C, Li Y, Gao J, Wang W, et al. High strength graphene oxide/polyvinyl alcohol composite hydrogels. Journal of Materials Chemistry. 2011;**21**(28):10399-10406

[89] Lu B, Li T, Zhao H, Li X, Gao C, Zhang S, et al. Graphene-based composite materials beneficial to wound healing. Nanoscale. 2012;**4**(9): 2978-2982

[90] Ku SH, Park CB. Myoblast differentiation on graphene oxide. Biomaterials. 2013;**34**(8):2017-2023

[91] Mahmoudi M, Akhavan O, Ghavami M, Rezaee F, Ghiasi SMA. Graphene oxide strongly inhibits amyloid beta fibrillation. Nanoscale. 2012;**4**(23):7322-7325

[92] Janib SM, Moses AS, MacKay JA. Imaging and drug delivery using theranostic nanoparticles. Advanced Drug Delivery Reviews. 2010;**62**(11):1052-1063

[93] Wang J, Mi P, Lin G, Wang YX, Liu G, Chen X. Imaging-guided delivery of Rnai for anticancer treatment. Advanced Drug Delivery Reviews. 2016;**104**(1):44-60

[94] Park K, Lee S, Kang E, Kim K, Choi K, Kwon IC. New generation of multifunctional nanoparticles for cancer imaging and therapy. Advanced Functional Materials. 2009;**19**(10):1553-1566

[95] Baker SN, Baker GA. Luminescent carbon nanodots: Emergent nanolights. Angewandte Chemie, International Edition. 2010;**49**(38):6726-6744

[96] Yang K, Zhang S, Zhang G, Sun X, Lee ST, Liu Z. Graphene in mice: Ultrahigh in vivo tumor uptake and efficient photothermal therapy. Nano Letters. 2010;**10**(9):3318-3323

[97] Sun Z, Huang P, Tong G, Lin J, Jin A, Rong P, et al. VEGF-loaded graphene oxide as theranostics for multi-modality imaging-monitored targeting therapeutic angiogenesis of ischemic muscle. Nanoscale. 2013;**5**(15):6857-6866

[98] Yang HW, Huang CY, Lin CW, Liu HL, Huang CW, Liao SS, et al. Gadolinium-functionalized nanographene oxide for combined drug and microrna delivery and magnetic resonance imaging. Biomaterials. 2014;**35**(24):6534-6542

[99] Liu Q, Guo B, Rao Z, Zhang B, Gong JR. Strong two-photon-induced fluorescence from photostable, biocompatible nitrogen-doped graphene quantum dots for cellular and deep-tissue imaging. Nano Letters. 2013;**13**(6):2436-2441

[100] Abdullah AN, Lee JE, In I, Lee H, Lee KD, Jeong JH, et al. Target delivery and cell imaging using hyaluronic acid-functionalized graphene quantum dots. Molecular Pharmaceutics. 2013;**10**(10):3736-3744

[101] Yoo JM, Kang JH, Hong BH. Graphene-based nanomaterials for versatile imaging studies. Chemical Society Reviews. 2015;**44**(14):4835-4852

[102] Li JL, Bao HC, Hou XL, Sun L, Wang XG, Gu M. Graphene oxide

nanoparticles as nonbleaching optical probe for two-photon luminescence imaging and cell therapy. Angewandte Chemie, International Edition. 2012;**51**(8):1830-1834

[103] Liu Q, Guo B, Rao Z, Zhang B, Gong JR. Strong two-photon-induced fluorescence from photostable, biocompatible nitrogen-doped graphene quantum dots for cellular and deep-tissue imaging. Nano Letters. 2013;**13**(6):2436-2441

[104] Park K, Lee S, Kang E, Kim K, Choi K, Kwon IC. New generation of multifunctional nanoparticles for cancer imaging and therapy. Advanced Functional Materials. 2009;**19**(10):1553-1566

[105] Yang K, Zhang S, Zhang G, Sun X, Lee ST, Liu Z. Graphene in mice: Ultrahigh *in vivo* tumor uptake and efficient photothermal therapy. Nano Letters. 2010;**10**(9):3318-3323

[106] Hong H, Yang K, Zhang Y, Engle JW, Feng L, Yang Y, et al. In vivo targeting and imaging of tumor vasculature with radiolabeled, antibody-conjugated nanographene. ACS Nano. 2012;**6**(3):2361-2370

[107] Sun Z, Huang P, Tong G, Lin J, Jin A, Rong P, et al. VEGF-loaded graphene oxide as theranostics for multi-modality imaging-monitored targeting therapeutic angiogenesis of ischemic muscle. Nanoscale. 2013;**5**(1):6857-6866

[108] Cornelissen B, Able S, Kersemans V, Waghorn PA, Myhra S, Jurkshat K, et al. Nanographene oxide-based radioimmunoconstructs for in vivo targeting and SPECT imaging of HER2-positive tumors. Biomaterials. 2013;**34**:1146-1154

[109] Jiang L, Fan Z. Design of advanced porous graphene materials: From graphene nanomesh to 3D architectures. Nanoscale. 2014;**6**(4):1922-1945

[110] Caravan P, Ellison JJ, TJ MM, Lauffer RB. Gadolinium(III) chelates as MRI contrast agents: Structure, dynamics, and applications. Chemical Reviews. 1999;**99**(9):2293-2352

[111] Yoo JM, Kang JH, Hong BH. Graphene-based nanomaterials for versatile imaging studies. Chemical Society Reviews. 2015;**44**(14):4835-4852

[112] Yang HW, Huang CY, Lin CW, Liu HL, Huang CW, Liao SS, et al. Gadolinium-functionalized nanographene oxide for combined drug and microrna delivery and magnetic resonance imaging. Biomaterials. 2014;**35**(24):6534-6542

[113] Yang K, Gong H, Shi X, Wan J, Zhang Y, Liu Z. In vivo biodistribution and toxicology of functionalized nano-graphene oxide in mice after oral and intraperitoneal administration. Biomaterials. 2013;**34**(11):2787-2795

[114] Wang YW, Fu YY, Peng Q, Guo SS, Liu G, Li J, et al. Dye-enhanced graphene oxide for photothermal therapy and photoacoustic imaging. Journal of Materials Chemistry B. 2013;**1**(42):5762-5767

[115] Huang J, Zong C, Shen H, Liu M, Chen B, Ren B, et al. Mechanism of cellular uptake of graphene oxide studied by surface-enhanced Raman spectroscopy. Small. 2012;**8**(16):2577-2584

[116] Lalwani G, Cai X, Nie L, Wang LV, Sitharaman B. Graphene-based contrast agents for photoacoustic and thermoacoustic tomography. Photoacoustics. 2013;**1**(3-4):62-67

[117] Patel MA, Yang H, Chiu PL, Mastrogiovanni DD, Flach CR, Savaram K, et al. Direct production of graphene nanosheets for near infrared

photoacoustic imaging. ACS Nano. 2013;**7**(9):8147-8157

[118] Sheng Z, Song L, Zheng J, Hu D, He M, Zheng M, et al. Protein-assisted fabrication of nano-reduced graphene oxide for combined in vivo photoacoustic imaging and photothermal therapy. Biomaterials. 2013;**34**(21):5236-5243

[119] Kim YK, Han SW, Min DH. Graphene oxide sheath on Ag nanoparticle/graphene hybrid films as an antioxidative coating and enhancer of surface-enhanced Raman scattering. ACS Applied Materials & Interfaces. 2012;**4**(12):6545-6551

[120] Liu Z, Guo Z, Zhong H, Qin X, Wan M, Yang B. Graphene oxide based surface enhanced Raman scattering probes for cancer cell imaging. Physical Chemistry Chemical Physics. 2013;**15**(8):2961-2966

[121] Ma X, Qu Q, Zhao Y, Luo Z, Zhao Y, Ng KW, et al. Graphene oxide wrapped gold nanoparticles for intracellular Raman imaging and drug delivery. Journal of Materials Chemistry B. 2013;**1**(47):6495-6500

[122] Song ZL, Chen Z, Bian X, Zhou LY, Ding D, Liang H, et al. Alkyne-functionalized superstable graphitic silver nanoparticles for Raman imaging. Journal of the American Chemical Society. 2014;**136**(39):13558-13561

[123] Park K, Lee S, Kang E, Kim K, Choi K, Kwon IC. New generation of multifunctional nanoparticles for cancer imaging and therapy. Advanced Functional Materials. 2009;**19**(10):1553-1566

[124] Huang P, Rong P, Jin A, Yan X, Zhang MG, Lin J, et al. Dye-loaded ferritin nanocages for multimodal imaging and photothermal therapy. Advanced Materials. 2014;**26**(37):6401-6408

[125] Ma J, Huang P, He M, Pan L, Zhou Z, Feng L, et al. Folic acidconjugated Laf3:Yb,Tm@SiO_2 nanoprobes for targeting dual-modality imaging of upconversion luminescence and X-ray computed tomography. The Journal of Physical Chemistry. B. 2012;**116**(48):14062-14070

[126] Cheng Z, Al Zaki A, Hui JZ, Muzykantov VR, Tsourkas A. Multifunctional nanoparticles: Cost versus benefit of adding targeting and imaging capabilities. Science. 2012;**338**(6109):903-910

[127] Rong P, Yang K, Srivastan A, Kiesewetter DO, Yue X, Wang F, et al. Photosensitizer loaded nanographene for multimodality imaging guided tumor photodynamic therapy. Theranostics. 2014;**4**(3):229-239

[128] Wu H, Shi H, Wang Y, Jia X, Tang C, Zhang J, et al. Hyaluronic acid conjugated graphene oxide for targeted drug delivery. Carbon. 2014;**69**(12):379-389

Chapter 12

Tumor Malignancy Characterization in Clinical Environments: An Approach Using the FYC-Index of Spiculation and Artificial Intelligence

Fernando Yepes-Calderón, Flor M. Medina, Nolan D. Rea and José Abella

Abstract

According to the World Health Organization, cancer is the second leading cause of death in the world. The myriad of variations, paths of development, and mutations make this abnormality challenging to treat. With the advent of medical imaging, complex qualitative information is collected with the aim of characterizing the pathology; however, the uncomfortable and time-consuming histology remains the state of care within hospitals. This manuscript presents a strategy to extract quantifiable features from the images. The method captures shape perturbation as variations in reference to a perfect circle that is used in a standardized dimensional space. A multifeatured scheme is created when the quantification is applied in all slices produced by imaging modalities such as computed tomography, magnetic resonance imaging, and tomosynthesis. Later, the numbers obtained by the introduced algorithm are used in an artificial intelligence pipeline that correlates spicularity with aggressiveness using the histology as supervising factor.

Keywords: medical image analysis, tumor grading, cancer, tumor characterization

1. Introduction

Classifying cancer lesions in form and intensity from the images is of interest in radiology units [1–3]. Currently, histology is the gold standard to define cancer type, stage, and grade; nevertheless, histology comes with its associated costs and delays and has been reported to increase morbidity [4, 5]. When diagnosing from the images, the desired classification is accurate and repeatable only if the operator includes the quantitative domain to the set of available tools that are mostly from the qualitative domain. The quantification is accomplished by separating the neomass from the anatomical parts in the image employing segmentation.

 IntechOpen

Regarding segmentation, authors have proposed assisting techniques that partially or fully accomplish the tasks with different levels of accuracy [6–8].

After segmentation, the challenge is finding a repeatable and performant method for all kinds of cancer manifestations. Some quantifying approaches target cancer in specific parts of the body [9, 10], while others focus on particular kinds of cancer [11, 12].

Although technology has invaded the medical facilities, currently assisting tools are not of help in diagnosing cancer. The tasks are still performed by human experts employing purely qualitative judgment. There is a need to quantify and thus abandon the uncertainty produced by human variability.

In practice, qualitative features suggested by X-rads [13, 14] such as roughness and stiffness are difficult to conceptualize with mathematical models; therefore, indexes based on these features are complicated to model [15]. However, the shape of the captured objects is a stable feature in the field of view [16, 17] and, conveniently, has the required sensibility across all cancer manifestations because it captures the core manifestations of the disease, the disordered growth pattern [18, 19]. More importantly, tumor shape is quantified in a feature-enriched scheme to favor further machine-learning implementation. In this document, we employ the FYC-Index of spiculation [20] to assert quantification on the edges of breast tumors imaged with tomosynthesis [21, 22]. The numbers yielded by the FYC-Index strategy are fed to an artificial intelligence classifier that initially differentiates between benign and malign neo-masses, showing a high degree of accuracy in supervised experiments. The presented strategy is equally performant in all imaging techniques that generate volumetric representations by slicing, including MRI, CT, and tomosynthesis.

2. Materials and methods

2.1 Clinical data

A cohort of 48 breast tomosynthesis images underwent segmentation performed by an expert radiologist. Histology was performed on the 48 masses yielding 29 malignant cases and 19 benign. The resulting masks hold the specifications of the original images regarding the field of view and spatial resolution. Since the algorithm explained in Section 2.2 is immune to resolution changes and the field of view is standardized, records of the images' specifications are not provided in this document.

2.2 The FYC-Index of spiculation

The reader is invited to refer to **Figure 1**. Recall that the procedure explained below is used on both views, axial and sagittal.

Block I. Images of CT, MRI, or tomosynthesis are suitable for this processing due to their slicing nature. The FYC-Index re-sample all masks to isometric

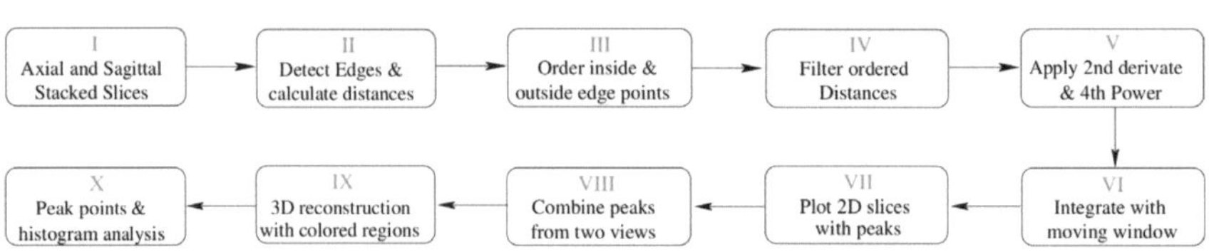

Figure 1.
Block diagrams for the FYC-Index pipeline.

voxels of 1 mm before selecting the biggest mask through area calculation. Next, the dimensions of the biggest bounding box are used as a dimensional template. Then, the other slices in the study—including those of other tumors in case we are working with a population—are scaled to the dimensions of the biggest bounding box. This process also centers the masks. Distortion in the mask growing process is avoided by using the adaptive supersampling method [23, 24]. After scaling, all the images share the same field of view (FOV) and therefore, the same planar coordinates for the center point.

Block II. Then, the edges of the masks are detected using the Canny edge detector [25].

Block III. As the Canny detector does not create single-pixel edges, the system detects two paths corresponding to the outer and inner edges. The Euclidean distance from the artificially created center of coordinates to each point in the edge is saved in two arrays, one corresponds to the outer edge and the other to the inner edge. The two arrays are averaged in an ordered array of distances (AoD). The run along the edge that creates the AoD is standardized by starting the distance calculation at the top center of the image and taking the edging points in a clockwise fashion until the starting point is located at a distance of $\sqrt{(2)}$ mm of the current point or below. Recall that voxels are all set to 1 mm.

Block IV. The AoD is Gaussian filtered creating the FAoD. This filtering is intended to eliminate the high-frequency components produced by the digital grid. The filter is implemented in the frequency domain, keeping 80% of the original spectral power. According to [26], maintaining the 80% of the signal spectral power assures that the important content of the signals is kept.

Block V. A five-point differentiation is applied to find the regions of rapid change; next, a second five-point differentiation is executed to recover the inflection points. These operations are generalized to each point in FAoD as shown in **Eq. 1**:

$$p'_n = [(d_n - d_{n-2}) + (d_n - d_{n-1}) + (d_{n+1} - d_n) + (d_{n+2} - d_n)]/4 \tag{1}$$

The second derivative “p”— obtained with the second pass of Eq. (1)—is where peaks are detected. The peak elements on FAoD are exalted, while regions of low dynamics in the same array are diminished when raising FAoD to the fourth power.

Block VI. A moving window integration selects peaks in the exponential second derivative. Given points $p(s) = (s, d)$, the area (A) under the curve section with a width (N) is calculated for step (s), as it is shown in Eq. (2). If $A(s) > T$ for a chosen value of T, s is added to this list of locations of peaks:

$$A(s) = \sum_{i=-\frac{N}{2}}^{\frac{N}{2}} p\left[\left(\frac{sN}{2}\right) - \left(\frac{N}{2} + i\right)\right] \tag{2}$$

Block VII. The spiculation quantifying process is executed in axial and sagittal views.

Block VIII. The location of the detected peaks is then crossed; we only kept the points that coincide in both views.

Block IX. These points when mapped back in the images uplift the regions where the tumor presents a highly disorganized growing pattern.

Block X. Each slice in the study contributes to the histogram signature of the tumor. The FYC-Index defines the span of the histograms by using the maximum and minimum amount of points found in the slices when working on a single mass or among all analyzed tumors when working on populations.

Under the FYC-Index domain, while more spiculation, the histogram profiles are more populated in the right side.

2.3 Proof of concept on synthetic data

Testing on extremes is a common practice in engineering. Unfortunately, finding extremes on clinical data is cumbersome. The difficulty relies on the nature of the information; in the clinics, where the patients are imaged on the presumption that some abnormality is present, the images often yield moderately spiculated masses, posing a problem overall for the lower extreme reference. Regarding the highly spiculated reference, one can use the histogram signature to pinpoint the slice yielding the most right-filling pattern. However, a sounded proof of concept should comply with the common complexity found in the clinics, where two masses can have similar volumes and have a different nature regarding malignancy; thus, conventional methods are unable to detect differences. To overcome this problem, we have created a synthetic framework where lower references are created by stacking the less spiculated slice among all the data analyzed. A mildly spiculated mass is created by stacking a mildly spiculated slice among the study, and, analogously, the extreme spiculated sample is created by stacking the most spiculated slice found in the study. For the three samples, the stacking is driven in a manner that the masses end by having a similar volume.

2.4 Artificial intelligence (AI) implementation

Every column in the histogram signature created by employing the procedure in Section 2.2 is seen as a feature in classification postulate that aims to distinguish between malign and benign samples. This is possible due to the independence of the peaks counting in a slice by slice fashion. In general, the perturbations on the slice n do not have any correlation with the perturbations on slice m; therefore, orthogonality is granted. In addition to the bins counting, the number of bins fulfilled—some bins may end empty—those filled from the middle bin to the right and those filled to the middle bin to the left, is also used in the featuring space.

Every tumor population has a different span in the histogram signature; however, the amount of peak-counting-derived features have been set constant by forcing seven equally spaced bins regardless of the peak-counting range. Thus, the experiments always create an analyzing matrix containing 11 columns, 10 columns for the features, and 1 column to register the supervising factor provided by the histology. The current exercise presents a boolean support vector machine (SVM) classifier, where the machine is trained to provide a benign or malign verdict.

The data matrix is scaled and normalized using Python-Pandas [27, 28]. The classifier estimators are proved by cross correlation where the train and test samples are gathered from the original dataset using $(0.7 : 0.3)$ (train:test) in a fivefold experimental scheme. For the classification experiments, Scikit-learn [29] is employed.

Listing 1: Python code use to run the SVM classifier while progressively adding features.

```
def run Features Testing Classification (features, mdata, lbls):
atregs = []
ascores = []
for i in length(features):
est = feature_selection.SelectKBest (k=i)
est . fit (mdata, lbls)
tregs = est . get_support (indices = True)
```

```
ndata = est . transform (mdata)
estsvm = svm . LinearSVC ()
gs = grid_search . GridSearchCV (estsvm, {'C' : np . logspace (–4,3)})
tscore = np . mean (cross_validation . cross_val_score (gs, ndata, lbls, n_jobs=5))
```

As it is shown in Listing 1, the SVM classification is done after progressively adding features which are grabbed from the *mdata* matrix using the indexes saved in the features' array. The accuracy records presented in Section 4 correspond to the experiment that yielded the highest accuracy values per folding.

3. Results

3.1 FYC-Index extraction

Figure 2 shows how the algorithm yields two different outcomes based on the tortuosity of the two analyzed shapes. The small shape refers to a mostly rounded region of interest (ROI), therefore, does not present abrupt changes in the distances from the edging points to the center of FOV. In contrast, the same measure yields rapidly changing distances in the big ROI. Those rapidly changing distances are captured by the first derivate and framed in their inflection points by the second derivate. Later, those points are amplified and made all positive by the fourth power function, while the same fourth power function diminishes changes in which the derivate yielded values in the range (−1, 1). As the moving window adds up all values encountered in its domain, the regions of rapid change represented by large values compute to higher numbers within the domain of the moving window, and that is where the enhanced points appear in the plot. As all the points are mapped with their original coordinates, a crossing of 3D positions among the selected points

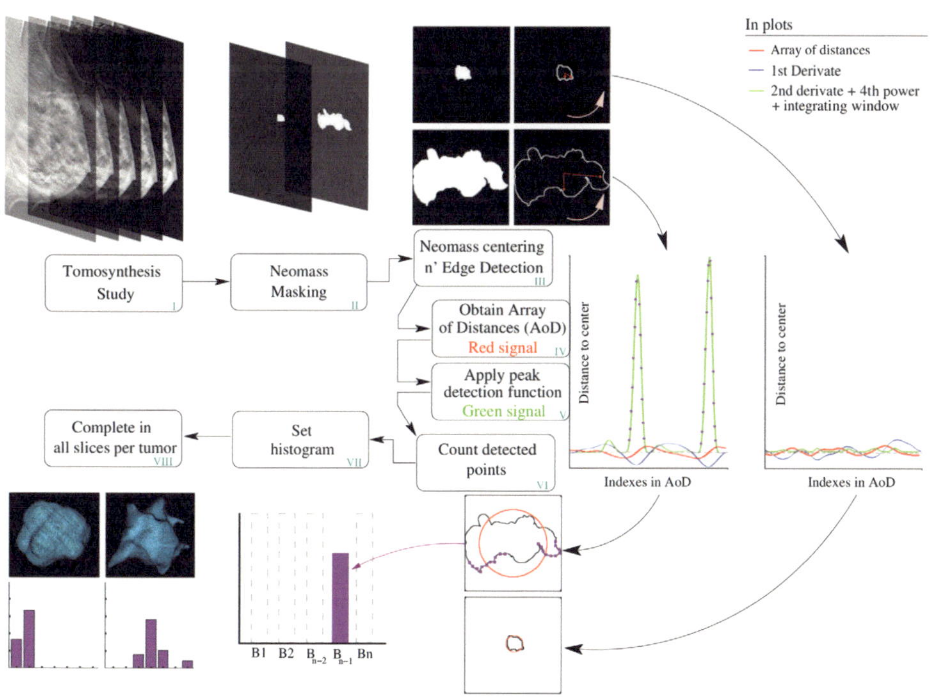

Figure 2.
FYC-Index extraction. The inner loop is the detailed block diagram similar to the one shown in ***Figure 1*** *but specific for tomosynthesis images. The outer loop shows sampling images on each block.*

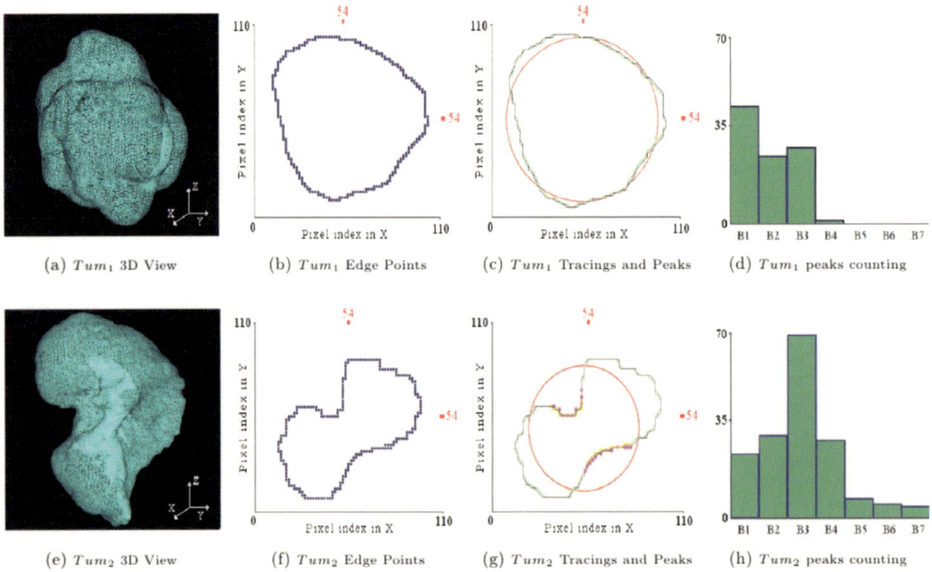

(a) Tum_1 3D View (b) Tum_1 Edge Points (c) Tum_1 Tracings and Peaks (d) Tum_1 peaks counting

(e) Tum_2 3D View (f) Tum_2 Edge Points (g) Tum_2 Tracings and Peaks (h) Tum_2 peaks counting

Figure 3.
Histogram signature of the FYC-Index on two tumors and intermediate steps (b, c, d, g) of processing. The circles in frames in (c) and (g) correspond to perfectly rounded regions where the area is equal to the one of the mask.

in two image views filters out positions erroneously selected. Finally, the presented procedure allocates an item of frequency in a histogram where the bins contain ranges of point counting. Naturally, highly spiculated slices contribute mostly to the right bins of the histogram. When all slices in a tumor have been analyzed, the operator could be sure that the histogram is descriptive of the degree of homogeneity of the mass which is also associated with aggressiveness (see **Figure 3**).

A sample of the process where the 3D reconstruction of the masses together with the respective normalized FYC-Index histogram is presented in **Figure 4**.

3.2 Analysis of synthetic data

As explained in Section 2.3, extreme references are created to demonstrate the span of the method and the capacity to deliver a representation of easy interpretation. The synthetic creations are shown in **Figure 5**.

The results obtained on synthetic data corroborates that the FYC-Index is sensible to the changes in the edges that distinguish between malign and benign masses. In contrast, commonly used geometrical indexes are not sensitive to changes. In this exercise, we have isolated the spiculation by equalizing the volumes of the studied software objects. A complete set of 3D geometrical functions are applied on the clinical data in use, with the aim of comparing the performance of standard of care tools in the clinics, and the FYC-Index is shown in **Figure 6**.

4. Verdicts dictated by (AI) implementation

The fivefolding SVM exercise proposed in Section 2.4 was executed using a Python-Pandas dataframe and Scikit-Learn SVM. The results are registered in **Table 1**.

The strong-force algorithm presented in Section 2.4 executed the supervised classification with a high degree of accuracy. The design of the experiments turns the classification into the capacity to differentiate whether a mass is benign or malign.

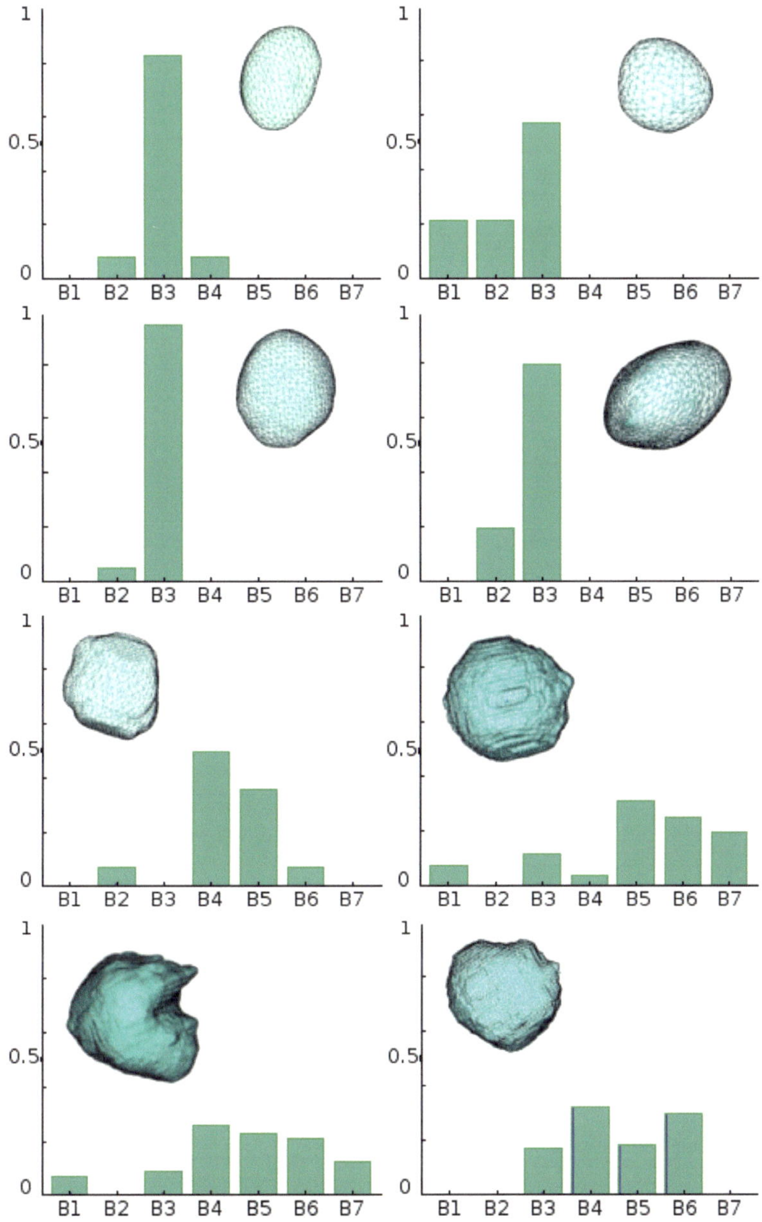

Figure 4.
A sample of the processed tumors and their FYC-Index signatures.

5. Discussion

The proposed method is sensitive to slight changes in the edges of the masses that are characteristically malignant. The same method includes a stage of quantification that has proven to be descriptive at a simple glance even for nonspecialized operators. Since the procedure has been automated, it is compliant with the confidentiality regulations and, therefore, can be easily implemented in hospitals and clinics. The FYC-Index is a flexible method equally performant when analyzing masses in individuals and populations. The method presents a signature which results in a measure of lobularity. This strategy works regardless of factors such as size and spatial resolution. Moreover, the results are direct and easy to interpret.

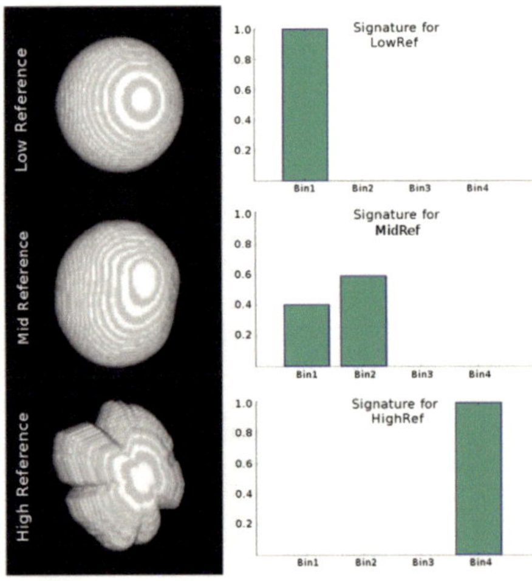

Index	lowRef	MidRef	highRef
Volume	235965	235956	235944
volBoundingBox	440896	445440	445440
volBoxRatio	0.53	0.53	0.53
Sphericity	0.66	0.66	0.66
VolEllipsoid	235974	237205	242666
Compactness	0.99	0.99	0.99
Ell-Elongation	1.00	1.11	1.04

Figure 5.
Performance of the FYC-Index in software-created references. On the right, a table with records of often used 3D geometrical indexes. Note that these indexes are not sensible within the characteristics that require to be quantified.

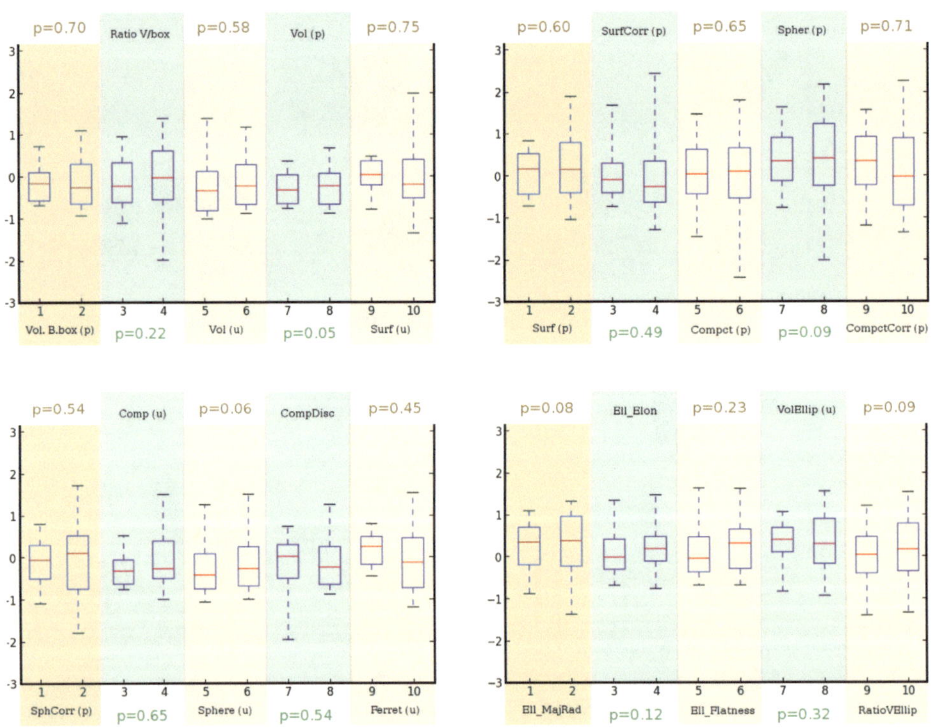

Figure 6.
The two boxes per colored column correspond to the clinical data detailed in Section 2.1. Normality was discarded by Kolmogorov test [30] done in the two groups separately. As normality was not met, the nonparametric Kruskal-Wallis test [31] was employed. The p-values are mapped back and forward in the chi-square distribution.

The specifications of the FYC-Index make it suitable to analyze all sort of cancer manifestations, regardless of localization or pathogenic roots. The presented strategy uses a machine-learning classifier to rapidly characterize the malignancy of a mass. However, the real challenge consists of defining malignancy together with aggressiveness. Such an approach requires more rounds of training/testing sessions

Folding	Accuracy (%)	Sensibility (%)	Specificity (%)
1	93.4	92.1	89.1
2	91.3	92.4	90.4
3	90.3	90.2	89.6
4	92.7	90.1	89.3
5	89.9	90.0	89.6

Results for the fivefolding experiments on histograms acquired with the FYC-Index of spiculation.

Table 1.
SVM-supervised classification.

with sufficient samples in all grading range. This multilevel classification should be designed to follow the classification directives presented in the X-RADS standards; thus, the existing automatic tools can also provide insights for selecting more accurate treatments. To the best of our knowledge, no other authors are integrating the tools as we have proposed. The use of the features we have proposed is a novel view of the solution; therefore, we do not include in this report a comparison with other methods.

6. Conclusion

Cancer is the second most threating disease which humanity has not been able to neutralize. Other diseases that were considered pandemics in the past, costing millions of human lives, have been eradicated through vaccination. Rapidly mutating diseases such as AIDS have been downgraded from mortal to chronic. Maladies like high blood pressure, stroke, or cirrhosis among several other chronic afflictions have been associated with race, genetics, habits, or exposition factors, providing a way to reduce the probability of acquiring them or a path of development where scientists still have space to explore. Cancer instead affects all humans regardless of any factor. The only aspect that increases the surviving expectations, without a doubt, is early detection, and it is here where the method presented in this manuscript gains relevance. Detection from the images is possible, and automatic diagnosis not only avoids the painful and uncomfortable biopsy, but it also contributes to faster and more accurate verdicts.

Author details

Fernando Yepes-Calderón[1]*, Flor M. Medina[2], Nolan D. Rea[1] and José Abella[2]

1 Children's Hospital Los Angeles, Los Angeles, CA, USA

2 Fundación Valle del Lili, Cali, Colombia

*Address all correspondence to: fernandoyepesc@gmail.com

References

[1] Catalano OA, Samir AE, Sahani V, Hahn PF. Pixel distribution analysis: Can it be used to distinguish clear cell carcinomas from angiomyolipomas with minimal fat? Genitourinary Imaging. 2007;**247**(3):11-38. URL: www.rsna.org/rsnarights

[2] Chaudhry HS, Davenport MS, Nieman CM, Ho LM, Neville AM. Histogram analysis of small solid renal masses: Differentiating minimal fat angiomyolipoma from renal cell carcinoma. Genitourinary Imaging. 2011;**1**:1-3. DOI: 10.2214/AJR.11.6887. URL: www.ajronline.org

[3] Arakeri MP, Reddy RM. A novel CBIR approach to differential diagnosis of liver tumor on computed tomography images. Procedia Engineering. 2012;**38**: 528-536. DOI: 10.1016/j.proeng.2012.06.066

[4] Stigliano R, Marelli L, Yu D, Davies N, Patch D, Burroughs AK. Seeding following percutaneous diagnostic and therapeutic approaches for hepatocellular carcinoma. What is the risk and the outcome? Seeding risk for percutaneous approach of HCC. Cancer Treatment Reviews. 2007;**33**(5): 437-447. DOI: S0305-7372(07)00041-2 [pii] 10.1016/j.ctrv.2007.04.001. URL: http://www.ncbi.nlm.nih.gov/pubmed/17512669

[5] Bedossa P. Liver biopsy. Gastroentérologie Clinique et Biologique. 2008;**32**:4-7

[6] dos Santos DP, Kloeckner R, Wunder K, Bornemann L, Düber C, Mildenberger P. Effect of kernels used for the reconstruction of MDCT datasets on the semi-automated segmentation and volumetry of liver lesions. Technique and Medical Physics. 2013; **19**:780-784. DOI: 10.1055/s-0033-1356178

[7] Guo Y, Feng Y, Sun J, Zhang N, Lin W, Sa Y, et al. Automatic lung tumor segmentation on PET/CT images using fuzzy Markov random field model. Computational and Mathematical Methods in Medicine. 2014;**2014**:8-10. DOI: 10.1155/2014/401201

[8] Schulz J, Skrøvseth SO, Tømmerås VK, Marienhagen K, Godtliebsen F. A semiautomatic tool for prostate segmentation in radiotherapy treatment planning. BMC Medical Imaging. 2014; **12**(1):1. DOI: 10.1186/1471-2342-12-25. URL: BMC Medical Imaging

[9] Ftterer J, Heijmink S, Scheenen T, Veltman J, Huisman HJ. Prostate cancer localization with dynamic contrast-enhanced MR imaging and proton MR spectroscopic imaging. RSNA Radiology. Nov 2006;**241**(2):449-458

[10] Oto A, Kayhan A, Jiang Y, Tretiakova M, Yang C, Antic T. Prostate cancer: Differentiation of central gland cancer from Benign prostatic hyperplasia by using diffusion-weighted and dynamic contrast-enhanced MR imaging. RSNA Radiology. 2010;**257**

[11] Mendez A, Tahoces P, Lado M, Souto M, Correa J, Vidal J. Automatic detection of breast border and nipple in digital mammograms. Computer Methods and Programs in Biomedicine; May 1996;**49**(3):253-262

[12] Doyle S, Rodriguez C. Detecting prostatic adenocarcinoma from digitized histology using a multi-scale hierarchical classification approach. In: 2006 International Conference of the IEEE EMB, New York, NY; 2006. pp. 4759-4752. DOI: 10.1109/IEMBS.2006.260188

[13] Dorsi EME, Sickles C, Morris E. ACR BI-RADS Atlas, Breast Imaging

Reporting and Data System. American College of Radiology; 2013

[14] Weinreb J, Barentsz J, Choyke P, Cornud F, Haider M, Macura K, et al. PI-RADS prostate imaging-reporting and data system: 2015 version 2. European Urology; Jan 2016;**69**(1): 16-40

[15] Yu H, Wilson SR. Liver masses with acoustic radiation force impulse technique. Ultrasound Quarterly. 2011; **27**:217-223. URL: www.ultrasound-quarterly.com

[16] Rangayyan RM, Mudigonda NR, Desautels JEL. Boundary modeling and shape analysis methods for classification of mammographic masses. Medical & Biological Engineering & Computing. 2000;**38**(5):487-496

[17] Guliato D, Rangayyan RM, Carvalho JD, Santiago SA. Polygonal modeling of contours of breast tumors with the preservation of spicules. IEEE Transactions on Biomedical Engineering; **55**(1). DOI: 10.1109/TBME.2007.899310

[18] Brown JM, Giaccia AJ. The unique physiology of solid tumors: Opportunities (and problems) for cancer therapy. Cancer Research. 1998; **7**:1408-1416

[19] Erasmus JJ, Connolly JE, McAdams HP, Roggli VL. Solitary pulmonary nodules: Part I. Morphologic evaluation for differentiation of benign and malignant lesions. Radiographics. 2000; **20**(1):43-58

[20] Yepes-Calderon F, Johnson R, Lao Y, Hwang D, Coloigner J, Yap F, et al. The 3D edge runner pipeline: A novel shape-based analysis for neoplasms characterization. In: SPIE 9788, Medical Imaging 2016: Biomedical Applications in Molecular, Structural, and Functional Imaging: 97882N; 29 March 2016. DOI: 10.1117/12.2217238

[21] Abdel R, Bakry RE. Breast tomosynthesis: A diagnostic addition to screening digital mammography. The Egyptian Journal of Radiology and Nuclear Medicine. 2018;**49**(2):529-535

[22] Eghtedari M, Tsai C, Robles J, Blair SL, Ojeda-Fournier H. Tomosynthesis in breast cancer imaging: How does it fit into preoperative evaluation and surveillance? Surgical Oncology Clinics of North America. 2018;**27**(1):33-49

[23] Whitted T. An improved illumination model for shaded display. Communications of the ACM. 1980;(4): 343-349

[24] Rigau J, Feixas M, Sbert M. New contrast measurements for pixel supersampling. In: Proceedings of CGI02. July 2002:439-451

[25] Canny J. A computational approach to edge detection. IEEE Transactions on Pattern Analysis and Machine Intelligence; PAMI-8. 1986:679-698. DOI: 10.1109/TPAMI.1986.4767851

[26] Shannon CE. A mathematical theory of communication. The Bell System Technical Journal. 1948;**27**:379-423, 623-656

[27] McKinney W. Data structures for statistical computing in python. In: van der Walt S, Millman J, editors. Proceedings of the 9th Python in Science Conference; 2010. pp. 51-56

[28] McKinney W. Pandas: A Foundational Python Library for Data Analysis and Statistics

[29] Pedregosa F, Varoquaux G, Gramfort A, Michel V, Thirion B, Grisel O, et al. Scikit-Learn: Machine learning in Python. The Journal of Machine Learning Research. 2011;**12**:2825-2830

[30] Massey FJ. The Kolmogorov-Smirnov test for goodness of fit. Journal of the American Statistical Association;

1951;**46**(253):68-78. DOI: 10.1080/01621459.1951.10500769

[31] Weaver KF, Morales V, Dunn SL, Godde K, Weaver PF. An Introduction to Statistical Analysis in Research: With Applications in the Biological and Life Sciences, Chapter 8. USA: John Wiley & Sons; 2017. DOI: 10.1002/9781119454205.ch8